MW01102253

NorKam Secondary School
730 12th St
Kamloops, BC V2B 3C1
Telephone: 250-376-1272

THE ENCYCLOPEDIA OF

WOMEN'S
REPRODUCTIVE CANCER

THE ENCYCLOPEDIA OF

WOMEN'S REPRODUCTIVE CANCER

Carol Turkington
Mitchell Edelson, M.D.

Facts On File, Inc.

The Encyclopedia of Women's Reproductive Cancer

Facts On File, Inc.
132 West 31st Street
New York NY 10001

Library of Congress Cataloging-in-Publication Data

Turkington, Carol.
The encyclopedia of women's reproductive cancer / Carol Turkington and Mitchell Edelson, M.D.
p. ; cm.
Includes bibliographical references and index.
ISBN 0-8160-5031-7 (hc. ; alk. paper)
1. Generative organs, Female—Cancer—Encyclopedias. 2. Cancer in women—Encyclopedias. I. Title.
[DNLM: 1. Genital Neoplasms, Female—Encyclopedias—English. WP 13 T939ea 2005]
RC280.G5T78 2005
616.99'465'03—dc22   2004043253

Facts On File books are available at special discounts when purchased in bulk quantities for businesses, associations, institutions, or sales promotions. Please call our Special Sales Department in New York at (212) 967-8800 or (800) 322-8755.

You can find Facts On File on the World Wide Web at http://www.factsonfile.com

Text and cover design by Cathy Rincon

Printed in the United States of America

VB Hermitage 10 9 8 7 6 5 4 3 2 1

This book is printed on acid-free paper.

CONTENTS

FOREWORD

Women's reproductive cancers account for 12 percent of all cancers in women. The treatments available for these cancers, which affect the cervix, uterus, ovary, fallopian tube, vulva, and vagina, have become more refined in recent years. The newer treatments we have today aim to cure women of these cancers while minimizing the short- and long-term side effects.

Modern surgical procedures are becoming less extensive, with the use of minimally invasive surgery and sentinel node biopsies. Radiation therapy treatments are focusing on treating the cancer cells but sparing the normal cells. Chemotherapy is evolving with the development of new drugs that are targeting the cancer cells and leaving the normal cells alone. Additionally, combinations of these modalities (surgery, radiation therapy, and chemotherapy) are being used to maximize the destructive effect on these cancer cells.

I know firsthand the difficulty of explaining these treatments in easy-to-understand language. The goal of this encyclopedia is to simplify the language that is used so that women can better understand the treatment options and better prepare themselves for surgery, radiation, or chemotherapy.

—Mitchell Edelson, M.D.

ACKNOWLEDGMENTS

The creation of a detailed encyclopedia involves the help and guidance of a wide range of experts, without which this book could not have been possible.

First of all, thanks to all the staff at Fox Chase Cancer Center in Philadelphia, and to Dr. Mitchell Edelson. Also thanks to the staffs of the National Institute of Mental Health, the National Institute of Nursing Research, the American Medical Association, National Institutes of Health, American Association of People with Disabilities, American College of Obstetricians and Gynecologists, American Heart Association, American Psychiatric Association, American Psychological Association, American Society of Hematology, the Cancer Information Service, Centers for Disease Control and Prevention, the Food and Drug Administration, the National Cancer Institute, and the American Board of Plastic and Reconstructive Surgeons.

Thanks also to the Look Good . . . Feel Better program, National Bone Marrow Transplant Link, National Marrow Donor Program, American Brachytherapy Society, Cancer Hope Network, Cancer Information and Counseling Line, Cancer Information Service, Cancer Net, Cancer Research Institute, Cancer Survivors Network, CanSur-mount, I Can Cope, International Union Against Cancer, CHEMOcare, Chemotherapy Foundation, National Association of Hospital Hospitality, Hereditary Cancer Institute, National Cancer Institute, Hospice Education Institute, HospiceLink, and the National Hospice and Palliative Care Organization.

Also, thanks to the National Hospice Foundation, Cancer Legal Resource Center, American College of Radiology, American Society of Clinical Oncology, Association of Community Cancer Centers, Society of Gynecologic Oncologists, American College of Radiology, American Institute for Cancer Research, Cancer Research Foundation of America, Cancer Research Institute, European Organisation for Research and Treatment of Cancer, National Asian Women's Health Organization, and the National Women's Health Information Center.

Thanks also to the librarians at the Hershey Medical Center medical library, the National Library of Medicine, the Reading Public Library, and the Pennsylvania State Library.

Finally, thanks to my agent, Gene Brissie, of James Peter Associates; to Bert Holtje; to my editor, James Chambers, and Vanessa Nittoli at Facts On File; and to Kara and Michael.

INTRODUCTION

More than 80,000 American women will be diagnosed with a reproductive, or gynecologic, cancer each year, including cancers of the cervix, uterus (endometrium), ovaries, fallopian tubes, vagina, and vulva. Although most women diagnosed with these cancers will survive their diagnoses for years, others will not. Since 1999, about 130,000 women in this country have died as a result of their diagnoses with a gynecologic cancer. This year, an estimated 26,000 women in the United States are expected to lose their lives to some form of gynecologic cancer.

Early detection and appropriate treatment of gynecologic cancers are key in lowering this death toll, because when diagnosed at their earliest stages, gynecologic cancers offer excellent prognoses for long-term survival. Unfortunately, a significant percentage of women diagnosed with these cancers are identified in the advanced stages of the disease, when five-year survival rates are far lower.

There is no single reason for these late-stage diagnoses, but a lack of knowledge regarding risk factors, symptoms, and diagnostic tools available to screen for these cancers is a contributing factor. Although public education efforts about breast cancer screening has made women keenly aware of the importance of mammograms, the same cannot be said for gynecologic cancer. Far too many patients say they did not know the warning signs or symptoms of various gynecologic cancers until

after they were diagnosed, and many did not know they had one or more known risk factors. Still others think they have nothing to worry about if their most recent Pap smear results are normal, assuming that a Pap smear screens for all gynecologic cancers. In fact, it only reliably screens for cervical cancer.

The Encyclopedia of Women's Reproductive Cancer is designed to answer these questions about reproductive cancer, and includes the most up-to-date information on cancers of the ovary, vagina, vulva, and uterus that may affect a woman during her lifetime. It has been designed as a guide and reference to a wide range of subjects important to the understanding of a woman's reproductive health, and includes a wide variety of contact information for organization and governmental agencies affiliated with cancer issues, including current Web site addresses and phone numbers.

However, the book is not designed as a substitute for prompt assessment and treatment by oncologic experts in the diagnosis and treatment of women's reproductive cancer.

In this encyclopedia, we have tried to present the latest information in the field, based on the newest research. Although information in this book comes from the most up-to-date medical journals and research sources, readers should keep in mind that changes occur very quickly in reproductive oncology. A bibliography has been included for those who seek additional sources of information.

ENTRIES A–Z

abdominal swelling An enlargement of the lower torso. As one of the primary symptoms of OVARIAN CANCER, abdominal swelling is usually caused by abnormal pooling of fluid in the abdomen (ascites). Swelling can occur in a normal premenstrual period, but if the symptom persists, it should be reported to a doctor.

Actiq (fentanyl) A painkilling narcotic in the form of a raspberry-flavored lollipop, prescribed for cancer patients whose pain cannot be controlled with oral narcotics. Pain relief begins while the lozenge is consumed and continues for several hours. To prevent accidental ingestion by children, the childproof package can be opened only with a pair of scissors.

The Actiq unit is placed between the cheek and gum. As it dissolves, a portion of the medication is absorbed quickly across the lining of the mouth into the bloodstream. The remaining medication is swallowed and slowly absorbed. As soon as the drug enters the bloodstream it is carried throughout the body. Pain relief begins within 15 minutes, but the full effect may not occur for up to 45 minutes.

Actiq must be used only for cancer pain not controlled by other pain medication, and only by people who are already taking and who are tolerant to prescription narcotic pain medicines. Actiq can be fatal if used by patients who are not already taking prescription narcotic pain medicines on a regular schedule because it may slow breathing to a dangerous level.

acupressure A technique in which pressure is applied to the skin by the fingers, as a way of treating a variety of conditions. In cancer patients, it is used to treat CHEMOTHERAPY-related nausea. Based on the same principles as ACUPUNCTURE, acupressure therapists press on acupuncture points with the fingers instead of using needles. (Other therapists use electrical impulses, heat, laser beams, sound waves, friction, suction, or magnets instead of their fingers at the acupressure points, to the same purpose.)

Acupressure cannot cure cancer, but numerous studies have shown it is effective in relieving the nausea that often follows chemotherapy treatment or surgery. The technique can be used alone or as part of a system of manual healing such as shiatsu massage.

See also ACUSTIMULATION.

acupuncture A technique, used to treat a variety of conditions, in which very thin needles of varying lengths are inserted through the skin into spots known as acupoints. Although there is no evidence that acupuncture is effective as a treatment for cancer, clinical studies have found it to be effective in treating nausea caused by chemotherapy drugs and surgical anesthesia. This finding was supported by a National Institutes of Health expert panel consisting of scientists, researchers, and health-care providers. There is also some evidence that acupuncture may lessen the need for conventional pain-relieving drugs.

Acupuncture has been practiced for the past 2,000 years and is an important component of Chinese medicine. Traditional Chinese practitioners believe that health depends on a vital energy called *qi* (pronounced "chee"), which they believe flows through pathways in the body called meridians. Practitioners believe that an obstruction along a meridian blocks the natural flow of energy, creating pain and disease. Also important in Chinese medicine is the idea of the opposing forces of yin and yang, which, when balanced, are said to work together with *qi* to promote physical and mental wellness. The insertion of needles into precise points on the skin is believed to unblock energy flow, balance yin and yang, and restore health. Originally, 365 acupoints were identified, corresponding to the number of days in a year; the number of acupoints gradually grew to more than 2,000.

Some practitioners in the West reject the traditional philosophies of Chinese medicine and claim that acupuncture works by stimulating the production of endorphins, natural painkiller substances found in the body. Because Western scientists have found it hard to study meridians (which do not correspond to nerve or blood circulation pathways), some do not believe that meridians exist. Despite differing philosophies, however, healthcare practitioners generally agree that when used along with mainstream medicine, acupuncture can produce real benefits.

Traditional acupuncture needles were made of bone, stone, or metal (including silver and gold); modern disposable acupuncture needles are made of very thin stainless steel. In 1996, the U.S. Food and Drug Administration approved the use of acupuncture needles by licensed practitioners. By law, needles must be labeled for one-time use only.

The procedure should cause little or no discomfort, because the needles are as thin as a strand of hair and are usually left in place for less than half an hour. Some acupuncturists twirl the needles or apply low-voltage electricity to them as a way to enhance the results. When conducted by a trained professional, acupuncture is generally considered safe. The number of complications reported have been relatively few, but there is a risk that a patient may be harmed by an acupuncturist who is not well trained.

There are more than 10,000 acupuncturists in the United States, and about 32 states have established training standards for licensing the practice of acupuncture. Medicare does not cover acupuncture, but it is covered by some private health insurance plans and health maintenance organizations (HMOs). Consumers should consult an experienced, qualified practitioner who is state licensed or board certified. The American Academy of Medical Acupuncture (http://www.medicalacupuncture.org) can refer patients to physicians (M.D.'s or D.O.'s) who practice acupuncture.

See also ACUPRESSURE; ACUSTIMULATION.

acustimulation Mild electrical stimulation of acupuncture points to control symptoms such as nausea and vomiting.

See also ACUPRESSURE.

adenocarcinoma A tumor that develops from a malignant change in the mucus- or hormone-secreting lining of an organ (the prefix *adeno-* refers to glandular cells). Most ovarian and endometrial cancers are adenocarcinomas, which also may occur in the vagina and cervix, among other areas.

adenomatous hyperplasia Overgrowth of cells relating to an adenoma (a benign epithelial tumor), a type of ENDOMETRIAL HYPERPLASIA that causes abnormal or heavy bleeding during menopause by the overgrowth of the uterine lining. Adenomatous hyperplasia may be the precursor to ENDOMETRIAL CANCER.

adjuvant treatment Therapy that is used in addition to primary treatment. Adjuvant treatment for cancer usually entails the use of CHEMOTHERAPY, HORMONAL THERAPY, or RADIATION THERAPY begun after surgery to increase the likelihood of killing all cancer cells. Adjuvant treatment is usually indicated if there is a suspicion that cancer cells have remained in the body after application of the primary method of treatment.

Studies have shown that adjuvant treatment can prevent the recurrence of cancer. Although some doctors believe that the benefits of adjuvant therapy are minimal and that such treatment is thus unnecessary, most experts believe the benefits outweigh the risks.

adnexal mass A mass that has grown in the uterine adnexa (a part of the reproductive organs that includes the fallopian tube and ovary). Adnexal masses may be caused by simple OVARIAN CYSTS, benign or malignant ovarian tumors, or irregularities in the fallopian tubes. The lesions, which are usually harmless cysts that disappear spontaneously, are extremely common during a woman's reproductive years. However, in a few cases they can become malignant; the chance of development of a cancerous adnexal mass is about 1.5 percent over a woman's lifetime.

Symptoms

Most of the time adnexal masses do not produce symptoms, which may include pelvic pain or irregular menstrual periods. When adnexal masses grow bigger than about two inches, they may begin to press on the bladder or rectum, increasing the frequency of urination or causing constipation. An adnexal mass may cause sudden, severe pain if it twists, cutting off the blood supply to the ovary. This ovarian torsion does not happen often.

Diagnosis

A physical exam and medical history can help a doctor determine the cause of these symptoms. Adnexal masses are usually found during a routine pelvic exam of women who have no symptoms. If the doctor feels an adnexal mass, or if a woman has pelvic symptoms, the doctor may order a pelvic ultrasound. If the woman has an adnexal mass, it appears on an ultrasound and the radiologist is able to describe its size, location, and appearance. It is important to determine whether the masses are filled with fluid (cystic), are solid, or are both. Fluid-filled cysts are less likely to be malignant than are solid masses.

Treatment

Treatment of an adnexal mass depends on its size and type, the woman's age, and the occurrence of symptoms. A small mass in a woman of reproductive age who has no symptoms almost always disappears without treatment within four to six weeks. In this case, a doctor usually recommends another ultrasound in four to six weeks to make sure the cyst has disappeared.

Occasionally, BIRTH CONTROL PILLS may be prescribed to help the cysts disappear more quickly—or at least to help prevent new cysts from growing. In about 75 percent of cases, these masses have disappeared by the second ultrasound.

If the mass is definitely a cyst that remains the same size, it can be followed by repeated ultrasounds and physical exams. However, if the mass does not disappear, surgery may be recommended.

Because girls do not ovulate before their first menstrual period and women do not ovulate after menopause, masses that occur in patients in these age groups are not likely to be harmless cysts. Normally, adnexal masses in prepubertal women should be removed surgically. In postmenopausal women, small cystic adnexal masses may be watched for a time, as these may also go away or remain stable over repeated evaluations.

Surgery A gynecologic oncologist can surgically remove suspicious ovarian masses. The decision of whether or not surgery should be performed for an adnexal mass depends on the risk of malignancy, the woman's worries about infertility, the ultrasound appearance of the mass, and the patient's history of abdominal surgery.

If the mass does not seem suspicious, a doctor may remove the ovarian cyst or the entire ovary by using LAPAROSCOPY. In this technique, the doctor inserts a viewing scope and surgical instruments through small incisions, watching the surgery on a video screen. Through this method, the entire ovary, or in some cases just the ovarian cyst, may be removed.

Some experienced gynecologic cancer specialists may choose to remove even suspicious adnexal masses laparoscopically. However, when there is a very high risk of malignancy, surgery is performed through a traditional abdominal incision.

After the ovary or the ovarian cyst is removed, it is sent for a frozen section BIOPSY. While the patient is asleep on the operating table, the pathologist examines the tissue to find out whether it is benign or malignant. If the adnexal mass is benign and the patient is young, removing only the ovarian cyst, and thus saving the remainder of the ovary, is often possible.

Otherwise, it is better to remove both ovaries and to perform a complete HYSTERECTOMY. This course is often a good option for women who do not want any more children, who are close to menopause, or who have other gynecologic problems, such as uterine fibroids or abnormal bleeding, that requires surgical treatment.

If the frozen section biopsy uncovers cancer, but the tumor does not seem to be spreading, the surgeon stages the cancer by examining the upper abdomen, taking a biopsy sample of the lymph nodes, removing the fatty tissue in the upper abdomen, and performing other biopsies to find out whether the cancer has spread. If ovarian cancer is found, the surgeon also removes the ovaries, the fallopian tubes, and the uterus. In young women who want to retain the ability to have children, the surgeon sometimes removes only the ovary and tube that are malignant. If an advanced ovarian cancer is found, the surgical treatment usually includes bilateral salpingo-oophorectomy, hysterectomy, and removal, as complete as possible, of areas where cancer has spread.

The surgeon will explain possible side effects to the patient before surgery. Side effects are related to the type and extent of the surgery being performed. Generally, side effects include the possibility of bleeding, infection, aesthetic problems, and injury to other organs. In most cases, the risk of serious surgical side effects is less than 1 percent.

Adriamycin (doxorubicin) A type of intravenous (IV) antibiotic CHEMOTHERAPY drug used to treat many types of cancer, including OVARIAN CANCER. Adriamycin disrupts the growth of cancer cells. This drug must be administered carefully because it can cause severe skin damage and scarring if it leaks outside the vein. Patients should alert the nurse immediately if there is any stinging or burning in the vein while this drug is being given.

Patients who take Adriamycin should drink high levels of fluids; the more urine that is produced, the less likely bladder or kidney problems will occur.

Side Effects

The most common side effects include nausea and vomiting, HAIR LOSS, decreased white blood cell and platelet levels, APPETITE LOSS, and temporary red urine. Rare side effects that require immediate attention include irregular heartbeat, shortness of breath, wheezing, pain at the injection site, and swelling of extremities.

The most significant side effect of this drug is the direct damage to individual muscle cells of the heart, called cardiomyopathy, which is related to total lifetime dosage. Women who may benefit from continued treatment with this drug may be given another drug, dexrazoxane (Zinecard), to help prevent heart damage.

Adrucil See FLUOROURACIL.

advance directives A written document, completed and signed when a person is legally competent, that explains what the person would or would not want if unable to make decisions about medical care. Common advance directives include the following:

- *HEALTH-CARE PROXY (or health-care power of attorney).* The document gives another person the authority to make decisions for a patient who is unable to do so.
- *Living will.* Used in the case of a dying patient, it directs a doctor to use, not start, or stop treatment when the patient cannot make his or her wishes known.
- *Nonhospital DO NOT RESUSCITATE ORDER.* The order directs emergency staff not to resuscitate a person who is not in a hospital or other health-care facility.

Advance directives are an important part of any patient's financial affairs, since such documents allow someone else to make treatment decisions on a patient's behalf when the person is no longer capable of making those decisions.

Patients should prepare and sign advance directives that comply with state law and give copies to family, friends, and doctors. The document should reflect the patient's wishes and appoint someone who is willing to comply with his or her wishes to make decisions.

African-American women For many complex reasons, African-American women suffer disproportionately from many reproductive cancers, and, in general, they have a lower five-year survival rate and are more likely to die of reproductive cancers than are white American women. As a result, the average life expectancy of African

Americans (70 years) is six years less than the national average.

Minorities receive substandard medical care because of racial discrimination in health-care settings, time pressures on health-care workers, and low-end health insurance plans, according to a recent landmark report by the U.S. Institute of Medicine. As a result, more African Americans and members of other minorities die of cancer than do white Americans. Lower-quality medical care occurred even when minority patients' income, age, medical condition, and insurance coverage were similar to those of white patients.

Early detection could lower the high cancer death rates among African Americans, since regular cancer-related checkups and other testing find cancer early, when treatment is more successful. About half of all cancers can now be discovered early by such screening methods, but many African Americans are not getting this preventive care.

Cervical Cancer

African-American women have the second highest incidence rates of cervical cancer (13.3 per 100,000 population, compared to 17.5 for Hispanics and 9.6 for whites). The cervical cancer death rate among African-American women is three times the rate of Caucasian women and twice the rate of Hispanics, according to statistics compiled in 2000. In addition, African-American women have at least a 50 percent higher incidence of uterine cancer than do white women.

Ovarian Cancer

African-American women with OVARIAN CANCER have a 30 percent greater risk of death from any cause and are more likely to die earlier when compared to Caucasian women with ovarian cancer. In general, African-American women are younger when they are diagnosed with ovarian cancer, tend to have tumors discovered at a more aggressive stage, and are less likely to undergo surgery.

Findings in a study published in the March 15, 2002, issue of *Cancer* indicate that ethnicity itself is a risk factor in ovarian cancer survival even after other risk factors are adjusted. Other studies have also shown that African Americans with ovarian cancer have higher death rates than Caucasians with ovarian cancer. While ethnicity is a risk factor,

little is known about the differences in risk factors between Caucasians and African Americans with ovarian cancer that could affect survival.

According to a study by the SURVEILLANCE, EPIDEMIOLOGY, AND END RESULTS (SEER) program, showed there are significant differences between Caucasian and African-American women in diagnosis and treatment of ovarian cancer. SEER is a population-based national cancer surveillance database that includes demographic, clinical, treatment, and survival information on men and women diagnosed with cancer. Data from 12,285 Caucasian women and 798 African-American women diagnosed with primary, malignant ovarian carcinoma, and factors analyzed include marital status, age at diagnosis, tumor stage, tumor histological characteristics and grade, LYMPH NODE involvement, site-specific surgical treatment, and death of any cause.

The study found that African-American women tend to be diagnosed at an age two years younger than Caucasian women and are more than twice as likely to be unmarried. African-American women are 50 percent more likely to be diagnosed at stage IV disease and more likely to have lymph node involvement and distant spread of the disease. African-American women also are 40 percent less likely to have surgery. Average survival time after diagnosis for African-American women was 22 months; Caucasian women on average survived almost a year longer—32 months.

See also ASIAN WOMEN; HISPANIC/LATINA WOMEN; RACE AND REPRODUCTIVE CANCERS.

age   In general, older women are more likely to be diagnosed with most types of reproductive cancers. For example, most women who have ENDOMETRIAL CANCER are postmenopausal, between the ages of 55 and 70. Likewise, invasive VULVAR CANCER is rarely diagnosed in women before age 55.

Unlike other types of reproductive cancers, however, CERVICAL CANCER usually affects women between the ages of 35 and 55 and is not uncommon among younger women. In fact, cervical cancer is the most common type of reproductive cancer in younger women.

Air Care Alliance (ACA)   A national league of humanitarian flying organizations dedicated to providing air travel for severely ill patients (such as cancer patients) who cannot afford air transportation. The ACA has member groups whose activities include health care, patient transport, and other kinds of public-benefit flying. For contact information, see Appendix I.

AirLifeLine The oldest and largest national volunteer pilot organization in the United States, dedicated to providing transportation to and from medical destinations for patients in financial need. For a quarter-century, AirLifeLine has helped to ensure equal access to health care and improve the quality of life for thousands of people throughout the United States. Flights are staffed with volunteer pilots who donate their time and all of the flight costs.

AirLifeLine is a charitable nonprofit organization funded by donations from individuals, foundations, corporations, and volunteer pilots. For contact information, see Appendix I.

alcohol and endometrial cancer Although alcohol has been linked to the development of breast cancer (a type of cancer influenced by estrogen) very few studies have found an association between alcohol use and endometrial cancer, which also depends on estrogens for survival. Some studies have found that alcohol intake increases the concentration of sex hormones, and a high level of estrogen appears to be related to endometrial cancer.

Of the 13 studies that have reported on the relationship between endometrial cancer and use of alcohol, only two have found a link. The rest of the studies have reported no definite association or an inverse association.

These data are in contrast to many reports relating a link between breast cancer and alcohol use, despite the fact that both cancers are believed to be estrogen dependent.

alendronate sodium A drug that affects bone metabolism. Alendronate sodium is being studied as a possible treatment for bone pain caused by cancer. It belongs to the family of drugs called bisphosphonates.

alkaline phosphatase An enzyme produced by bone tissue that may appear in high levels in the blood of women who have cancer that has spread to the bone, among other conditions.

See also ALKALINE PHOSPHATASE TEST.

alkaline phosphatase test A test that measures the level of an enzyme called ALKALINE PHOSPHATASE (ALP) in the blood. This enzyme is found in all tissues, especially in the liver, bile ducts, placenta, and bone. Since damaged or diseased tissue releases enzymes into the blood, ALP measurements can be abnormal in many conditions, including cancer. But the serum ALP level is also high in some normal circumstances, such as during normal bone growth or in response to a variety of drugs.

The ALP test is one of several that may be used to help diagnose cancers that typically spread to the bone. The normal range is 44 to 147 IU/l. Higher-than-normal levels may indicate leukemia or bone cancer.

alkylating agents Drugs that cause a chemical process to disrupt cell division, especially in fast-growing cells. Types of alkylating agents include alkyl sulfonates, ethylenimines, nitrogen mustards, nitrosoureas, and triagenes.

allicin A phytochemical found in onions and GARLIC that experts suspect may help protect against cancer. Allicin is most widely recognized for its action as an antiviral, antifungal, and antibacterial agent with the ability to block the toxins produced by bacteria and viruses. It is also an ANTIOXIDANT and helps to eliminate toxins from the body.

alopecia See HAIR LOSS.

alpha-fetoprotein test A tumor marker test that checks for high levels of alpha-fetoprotein (AFP), which is typically found in embryonic tissue and blood. Although alpha-fetoprotein is generally found during periods of fetal development, it rarely appears in nonpregnant, healthy adults. High levels of AFP in the blood can signal the appearance of certain cancers, including OVARIAN CANCER, and can be used to help determine whether a particular treatment is working.

altretamine (Hexalen, hexamethylmelamine) An ALKYLATING AGENT type of oral CHEMOTHERAPY used to treat OVARIAN CANCER. It works by disrupting and killing cancer cells. Side effects include nausea and vomiting, decreased white blood cell and platelet counts, FATIGUE, DIARRHEA, mood changes, and APPETITE LOSS.

American Association for Cancer Education (AACE) A professional organization of educators in many disciplines who are working to improve the quality of education in the field of cancer. The association provides a forum for those concerned with the education of health professionals, working to advance the prevention of cancer, expedite early cancer detection, promote individualized therapy, and develop rehabilitation programs for cancer patients.

AACE efforts extend to the faculties of schools of medicine, dentistry, osteopathy, education, pharmacy, nursing, public health, and social work. The association encourages projects for the training of paramedical personnel as well as educational programs for the general public, populations at risk, and patients with cancer.

The group was founded in 1947 as the Cancer Coordinators, an association of cancer educators from U.S. medical and dental schools that met annually to discuss issues in the field. The mission of the association today is to foster cancer education throughout the world. It provides a forum for health-related professionals concerned with the study and improvement of cancer education at the undergraduate, graduate, continuing professional, and paraprofessional levels. Active members include physicians, dentists, nurses, health educators, social workers, occupational therapists, and other professionals interested in cancer education. For contact information, see Appendix I.

American Cancer Society (ACS) A nationwide community-based organization dedicated to eliminating cancer as a major health problem by preventing cancer, saving lives, and easing suffering through research, education, advocacy, and service. It is one of the oldest and largest voluntary health agencies in the United States: more than two million Americans are involved in programs of research, education, patient service, advocacy, and rehabilitation. Headquartered in Atlanta, Georgia, the ACS has state divisions throughout the country and more than 3,400 local offices.

To ease the impact of cancer on patients and their families, the American Cancer Society provides service and rehabilitation programs as well as patient and family education and support programs. The ACS provides printed materials and conducts educational programs. Cancer Society staff members also accept calls and distribute publications in Spanish and sponsor a number of related support groups, including CANCER SURVIVORS NETWORK and LOOK GOOD . . . FEEL BETTER. A local ACS group may be listed in the white pages of the telephone directory.

To date, the society has invested more than $2.4 billion in cancer research and has provided grant support to 32 Nobel Prize winners early in their career. The society's overall annual expenditure in research grew steadily from $1 million in 1946 to more than $125 million in 2002. The research program focuses primarily on peer-reviewed projects initiated by beginning investigators working in leading medical and scientific institutions across the country. It consists of three components: extramural grants, intramural epidemiology and surveillance research, and the intramural behavioral research center. The society's prevention programs focus primarily on tobacco control, the relationship between diet and physical activity and cancer, promotion of comprehensive school health education, and reduction of the risk of skin cancer. The society also tries to provide patients and professionals with information via its early detection guidelines and its detection education and advocacy programs, in order to ensure that all cancers are found at the earliest possible stage when there is the greatest chance for successful treatment. The society sponsors national conferences and workshops, audiovisual and print publications, the American Cancer Society Web site, and the National Call Center, as well as clinical awards, professorships, and scholarships.

The American Cancer Society Web site (www. cancer.org) is sponsored by the ACS to provide life-saving information to the public. The site includes an interactive cancer resource center, containing in-depth information on every major cancer type. Through the resource center, visitors can order American Cancer Society publications, gain access to recent news articles, and find additional on- and off-line resources. Other sections on the Web site include a directory of medical resources, links to other sites organized by cancer type or topic, resources for media representatives, and information on the society's research grants program, advocacy efforts, and special events. For contact information, see Appendix I.

American Chronic Pain Association (ACPA) A nonprofit, tax-exempt organization that has more than 400 chapters in the United States, Canada, Australia, New Zealand, Mexico, England, Ireland, Wales, Scotland, India, Jordan, and Russia. Since 1980, the association has provided a support system, for people with chronic pain, through education in pain-management skills and self-help group activities. Groups are open to anyone who has chronic pain, regardless of race, creed, sexual orientation, or source of the pain.

The ACPA facilitates peer support and education for individuals who have chronic pain and their families so that these individuals may live more fully in spite of pain. The association also works to raise awareness among the health-care community, policy makers, and the public about issues of living with chronic pain. For contact information, see Appendix I.

American College of Radiology (ACR) A medical specialty society established in 1923 that promotes high-quality medical imaging. With more than 31,000 members, the college has been a leader in radiation oncology for the past 25 years. The ACR recently created the American College of Radiology Imaging Network, a multicenter network that conducts diagnostic imaging studies comparing standard techniques and equipment with newer technology.

The members of the American College of Radiology include radiologists, radiation ONCOLOGISTS, and medical physicists. For more than three-quarters of a century, the ACR has devoted its resources to making imaging safe, effective, and accessible to those who need it.

The ACR supports a number of accreditation programs, including ultrasound, magnetic resonance imaging, nuclear medicine, radiation oncology, radiography/fluoroscopy, and computer tomography. Patients can search for accredited facilities near their home by visiting the ACR Web site. For contact information, see Appendix I.

American Institute for Cancer Research (AICR) A nonprofit group that provides information about cancer prevention, particularly through diet and nutrition, and supports research at sites throughout the United States. The institute also offers a toll-free nutrition hotline, a pen pal support network, and a wide array of consumer and health-professional brochures, plus information about nutrition and its link to cancer and cancer prevention.

The AICR also supports CancerResource, an information and resource program for cancer patients. A limited selection of Spanish-language publications is available.

Since its founding in 1982, the American Institute for Cancer Research has grown into the nation's leading charity in the field of diet, nutrition, and cancer. AICR also offers a wide range of cancer-prevention education programs and publications for health professionals and the public. Through these pioneering efforts, AICR has helped focus attention on the link between cancer and lifestyle choices. For contact information, see Appendix I.

American Joint Committee on Cancer (AJCC) An organization established in 1959 to publish systems of classification of cancer, including staging and end results reporting, for doctors. This information is used to select the most effective treatment, determine prognosis, and continue evaluation of cancer-control measures.

The organization is comprised of six founding organizations, four sponsoring organizations, and seven liaison organizations. Membership is reserved for those organizations whose missions or goals are consistent with or complementary to those of the AJCC.

These organizations generally demonstrate involvement or activity in one or more of the following areas: cancer epidemiology, patient care, cancer control, cancer registration, professional education, research, and biostatistics.

Sponsoring organizations include the AMERICAN CANCER SOCIETY, the American College of Surgeons, the AMERICAN SOCIETY OF CLINICAL ONCOLOGY, and the Centers for Disease Control and Prevention. For contact information, see Appendix I.

American Pain Society A multidisciplinary organization of basic and clinical scientists, practicing clinicians, policy analysts, and others interested in advancing pain-related research, education, treatment, and professional practice. The American Pain Society was founded in 1977 in Chicago. Through its Pain Facilities Directory, the society offers information on more than 500 specialized pain treatment centers across the country. It also offers counseling for pain, referrals, and education programs. For contact information, see Appendix I.

American Society for Colposcopy and Cervical Pathology A nonprofit organization of healthcare professionals, founded in 1964 and committed to improving health care through the study, prevention, diagnosis, and management of lower genital tract disorders. For contact information, see Appendix I.

American Society of Clinical Oncology (ASCO) A nonprofit organization dedicated to supporting all types of cancer research, especially patient-oriented clinical research. ASCO's mission is to facilitate the delivery of high-quality health care, foster the exchange of information, further the training of researchers, and encourage communication among the various cancer specialties.

ASCO has more than 16,000 professional members worldwide, including clinical oncologists in medical oncology, therapeutic radiology, surgical oncology, pediatric oncology, gynecologic oncology, urologic oncology, and hematology; students; oncology nurses; and other health-care practitioners. International members make up 20 percent of the total membership and represent 75 countries worldwide. For contact information, see Appendix I.

aminoglutethimide (Cytadren, Elipten) A type of CHEMOTHERAPY drug that belongs to a class of hormone and hormone-inhibiting drugs called adrenal steroid inhibitors. These drugs stop the adrenal glands from making steroid HORMONES, including ESTROGEN. This drug is given orally and must be taken with hydrocortisone.

analgesic pump A device, containing narcotic medication, that can be operated by a patient to control pain. First available in 1974, the pump is hooked up to an intravenous line so that patients can obtain immediate pain relief on demand. When a button is pressed, the patient self-administers a preset dose of medication as often as needed (within preset limits to protect against excessive dosage). The analgesic pump has the psychological advantage of allowing the patient to exercise some control over pain, rather than wait for a nurse to administer an injection.

anastrozole An anticancer drug that belongs to the family of nonsteroidal aromatase inhibitors. Anastrozole is used to decrease estrogen production and suppress the growth of tumors that require ESTROGEN for growth.

anemia A lack of red cells in the blood. Anemia is a common problem among patients with cancer, causing debilitating FATIGUE. It is often produced by a decline in the level of hemoglobin (the part of blood that carries oxygen) or a reduction in the number of red blood cells.

Hemolytic anemia occurs when red blood cells are destroyed too early in their life cycle, possibly as a result of CHEMOTHERAPY or radiation.

Aplastic anemia occurs when the BONE MARROW makes too few red blood cells, as a result of either chemotherapy or radiation. Levels of white blood cells and platelets also decline.

Iron-deficiency anemia occurs when there is too little iron in the blood; the low level leads to a lack of hemoglobin, which in turn causes anemia. In those who have cancer, iron deficiency also may be caused by bleeding from a tumor.

Pernicious anemia occurs when there is a lack of vitamin B_{12} in the diet. Often cancer patients have a poor appetite and may not eat enough foods that contain vitamin B_{12}. Anemia also may occur with cancer spread to bone or in response to hormone therapy.

Symptoms

Regardless of the cause, the symptoms of anemia typically appear gradually. As blood counts tend to drop slowly, initial symptoms may not be readily apparent. Once anemia becomes significant, it may cause blood pressure to decrease when a person stands up quickly. Anemia may also cause weakness, dizziness, pallor, shortness of breath, heart palpitations, feeling of cold, or fatigue.

Treatment

Anemia that results from chemotherapy may be treated by iron and vitamin supplements, bone marrow stimulants such as ERYTHROPOIETIN (a medication that stimulates the production of blood cells), or transfusion therapy.

aneuploid   Cells with an abnormal number of DNA (either too much or not enough). Cancers with the same amount of DNA as normal cells are called "diploid"; those with too much or not enough DNA are called aneuploid. About two-thirds of breast cancers are aneuploid. Several studies suggest aneuploid cancers may be more aggressive.

Assessing the malignancy of a cell is done with FLOW CYTOMETRY, a procedure that measures the amount of cellular DNA.

angiogenesis   The formation of a network of blood vessels that penetrates into cancerous growths, supplying nutrients and oxygen and removing waste products, helping cancer to spread.

The walls of blood vessels are formed by cells that divide only about once every three years. However, when conditions require it, angiogenesis can stimulate them to divide sooner than that.

Angiogenesis is regulated by molecules that either activate or inhibit the process of growth. Normally the inhibitors predominate, blocking growth. Should a need for new blood vessels arise (such as to repair a wound), angiogenesis activators increase in number and inhibitors decrease. This reaction prompts the formation of new blood vessels.

Tumor angiogenesis begins when cancerous tumor cells release molecules that send signals to surrounding normal tissue, activating certain genes that in turn make proteins to encourage growth of new blood vessels. Other chemicals, called ANGIO-GENESIS INHIBITORS, signal the process to stop.

Because cancer cannot grow or spread without the formation of new blood vessels, scientists are trying to find ways to stop angiogenesis. They are studying natural and synthetic angiogenesis inhibitors (also called antiangiogenesis agents) in the hope that these chemicals will block the formation of new blood vessels. In animal studies, angiogenesis inhibitors have successfully stopped the formation of new blood vessels, causing the cancer to shrink and die.

When researchers realized that cancer cells can release molecules to activate the process of angiogenesis, the challenge became to find and study these angiogenesis-stimulating molecules in animal and human tumors. From such studies more than a dozen different proteins, as well as several smaller molecules, have been identified as *angiogenic,* meaning that they are released by tumors as signals for angiogenesis. Among these molecules, two proteins appear to be the most important for sustaining tumor growth: vascular endothelial growth factor (VEGF) and basic fibroblast growth factor (bFGF). VEGF and bFGF are produced by many kinds of cancer cells and by certain types of normal cells, too.

Although many tumors produce angiogenic molecules such as VEGF and bFGF, their presence is not sufficient to begin blood vessel growth. Angiogenesis begins if these activator molecules overcome a variety of angiogenesis inhibitors that normally restrain blood vessel growth. Almost a dozen naturally occurring proteins can inhibit angiogenesis, including proteins called angiostatin, endostatin, and thrombospondin. A finely tuned balance between the concentration of angiogenesis inhibitors and that of activators such as VEGF and bFGF determines whether a tumor can induce the growth of new blood vessels. To trigger angiogenesis, the production of activators must increase as the production of inhibitors decreases.

The discovery that angiogenesis inhibitors such as endostatin can restrain the growth of primary tumors raises the possibility that such inhibitors may also be able to slow tumor spread.

It has been known for many years that cancer cells that originate in a primary tumor can spread to other organs and form tiny, microscopic tumor masses that can remain dormant for years. A likely explanation for this tumor dormancy is that no angiogenesis occurred, so the small tumor lacked the new blood vessels needed for continued growth. One possible reason for tumor dormancy may be that some primary tumors secrete into the bloodstream the inhibitor angiostatin, which then circulates throughout the body and inhibits blood vessel growth at other sites. This process could prevent microscopic cancer cells from growing into visible tumors.

Almost two dozen angiogenesis inhibitors are currently being tested for patients who have cancers of the breast. If the results of clinical trials show that angiogenesis inhibitors are both safe and effective in treating cancer in humans, these agents may be approved by the U.S. Food and Drug Administration and made available for widespread use. The process of producing and testing angiogenesis inhibitors is likely to require several years.

angiogenesis inhibitor Substance (also called antiangiogenesis agent) that can prevent the growth of blood vessels from surrounding tissue to a solid tumor (ANGIOGENESIS). Preventing the growth of blood vessels in this way can eventually starve and kill tumors.

anorexia See APPETITE LOSS.

anthocyanins A group of plant chemicals, within the larger category of PHYTOCHEMICALS called PHENOLICS, that give intense color to certain red and blue fruits and vegetables (especially blueberry). These plant pigments are powerful ANTIOXIDANTS that have been studied extensively for their ability to fight cancer.

antibody therapy Treatment with a substance that can directly kill specific tumor cells or stimulate the immune system to kill tumor cells.

See also MONOCLONAL ANTIBODY THERAPY.

anti–carcinoembryonic antigen antibody An antibody against CARCINOEMBRYONIC ANTIGEN (CEA), a protein present in certain types of cancer cells.

antiemetics See ANTINAUSEA MEDICATION.

antiestrogens Substances that block the activity of ESTROGENS, the family of HORMONES that promote the development and maintenance of female sex characteristics. Several antiestrogen drugs such as TAMOXIFEN, have been developed to treat cancers that are affected by hormones, including breast cancer and ENDOMETRIAL CANCER.

Endometrial cancer cells seem to grow best in the presence of high levels of the female hormone estrogen. Women who have an intact uterus who take HORMONE REPLACEMENT THERAPY that includes estrogen but not progesterone are at risk for developing endometrial cancer if therapy is continued for many years. Experts suspect the same process can occur in women who are overweight, since fat cells produce a form of estrogen. On the other hand, treating women who have endometrial cancer with antiestrogen hormones may impede the growth of endometrial cancer cells.

Unlike chemotherapy or radiation therapy, hormone treatment does not kill cells directly, but it does make their environment less hospitable. Experts hope that eventually starved cells will die.

Side Effects
Antiestrogens used to treat endometrial cancer can cause increased appetite, water retention, nausea, weight gain, mood changes, and HAIR LOSS as well as less common side effects. Some women who have a history of blood clots or liver problems may be at increased risk for more serious side effects with these medications.

antigen A substance that is foreign to the body and capable of stimulating an immune response. Antigens are involved in several different studies investigating the use of VACCINES AGAINST CANCER. In these studies, researchers inject an antigen into a patient and wait for it to stimulate the person's IMMUNE SYSTEM to produce cells to fight it off—thereby killing cancer cells in the process.

antimetabolites Anticancer drugs that closely resemble substances needed by cells for normal growth and that interfere with normal metabolic processes within cells.

The chemotherapy drugs FLUOROURACIL, methotrexate, and mercaptopurine are all antimetabolites that prevent cell growth during a short specific interval in the cell's reproduction cycle by interfering with important enzyme reactions within the cell.

In order for antimetabolites to be effective, it may be necessary to administer them over the course of hours, days, or weeks. Side effects of antimetabolites can be severe, including blood cell disorders or stomach problems; sometimes, cancer cells can become resistant to a particular metabolite.

antinausea medication A type of drug that can prevent or reduce nausea and vomiting, common side effects of CHEMOTHERAPY and RADIATION THERAPY. Popular antinausea drugs include dexamethasone (DECADRON), prochlorperazine (COMPAZINE), thiethylperazine (Torecan), chlorpromazine (Thorazine), metoclopramide, lorazepam (Ativan), diazepam (Valium), dronabinol (MARINOL), granisetron (Kytril), dolasetron (Anzemet), and ondansetron (Zofran). Often a combination of these drugs is prescribed; if the first combination does not work, others may work better. Antinausea medications are often administered along with chemotherapy drugs to prevent nausea. Typically, it is much easier to prevent nausea and vomiting than to treat them once they occur.

antioxidants Compounds that fight cell damage caused by FREE RADICALS, rogue oxygen molecules that can attack cells throughout the body. Although free radicals serve important functions, such as helping the immune system fight disease, at excessive levels they can cause problems.

Highly reactive oxygen radicals (free radicals) are formed both during normal metabolism and in response to infection and some chemicals. They cause damage to fatty acids in cell membranes, and the products of this damage can then cause damage to proteins and DNA. The most widely accepted theory of the biochemical basis of many types of cancer is that cancer is triggered by free radical damage to tissues.

A number of nutrients are involved in protection against, or repair after, free radical damage—especially vitamin E, beta-carotene, vitamin C, and selenium. Collectively these are known as antioxidant nutrients, and they limit the cell and tissue damage caused by toxins and pollutants.

Because high dosages of antioxidant supplements can cause side effects, it is safer to consume antioxidants as part of a healthy diet. Antioxidants are found in fruits and vegetables (especially blueberries and yellow fruits and vegetables), brown rice, whole grains, meats, eggs, and dairy products.

Side Effects
Supplements that contain high doses of antioxidants can cause severe side effects including internal bleeding and may be toxic in patients who are taking anticoagulant medication. No one should use these or any supplements without consulting a doctor. In addition, high doses of vitamin E are potentially harmful if combined with blood-thinning drugs.

antitumor antibiotics A type of CHEMOTHERAPY that attacks microbes and is also toxic to cells, interfering with DNA. They are widely used to treat cancer. Examples of antitumor antibiotics include bleomycin and doxorubicin (Adriamycin).

AP A combination of the CHEMOTHERAPY drugs doxorubicin (ADRIAMYCIN) and CISPLATIN sometimes used to treat OVARIAN CANCER.

apoptosis Programmed cell death that occurs naturally during the development of a person's tissues and organs. During fetal development, apoptosis plays a vital role in determining the final size and form of tissues and organs. As more cells are produced than are required to form tissues and organs, unwanted cells are programmed to die, either because the chemical signals that direct them to go on living are suppressed or because they receive a specific signal to die. Experts believe that the suppression of apoptosis is associated with the uncontrolled cell growth in leukemia and other cancers. Apoptosis also occurs when viruses infect cells. Apoptosis differs from cell necrosis, in which cell death may be triggered by a toxic substance.

appetite loss   Lack of interest in eating is a problem frequently experienced by cancer patients as a direct result of advancing disease and as a side effect of treatment. Most types of CHEMOTHERAPY drugs cause some degree of appetite loss. People may lose their appetite while struggling with cancer because chemotherapy-related nausea, or mouth or stomach pain, alters appetite—or because pain itself can trigger appetite loss.

Appetite loss is a serious problem among cancer patients because it can lead to poor nutrition, which can interfere with recovery. Loss of appetite and weight loss can lead to CACHEXIA, a form of malnutrition.

Because good nutrition is essential to recovery, maintaining a healthy diet during treatment is important.

Treatment
Drugs such as megestrol (Megace) or dronabinol (MARINOL or marijuana) may be used to improve appetite. In addition, patients should try to eat

- Small, frequent meals
- Nutritious snacks
- Milk or butter with food
- High-calorie, high-protein food
- Attractive, appetizing meals

Other ways patients can encourage themselves to consume enough food include eating when they feel most comfortable; stimulating their appetite with light exercise; taking their medications with high-calorie drinks; and dining at a friend's home or a good restaurant. Patients may also try drinking lemon-flavored drinks; or eating cold, white food (such as ice cream, milkshakes, or boiled chicken) and rinsing the mouth before eating. Many patients find that eating red meat becomes unpleasant at this time; patients should substitute other high-protein meals they find more palatable. Normal appetite usually resumes after chemotherapy ends, although appetite may not be completely normal for several weeks.

aromatase inhibition   A type of HORMONE THERAPY, used for postmenopausal women who have hormone-dependent ENDOMETRIAL CANCER, in which production of the female HORMONE estradiol is blocked.

Asian women   Cancer affects women of all racial and ethnic groups, but in general, Asian women tend to have some of the lowest incidence and death rates of cancer in the world. In addition, Asian-American women have the highest life expectancy (85.8 years) of any ethnic or racial group in the United States. Yet there are disparities among Asian subgroups: Samoan (74.9 years), Native Hawaiian (77.2 years), Filipino (81.5 years), Japanese (84.5), and Chinese women (86.1 years).

However, once Asian women come to the United States, their rates of cancer tend to rise. Experts suggest this finding may indicate that cancer rates are more directly related to diet and environmental factors than to race.

Many of the differences in cancer incidence and mortality rates among racial and ethnic groups may be due to factors associated with social class rather than ethnicity. Socioeconomic status in particular appears to play a major role in the differences in cancer incidence and mortality rates, risk factors, and screening prevalence among racial and ethnic minorities. In part, this may occur because socioeconomic status predicts the likelihood of access to education, certain jobs, and health insurance, as well as income level and living conditions. All of these factors are associated with a person's chance of development of cancer and survival.

Asian women have a low rate of CERVICAL CANCER compared to that of other groups. It is also well established that Asian women in Asia have a much lower incidence of ENDOMETRIAL CANCER than do Caucasian women, although the cancer rate rises when Asian women immigrate to the United States. This finding is believed to be related to DIET in their home country; Asian women living in Asia consume much more tofu and other SOY PRODUCTS in their diet than in the United States.

As of 2000, Asian women had an incidence rate of 11.7 per 100,000, compared to 17.5 for Hispanics and 13.3 for African Americans. The rate of death from cervical cancer was also lower for Asian women—at 3.1 per 100,000. The exception to this generality is that cervical cancer incidence rates among Vietnamese women is extremely high.

aspiration The removal of fluid or cells from tissue by inserting a needle into an area and drawing the fluid into a syringe.

Association of Cancer Online Resources (ACOR)
A collection of online communities designed to provide timely and accurate information about cancer in a supportive environment. ACOR offers access to mailing lists that provide support, information, and community to everyone affected by cancer and related disorders.

In addition to supporting the mailing lists, ACOR develops and hosts state-of-the-art Internet-based knowledge systems that allow the public to find and use credible information relevant to their illness. In addition to mailing lists, ACOR aims to provide patients with access to varied and accurate information sources through Internet resource development and partnership with trusted content providers. ACOR also strives to improve communication between patients and health-care professionals through advocacy in a variety of public forums, including general media and professional journals.

Association of Community Cancer Centers (ACCC) The leading oncology policy organization in the United States for the cancer care team, dedicated to helping cancer professionals adapt to the complex challenges of program management, reimbursement, legislation, and regulations. In the 1970s the ACCC organized the first U.S. meeting to discuss hospital oncology units and HOSPICE care; throughout the 1990s, association support resulted in passage of ACCC's off-label drug legislation in 39 states. The association focuses on helping to assure that cancer programs are adequately funded, and develops guidelines for standard patient care.

ACCC members include medical and radiation oncologists, surgeons, cancer program administrators, hospital executives, practice managers, oncology nurses and social workers, and cancer program data managers. ACCC Institution/Group Practice members include more than 650 medical centers, hospitals, oncology practices, and cancer programs across the United States. For contact information, see Appendix I.

atypical cells Cells that are abnormal or not usual. Cancer is the result of the division of atypical cells.

back pain Low back pain can signal OVARIAN CANCER, UTERINE CANCER, or other abnormalities in those organs. There are many noncancerous conditions that cause low back pain; low back pain that occurs together with other symptoms of gynecological cancer should be investigated.

B cell A type of white blood cell produced in the BONE MARROW. The B cell is one of two types of white blood cells that play an important part in the immune system.

beta-carotene A common plant chemical in a group of more than 600. Beta-carotene is converted by the body into vitamin A, which performs many vital functions including the growth and repair of body tissues, formation of bones and teeth, resistance of the body to infection, and development of healthy eye tissues. Epidemiologic studies have linked high intake of foods rich in beta-carotene and high blood levels of the micronutrient to a lower risk of cancer.

Beta-carotene acts as an ANTIOXIDANT and immune system booster; it is found in bright orange–colored fruits and vegetables such as carrots, pumpkins, peaches, and sweet potatoes. Some experts suspect it may be possible to shield the body's immune system from the risk of cancer by supplementing the diet with beta-carotene.

Most but not all beta-carotene found in supplements is synthetic, consisting of only one molecule (natural beta-carotene in food is made of two molecules). Researchers originally saw no meaningful difference between natural and synthetic beta-carotene, but this view was questioned when the link between beta-carotene-containing foods and lung cancer prevention was not duplicated in studies that used synthetic beta-carotene. The most common beta-carotene supplement is 25,000 IU (15 mg) per day, though some people take as much as 100,000 IU (60 mg) per day. Excessive (more than 100,000 IU, or 60 mg per day) beta-carotene intake sometimes tints the skin yellow-orange. Individuals who take beta-carotene for long periods should also supplement their diet with vitamin E, as beta-carotene may reduce vitamin E level.

bioconjugate drug A new type of medication, currently being investigated, that combines a CHEMOTHERAPY drug (such as doxorubicin) with a sugar (such as hyaluronic acid [HA]) that normally helps cancer move through the human body. A bioconjugate drug can track down, invade, and destroy tumor cells as they spread. This drug, which also contains a large molecule (copolymer) that ensures that the drug enters only cancer cells, has been effective in killing OVARIAN CANCER, breast cancer, and colon tumor cells grown in the lab.

Some other methods of targeting cancer cells (such as using MONOCLONAL ANTIBODIES) fail because they attack the outside of a cancer cell but do not enter and destroy it.

Doxorubicin is administered as an intravenous drip to treat ovarian cancer; HA is found in human cartilage and helps cells stick to each other, grow, and migrate. HA binds to certain receptors on cells. There are high levels of HA receptors on many tumor cells, including ovarian cancer cells; these help the cancer spread. Tumor cells use these receptors to move out of the tumor and through the blood, reinvading elsewhere in the body.

When HA is combined with doxorubicin, the tumor cells bind to the HA and the doxorubicin is released into the tumor cells but nowhere else. Patients can tolerate only a limited amount of the drug because it is toxic to other cells, such as heart cells, and can cause heart attacks. While the HA targets the cancer cell, the third ingredient in this combination drug—a copolymer—contains a peptide that delivers the drug combination to a specific part of each cancer cell. Human tests of the triple combination are not scheduled to begin until at least 2005, but tests on mice will begin much sooner.

bioflavonoids   Chemical compounds related to vitamin C that have demonstrated an ability to slow cancer growth. These naturally occurring plant compounds act primarily as plant pigments and ANTIOXIDANTS, substances that fight cell damage caused by free radicals (rogue oxygen molecules that can attack cells throughout the body).

Lemons, grapes, plums, grapefruit, cherries, blackberries, and rosehips are some of the richest dietary sources of bioflavonoids. Other sources include citrus fruits, green peppers, broccoli, tomatoes, green tea, and some herb teas (especially stinging nettle tea). Bioflavonoids belong to a large group of more than 2,000 PHYTOCHEMICALS called phenols that are known to be very powerful antioxidants. Many studies have identified their unique role in protecting vitamin C from oxidation in the body, thereby allowing the body to reap more benefits from vitamin C.

Different bioflavonoids tend to have different health effects on the body, but in general, a diet high in bioflavonoids is associated with a lower incidence of many diseases, including cancer. Anyone taking bioflavonoid supplements should inform a doctor before undergoing surgery, because they may interfere with the results of some blood and urine tests.

biological response modifier (BRM)   Substances developed by researchers to strengthen the ability of the IMMUNE SYSTEM to find and destroy cancer. Treatment with a BRM alters the body's natural antitumor response by stimulating the BONE MARROW to make specific tumor-killing blood cells. These substances may serve directly as tumor-killing agents or chemical messengers, decrease the body's normal methods of suppressing the immune response, or change tumor cells so they are more likely to trigger an immune response to or be damaged by the immune system. Biological response

modifiers may also improve the body's tolerance to RADIATION THERAPY or to CHEMOTHERAPY.

There are many types of these modifiers, some produced by the body and others created in the lab. Many ongoing studies are investigating the use of the substances in BIOLOGICAL THERAPY to treat a wide variety of cancers.

The primary biological response modifiers include antibodies, COLONY-STIMULATING FACTORS, CYTOKINES (including interferons and interleukins), MONOCLONAL ANTIBODIES, and vaccines. Interferon is the best-known and most widely used biological response modifier. Although most human cells produce interferon, interferon also can be made by using recombinant molecular biological techniques. Although experts are not sure exactly how they work, interferons can play a role in the treatment of several cancers.

Researchers continue to discover new BRMs, learn more about their function, and develop ways to use them in cancer therapy. All of these substances alter the interaction between cancer cells and the body's immune defenses, restoring the body's ability to fight cancer. Biological therapies may be used to stop or control processes that allow cancer cells to grow, make cancer cells more recognizable to the immune system, boost the killing power of immune system cells, and alter the malignant growth patterns to make them more like those of healthy cells. BRMs also block or reverse the process that triggers abnormal cell growth that leads to a cancerous cell. They enhance the body's ability to repair normal cells damaged by other forms of cancer treatment, such as chemotherapy or radiation therapy. BRMs also stop cancer cells from spreading to other parts of the body.

Some BRMs are a standard part of treatment for certain types of cancer; others are being studied as new types of treatments, either alone or in combination. They are also being used with other treatments, such as radiation therapy and chemotherapy.

biological therapy   A relatively new type of cancer treatment, sometimes called immunotherapy, biotherapy, or BIOLOGICAL RESPONSE MODIFIER (BRM) therapy, that is designed to enhance the body's natural defenses against cancer. Biological therapies may be used to stop or suppress processes that allow cancer growth and to make cancer cells more recognizable and therefore more susceptible to destruction by the immune system. Biological therapies also boost the killing power of immune system cells and alter cancer cells' growth patterns to promote healthy behavior. They can be used to block or reverse the process that triggers a normal cell to grow abnormally and enhance the body's ability to repair normal cells damaged by other forms of cancer treatment, such as chemotherapy or radiation therapy. Biological therapy also can help prevent cancer cells from spreading to other parts of the body.

Biological Response Modifiers

BRMs are antibodies, cytokines, and other immune system substances produced in the lab for use in cancer treatment that alter the interaction between the body's immune defenses and cancer cells to boost the body's ability to fight the disease. They include interferons, interleukins, COLONY-STIMULATING FACTORS, MONOCLONAL ANTIBODIES, and vaccines.

Interferons

There are three major types of interferons, which are naturally occurring cytokines: interferon alfa, interferon beta, and interferon gamma. Interferon alfa is the type most widely used in cancer treatment.

Interferons can improve the way a cancer patient's immune system fights cancer cells and may slow the growth of cancer cells or promote their transformation into cells that behave more normally. Researchers believe that some interferons may also stimulate natural killer (NK) cells, T cells, and macrophages, boosting the immune system's anticancer function.

Interleukins

Interleukins are also cytokines that occur naturally in the body and can be produced synthetically. There are many different kinds of interleukins; interleukin-2 (IL-2 or aldesleukin) has been the most widely studied in cancer treatment. IL-2 stimulates the growth and action of cancer-killing immune cells such as lymphocytes.

Colony-Stimulating Factors (CSFs)

CSFs (sometimes called hematopoietic growth factors) usually do not directly affect tumor cells; rather, they encourage BONE MARROW stem cells to divide and develop into white blood cells, platelets, and red blood cells. Bone marrow is critical to immune system function because it is the source of all blood cells. The CSFs' stimulation of the immune system may benefit patients who are having cancer treatment. Because anticancer drugs can damage the body's ability to make white blood cells, red blood cells, and platelets, those who receive anticancer drugs have an increased risk of developing infections, becoming anemic, and bleeding more easily.

By using CSFs to stimulate blood cell production, doctors can increase dosages of anticancer drugs without increasing the risk of infection or the need for transfusion with blood products. As a result, researchers have found CSFs particularly useful when combined with high-dose chemotherapy.

CSFs include the following:

- *Granulocyte colony-stimulating factor (G-CSF) (filgrastim) and granulocyte-macrophage colony-stimulating factor (GM-CSF) (sargramostim)* can increase the number of white blood cells, thereby reducing the risk of infection in patients who are receiving chemotherapy. G-CSF and GM-CSF can also stimulate the production of stem cells in preparation for stem cell or bone marrow transplantation.

- *Erythropoietin* can increase the number of red blood cells and reduce the need for red blood cell transfusions of patients who receive chemotherapy.

- *Oprelvekin* can reduce the need for platelet transfusions in patients who receive chemotherapy.

Researchers are studying CSFs in clinical trials to treat some types of leukemia, metastatic colorectal cancer, melanoma, lung cancer, and other types of cancer.

Monoclonal Antibodies (MOABs)

MOABs are antibodies made in the laboratory that are produced by a single type of cell and are specific for a particular antigen. Researchers are trying to figure out how to create MOABs specific to the antigens found on the surface of the cancer cell being treated. MOABs that react with specific types of cancer may enhance the immune response to the cancer. MOABs can be programmed to interfere with the growth of cancer cells. In addition, they may be linked to CHEMOTHERAPY drugs, radioactive substances, other biological response modifiers, or other toxins so that when the antibodies latch onto cancer cells, they deliver these poisons directly to the tumor, helping to destroy it.

MOABs may help destroy cancer cells in bone marrow that has been removed from a patient in preparation for bone marrow transplantation. MOABs carrying radioisotopes may also prove useful in diagnosis of certain cancers.

Cancer Vaccines

Researchers are developing vaccines for cancer treatments that may encourage the immune system to recognize and reject cancer cells, preventing cancer recurrence. In contrast to vaccines against infectious diseases, VACCINES AGAINST CANCER are designed to be injected after the disease is diagnosed, rather than before it develops.

Cancer vaccines given when the tumor is small may be able to cure the cancer. Early cancer vaccine studies focused on patients with melanoma, but today vaccines are also being studied in the treatment of many other types of cancer, including lymphomas and cancers of the breast. Researchers are also investigating ways that cancer vaccines can be used in combination with other BRMs.

Side Effects

Biological therapies can cause a number of side effects, including rashes or swelling at the site where they are injected. Several biological response modifiers, including interferons and interleukins, may cause flulike symptoms including fever, chills, nausea, vomiting, and APPETITE LOSS. FATIGUE is another common side effect, and blood pressure may be affected. The side effects of IL-2 can often be severe, depending on the dosage given. Patients need to be closely monitored during treatment. Side effects of CSFs may include bone pain, fatigue, fever, and appetite loss. The side effects of MOABs vary, and serious allergic reactions may occur. Cancer vaccines can cause muscle aches and fever.

biomarkers   See CA 15-3; CA 125; CARCINOEMBRYONIC ANTIGEN (CEA); TUMOR MARKER.

biopsy   The surgical removal of a small piece of tissue or a small tumor for microscopic examination to determine whether cancer cells are present. In a traditional biopsy, a large hollow needle removes a core or plug of the tissue. In a FINE NEEDLE ASPIRATION, the tissue is sucked out of the suspected area. In needle biopsy, the surgeon removes a sample of tissue from the tumor with a needlelike instrument. In an INCISIONAL BIOPSY, the surgeon cuts into the tumor and removes a sample of tissue.

See also BONE MARROW ASPIRATION; CONE BIOPSY; CORE BIOPSY; EXCISIONAL BIOPSY.

biotherapy   Treatment to stimulate or restore the ability of the IMMUNE SYSTEM to fight infection and disease, and to lessen side effects caused by some cancer treatments. Biotherapy is also known as immunotherapy, biological therapy, or BIOLOGICAL RESPONSE MODIFIER therapy.

birth control pill   Oral contraceptives, also known simply as "the Pill," a birth control device that revolutionized contraception in the 1960s. The birth control pill, in various forms, has been on the market for more than 35 years and is the most popular form of reversible birth control in the United States.

The Pill works by suppressing ovulation (the monthly release of an egg from the ovaries) as a result of the combined actions of the hormones ESTROGEN and PROGESTIN. If taken daily as directed, it protects a woman almost completely from becoming pregnant. Oral contraceptives can reduce the risk of OVARIAN CANCER by half if used for five or more years. The use of birth control pills offers some protection against UTERINE CANCER as well.

Risks   Although birth control pills are safe for most women, they do carry some risks for some women. The Pill may contribute to high blood pressure, blood clots, and blockage of the arteries.

One of the major questions has been whether the Pill increases the risk of breast cancer in past and current Pill users. An international study published in the September 1996 issue of the journal *Contraception* concluded that women's risk of breast cancer 10 years after ending use of birth control pills was no higher than that of women who had never used the Pill. During use of the Pill and for the first 10 years after stopping, risk of breast cancer was only slightly higher in Pill users than in nonusers.

Most health experts advise that some women should not take the Pill:

- Women who smoke—especially those older than age 35
- Women who have a history of blood clots
- Women who have a personal history of breast or ENDOMETRIAL CANCER
- Women who have heart disease
- Women who are older than age 45

Minipill Another type of oral contraceptive, called the minipill, is taken daily but contains only the hormone progestin and no estrogen. These pills work by reducing and thickening cervical mucus to prevent sperm from reaching the egg. They also prevent the uterine lining from thickening, thereby preventing a fertilized egg from implanting in the uterus. Because they lack estrogen, these pills are slightly less effective than combined oral contraceptives. Women who take the minipill late (even by as little as three hours) have a higher chance of pregnancy.

Minipills can still decrease the risk of endometrial and ovarian cancer and pelvic inflammatory disease, and because they contain no estrogen, minipills do not present the risk of blood clots associated with estrogen in combined pills. They are a good option for women who can not take estrogen because they are breast-feeding or because estrogen-containing products cause them to have severe headaches or high blood pressure. Side effects of minipills include menstrual cycle changes, weight gain, and breast tenderness.

bisphosphonates Chemicals that block bone breakdown, typically used to treat osteoporosis. They can also be used to treat high calcium levels that may occur with some cancers, and to ease bone pain that occurs when CANCER spreads to the bones. Although bisphosphonates appear to improve bone symptoms in women with cancer, their use is still experimental.

bleeding, abnormal The most common warning sign of UTERINE CANCER. Cervical and VAGINAL CANCER, also may cause abnormal bleeding. FALLOPIAN TUBE CANCER, although rare, causes abnormal bleeding as one of its main symptoms.

Bleeding after menopause is abnormal and should be reported to a doctor immediately. Endometrial HYPERPLASIA, which can be the forerunner of uterine cancer, also causes abnormal bleeding.

Women in their childbearing years (and particularly in the premenopausal period) sometimes experience bleeding between menstrual periods. A woman who has more than two or three of these experiences should report them to a doctor. Bleeding after menopause or between periods may occur as a result of minor trauma (such as sex or douching). This also can be a sign of cervical or vaginal cancer and should be immediately reported to a doctor.

Occasionally, endometrial hyperplasia or uterine cancer can cause unusually heavy menstrual periods. A woman should notify her doctor of any sudden change in periods that continues longer than one or two cycles. Although it is not usually a sign of cancer, sudden heavy bleeding that requires a change of sanitary protection more than once per hour, that occurs more than once, or that lasts more than 24 hours should be reported.

Of course, not all bleeding is caused by malignant conditions. Noncancerous causes of bleeding include fibroid tumors, oral contraceptives, polyps, cervical inflammation, thyroid problems, and bleeding disorders.

blood count, complete (CBC) A test to measure the number of red blood cells, white blood cells, and platelets in a blood sample. Other factors also included in a CBC include hemoglobin (the level of oxygen-carrying protein) and hematocrit (percentage of red blood cells). A separate count of young red cells (called a retic or reticulocyte count) can be performed on the same blood sample, although it must be requested separately.

CBC results can reveal ANEMIA, a blood clotting problem, or an infection. A CBC is usually performed before each episode of CHEMOTHERAPY to measure the blood cell count, since chemotherapy often causes a drop in these levels. If the blood count is too low, the ONCOLOGIST may postpone chemotherapy treatment until it begins to rise.

bone marrow The soft, fatty substance filling the cavities of the bones, which contains immature cells called STEM CELLS. Stem cells produce

- White blood cells (leukocytes), which fight infection
- Red blood cells (erythrocytes), which carry oxygen to and remove waste products from organs and tissues
- Platelets (thrombocytes), which enable the blood to clot

CHEMOTHERAPY can affect bone marrow, causing a temporary decrease in the number of cells in the blood.

bone marrow aspiration A procedure in which a needle is inserted into the center of a bone, usually the hip, to remove a small amount of bone marrow for microscopic examination. BONE MARROW is the spongy substance on the inside of the bone in which blood cells are manufactured.

After the test, there is some pain or soreness at the site. The sample is analyzed for iron stores, red blood cell and white blood cell production and maturation, and number of megakaryocytes (cells that produce platelets).

A bone marrow aspiration is used to determine the cause of an abnormal result of a blood test; to confirm the diagnosis of anemia, an increase or drop in number of white blood cells, or a reduction of platelets in the blood; or to evaluate response to cancer treatments.

bone marrow biopsy See BONE MARROW ASPIRATION.

Bone Marrow Foundation A nonprofit organization dedicated to improving the quality of life for BONE MARROW TRANSPLANT patients and their families by providing financial aid, education, and emotional support. The foundation was created in 1992 to respond to the critical gap in financial coverage for patient support services.

Its Patient Aid Program has assisted hundreds of patients with the cost of donor searches, compatibility testing, bone marrow harvesting, medications, home and child-care services, medical equipment, transportation, cord blood banking, and housing expenses associated with the transplant.

The foundation currently accepts applications for aid from more than 70 bone marrow transplant centers throughout the United States. To fulfill the growing need for information and support of patients and their families, the foundation established the Marie M. Reynolds Resource and Educational Center to provide immediate information in a convenient format to patients, their families, and the clinicians who provide for their care. The center also seeks to provide support and encouragement to patients and families who are dealing with the challenge of a life-threatening disease. For contact information, see Appendix I.

bone marrow transplant A procedure to replace bone marrow that has been destroyed by high dosages of CHEMOTHERAPY drugs or by RADIATION THERAPY. In the past, bone marrow transplants had been tried in the treatment of breast and OVARIAN CANCER, but are no longer performed because the treatment is of no value.

Bone Marrow Transplant Family Support Network A national telephone support network for bone marrow transplant patients and their families that provides referrals, information, counseling, and health insurance information. For contact information, see Appendix I.

Bone Marrow Transplant Information Network (BMT InfoNet) A nonprofit organization dedicated exclusively to serving the needs of people who are facing a BONE MARROW, blood STEM CELL, or umbilical cord blood transplant. Founded in 1990 by a bone marrow transplant survivor, Susan Stewart, BMT InfoNet strives to provide high-quality medical information in easy-to-understand language so that patients can be active, knowledgeable participants in their health-care planning and treatment.

In addition to publications, BMT InfoNet offers patients and survivors emotional support. Its volunteer network of more than 200 transplant survivors is available to help newly diagnosed patients and their loved ones cope with the stress of a life-threatening diagnosis and the prospect of a bone marrow, stem cell, or cord blood transplant. For contact information, see Appendix I.

bone metastasis   The spread of cancerous cells to the bone, where they can cause severe pain.

Symptoms

Pain is the most common symptom of bone cancer, but symptoms vary with the location and size of the cancer. Tumors that occur in or near joints may cause swelling or tenderness in the affected area. Some women may experience continuous pain, whereas others may have only occasional discomfort, at least at first. If there is pain, it may be restricted to one area or may appear in different spots.

Bone cancer can interfere with normal movements and can weaken the bones, occasionally leading to fracture. Bone pain may change at different times of the day, or in response to rest or activity.

The most common sites of bone metastasis are the back, ribs, shoulder, and hips. If the cancerous cells spread to the spine, the patient may be paralyzed if the tumor compresses the nerves.

Other symptoms may include FATIGUE, fever, weight loss, and ANEMIA.

Diagnosis

In addition to a complete medical exam, the doctor may suggest a blood test to determine the level of an enzyme called ALKALINE PHOSPHATASE. A high level of alkaline phosphatase can be found in the blood when the cells that form bone tissue are active—such as when a broken bone is mending or when a tumor triggers the production of abnormal bone tissue.

X-rays can show the location, size, and shape of a bone tumor. If X-rays suggest that a tumor may be cancer, the doctor may recommend special imaging tests such as a bone scan, computed tomography (CT) scan, magnetic resonance imaging (MRI), or an angiogram.

Either a needle BIOPSY or an incisional biopsy can detect bone cancer. During a needle biopsy, the surgeon makes a small hole in the bone and removes a sample of tissue from the tumor with a needlelike instrument. In an incisional biopsy, the surgeon cuts into the tumor and removes a sample of tissue.

Treatment

Treatment options depend on the type, size, location, and stage of the original cancer, as well as the person's age and general health. Surgery is often the primary treatment; although amputation is sometimes necessary, pre- or postoperative chemotherapy may mean the limb can be spared. When possible, surgeons avoid amputation by removing only the cancerous section of the bone and replacing it with a prosthesis. CHEMOTHERAPY and RADIATION THERAPY may also be used alone or in combination.

Bone pain may be treated by irradiation, BISPHOS-PHONATES (clodronate or pamidronate), steroids such as oral prednisone, chemotherapy (mitoxantrone or a combination of docetaxel [Taxotere] and estramustine), or painkillers such as narcotics or nonsteroidal anti-inflammatory drugs.

bone scan   A specialized test that detects areas of altered bone metabolism by determining the level of a radioactive isotope that collects in the bones. During the test, a small amount of radioactive chemical is injected through a vein into the blood and circulates throughout the body; it is absorbed by areas of fast bone growth that may be associated with cancer.

As it decays, the chemical emits radiation, which is detected by a camera. When the tracer, or radioactive chemical, has collected in the bones a few hours after the injection, the scan is performed. Information from the camera is recorded in a computer, which then processes the data and creates an image. (Although the chemical used in the study is radioactive, it is not considered to be harmful.)

Normal distribution areas appear uniform and gray. "Hot spots" are areas where there is increased accumulation of tracer in the bone; these appear black. "Cold spots" are areas where there is less uptake of the radiotracer. These appear light or white.

The bone scan is the most sensitive way to identify cancer that has spread to the bone. Although the scan is quite sensitive, it can still miss small numbers of malignant cells in the bone. About 8 percent of the time the scan may miss bone cancer. On the other hand, certain other bone problems (such as a history of broken bones, Paget's disease, or arthritis) can cause an increase in the uptake of the radioactive substance.

borderline ovarian tumors   See TUMORS OF LOW MALIGNANT POTENTIAL.

BRCA1/BRCA2   The abbreviation for the genes (BReast CAncer 1 and BReast CAncer 2), found on chromosome 17 and chromosome 13, respectively. *BRCA1* and *BRCA2* normally help to suppress cell growth. Although these inherited gene mutations were originally found in women who had breast cancer, they are also responsible for about 9 percent of ovarian cancers (see OVARIAN CANCER–BREAST CANCER LINK). The lifetime ovarian cancer risk for women who have *BRCA1* or *BRCA2* mutations has been estimated to be between 17 percent and 44 percent. These estimates vary considerably because they are based on studies of women of various racial and ethnic groups living in different countries.

A woman who inherits either gene in an altered form has a higher risk of breast or ovarian cancer. Experts believe the *BRCA1* and *BRCA2* genes are responsible for nearly all cases of familial ovarian cancer, and about half of all cases of familial breast cancer.

Genes are small pieces of DNA, the material that acts as a master blueprint for all the cells in the body. A person's genes determine such traits as hair and eye color, height, skin color. Any mistakes in a gene that interfere with its function can lead to disease.

The *BRCA1* and *BRCA2* genes produce a protein that prevents genes from growing abnormally. Most women have two normal copies of the *BRCA1* gene, which produces this cancer-preventing substance. However, some women have inherited a genetic defect in one copy of their two *BRCA1* genes; as a result, their body does not produce a normal amount of this cancer-fighting substance. These women are at higher risk of breast or ovarian cancer.

Women inherit one copy of each of their genes from their mother and a second copy of each gene from their father. If one parent has a defective *BRCA1* gene, there is a 50 percent chance the child may inherit the defective copy, and a 50 percent chance the child may inherit the normal copy. If a person inherits a defective *BRCA1* gene, then each of that person's children likewise has a 50 percent chance of inheriting it. Because family members share a proportion of their genes and, often, their environment, it is possible that the large number of cancer cases seen in these families may be partly due to other genetic or environmental factors. Therefore, risk estimates that are based on families with many affected members may not accurately reflect the levels of risk in the general population.

Specific gene alterations have been identified in various ethnic groups. In Ashkenazi Jewish families, about 2.3 percent (23 of 1,000 persons) have an altered *BRCA* gene—about a five times higher incidence than that of the general population. Among people who have alterations in *BRCA1*, three particular alterations have been found to be most common in the Ashkenazi Jewish population. Other ethnic and geographic populations, such as Norwegian, Dutch, and Icelandic people, also have a higher rate of certain genetic alterations in *BRCA1*. This information about genetic differences between ethnic groups may help health-care providers to select the most appropriate genetic test.

Genetic Testing

It is possible to detect an altered *BRCA1* and *BRCA2* genes with a blood test; the cost of genetic testing can range from several hundred to several thousand dollars, and not all insurance policies cover the test. Some people may choose to pay for the test, even when their insurer would be willing to cover the cost, to protect their privacy. From the date that blood is drawn, several weeks or months may pass before test results are available. It may be possible to have the genetic test performed free as part of a clinical study at a comprehensive cancer center.

If the Test Result Is Positive

If a woman has a positive finding for an altered *BRCA1* or *BRCA2* gene, it does not mean she will definitely develop cancer, but her risk is much higher. Several possible preventive approaches may be effective. Careful monitoring for symptoms of cancer may reveal disease at an early stage, when treatment is more effective. Some women choose to have their healthy ovaries removed before cancer is diagnosed. Removal of ovaries for these women reduces their risk of breast or ovarian cancer to almost zero but does not absolutely prevent development of cancer.

breakthrough pain Intense increases in pain that occur with rapid onset even when painkillers are being used. Breakthrough pain can occur spontaneously or in relation to a specific activity.

breast cancer and ovarian cancer See OVARIAN CANCER–BREAST CANCER LINK.

breast cancer genes See *BRCA1/BRCA2*.

Brief Pain Inventory A questionnaire used to measure pain.

CA 15-3 A TUMOR MARKER found in the blood that is most useful in following the course of treatment of women diagnosed with advanced breast cancer. However, OVARIAN CANCER may also cause an increase in CA 15-3 levels. High levels of CA 15-3 also may be associated with noncancerous conditions, such as benign breast or ovarian disease, endometriosis, pelvic inflammatory disease, and hepatitis. Finally, pregnancy and lactation also can cause CA 15-3 levels to rise.

See also ONCOGENES.

CA 125 A protein sometimes found in an increased level in the blood, other body fluids, or tissues and that may suggest the presence of OVARIAN CANCER, among other types of cancer. CA 125 is considered to be a TUMOR MARKER or biomarker—a substance found in high levels in 80 percent of women who have advanced ovarian cancer. This level is also high in about half of those in the early stages of this disease. However, some women who have ovarian cancer never have an elevated CA 125 level. Other examples of tumor markers include CA 15-3 (breast cancer), CARCINOEMBRYONIC ANTIGEN (CEA) (ovarian, lung, breast, pancreas, and gastrointestinal tract cancers), and prostate-specific antigen (PSA) (prostate cancer).

The CA 125 level can be above normal in a variety of conditions besides ovarian cancer. But because most patients with ovarian cancer have a high CA 125 level, doctors use the test to follow a patient's response to a particular treatment (the CA 125 level drops if a treatment is working, or rises if the tumor is growing).

Experts have hoped that the CA 125 blood test also could be applied as a screening test to detect ovarian cancer at an early stage. Unfortunately, a number of studies with many thousands of patients have not shown CA 125 to be beneficial as a screening test for several reasons. First, many common benign conditions may cause an increase in level of CA 125, including menstrual periods, pregnancy, fibroids, endometriosis, and pelvic inflammatory disease. Nongynecologic conditions that increase the CA 125 level include inflammation of the pancreas (pancreatitis), cirrhosis of the liver, recent abdominal surgery, and RADIATION THERAPY. Other malignant tumors, such as those in the breast, lung, colon, and pancreas, also can increase the level of CA 125. Because so many other conditions can boost CA 125 level, this test yields a significant number of false-positive results. If every patient who had a positive result had additional diagnostic evaluations, many patients would require a surgical exploration of the abdomen to rule out a diagnosis of ovarian cancer definitively.

Moreover, studies have shown that using CA 125 as a screening tool has had no impact on the rate of death. Thus, the risks of the test outweigh the benefits. This is why routine CA 125 screening of patients who have no symptoms is not currently recommended.

However, in some cases a CA 125 test is a good idea. Some physicians still favor the test for patients with a strong family history of ovarian cancer and combine screening for ovarian cancer with pelvic and ultrasound examinations. Regular CA 125 blood tests are clearly indicated for monitoring patients previously diagnosed with ovarian cancer after treatment or detecting a recurrence at an early stage.

A large-scale study, the PROSTATE, LUNG, COLORECTAL AND OVARIAN (PLCO) CANCER SCREENING TRIAL, is currently reevaluating the usefulness of a blood test for CA 125 and studying a test called transvaginal ultrasound for ovarian cancer screening.

cachexia   A loss of body weight and muscle mass common among cancer patients.

cancer   A general term used to describe more than 100 different uncontrolled growths of abnormal cells in the body. A cancer cell divides and reproduces abnormally. These cells invade and destroy surrounding tissue, leaves the original site, and travels via the lymph or blood systems to other parts of the body, where it begins new cancerous tumors—a process referred to as metastasis.

Cancer Care   A national nonprofit agency, founded in 1944, that offers free support, information, financial assistance, and practical help to people who have cancer and their loved ones. Services are provided by oncology social workers and are available in person, over the telephone, and through the agency's Web site.

Since 1944, Cancer Care has been dedicated to providing emotional support, information, and practical help to people with cancer and their families. As the oldest and largest national nonprofit agency devoted to offering professional services, Cancer Care has helped more than 2 million people nationwide through its toll-free counseling line and teleconference programs, its office-based services, and Internet support. Services are offered to people of all ages, with all types of cancer, at any stage of the disease. Cancer Care's reach, including its cancer awareness initiatives, also extends to family members, caregivers, and professionals.

A section of the Cancer Care Web site and some publications are available in Spanish, and staff can respond to calls and e-mails in Spanish. For contact information, see Appendix I.

cancer center   A type of institution dedicated to treating and researching cancer, as designated by the NATIONAL CANCER INSTITUTE (NCI). A cancer center may have a narrow research focus in basic science, population research, epidemiology, diagnosis, immunology, or other areas. It is distinguished from both a *clinical cancer center,* which conducts research in clinical oncology and may or may not do basic and prevention research, and a *comprehensive cancer center,* which conducts basic research, clinical research, and prevention, control, behavioral, and population-based research.

The Cancer Centers Program of the NCI supports cancer research programs in about 60 institutions across the United States through Cancer Center support grants.

CancerFax   A service sponsored by the NATIONAL CANCER INSTITUTE (NCI) that provides NCI fact sheets on various cancer topics, as well as other NCI literature (in English or Spanish), via fax machine.

CancerFax can be accessed 24 hours a day, seven days a week, by anyone in the United States by dialing (800) 624-2511 on a touch-tone phone or on a telephone on a fax machine and following the recorded instructions. Anyone calling from outside the United States may use the local number (301-402-5874). For a fact sheet that explains how to use CancerFax, consumers may call the CANCER INFORMATION SERVICE at (800) 4-CANCER.

Cancer Fund of America (CFA)   A national nonprofit agency dedicated to helping cancer patients who are having financial difficulty. Its priority is patient care rather than research. Through its patient assistance programs, CFA provides supplies and items such as food, crutches, lotions and ointments, dressings, seasonal gift boxes, adult diapers, and bed pads.

Cancer Fund of America's mission differs greatly from that of many of the more than 200 U.S. charities that provide cancer-related services as its principal mission is to provide aid to the ill and needy rather than to conduct research. CFA provides support and services to financially indigent patients, disseminates information about early detection and prevention of cancer, provides commodities and gifts-in-kind to hospices and other health-care providers, and distributes donated merchandise to various nonprofit community service organizations that aid the ill, the needy, and infants. For contact information, see Appendix I.

Cancer Genetics Network   A national network of centers specializing in the study of inherited predisposition to cancer. It supports collaborative investigations on the genetic basis of cancer susceptibility, ways to integrate this new knowledge into medical practice, and methods to address the psychosocial, ethical, legal, and public health issues.

The network includes the following:

- Carolina-Georgia Cancer Genetics Network Center (Duke University Medical Center, Emory University, and the University of North Carolina/Chapel Hill)
- Georgetown University Medical Center's Cancer Genetics Network Center (Georgetown University Lombardi Cancer Center, Washington, D.C.)
- Mid-Atlantic Cancer Genetics Network Center (Johns Hopkins University and the Greater Baltimore Medical Center)
- Northwest Cancer Genetics Network (Fred Hutchinson Cancer Research Center in Seattle and the University of Washington School of Medicine in Seattle)
- Rocky Mountain Cancer Genetics Coalition (University of Utah, University of New Mexico, and University of Colorado)
- Texas Cancer Genetics Consortium (M. D. Anderson Cancer Center, Health Science Center at San Antonio, Southwestern Medical Center at Dallas, and Baylor College of Medicine)
- University of Pennsylvania Cancer Genetics Network
- UCI-UCSD Cancer Genetics Network Center (University of California/Irvine and the University of California/San Diego)
- Informatics Technology Group (provides supporting information)

Cancer Hope Network   A nonprofit organization that provides support to cancer patients and their families by matching them with trained volunteers who have undergone and recovered from a similar cancer experience. Matches are based on the type and stage of cancer, treatments used, side effects experienced, and other factors such as age and gender.

This program is available to all cancer patients and their loved ones anywhere in the United States at no cost. After patients contact the organization and discuss their situation, they are matched with an appropriate volunteer. Staff make a match based on the type of cancer, the similarity of treatment(s), the side effects experienced, and overall demographics, such as age or gender.

Patients may contact the group at any point, but ideally they should be matched with a volunteer before treatment, to give them a chance to discuss any fears and questions about treatment.

Volunteers are former patients who have survived a cancer experience and who want to help others as they deal with the disease; they have been off treatment for at least one year and have gone through extensive training before their first patient visit. For contact information, see Appendix I.

Cancer Information and Counseling Line   A toll-free telephone service that is part of the psychosocial program of the AMC Cancer Research Center. Professional counselors provide up-to-date medical information, emotional support through short-term counseling, and resource referrals to callers nationwide between the hours of 8:30 a.m. and 5 p.m. MST. Individuals may also submit questions about cancer and request resources via e-mail. For contact information, see Appendix I.

Cancer Information Service (CIS)   A service sponsored by the NATIONAL CANCER INSTITUTE (NCI) to interpret research findings for the public and to provide personalized responses to specific questions about cancer. As a resource for information and education about cancer, the CIS helps people become active participants in their own health care by providing the latest information on cancer in understandable language.

Through its network of regional offices, the CIS serves the United States, Puerto Rico, the U.S. Virgin Islands, and the Pacific Islands. For 25 years, the CIS has provided the latest and most accurate cancer information to patients and families, the public, and health professionals. Its Partnership Program participates in research efforts to find the best ways to help people adopt healthier behaviors and provides access to NCI information over the Internet.

Through the CIS toll-free telephone service, callers can speak to knowledgeable, caring staff who are experienced in explaining medical information in easy-to-understand terms. CIS information specialists can answer calls in English and Spanish and provide cancer information to deaf and hard-of-hearing callers through a toll-free TTY number (1-800-332-8615).

CIS staff have access to comprehensive, accurate information from the NCI on a range of cancer topics, including the most recent advances in cancer treatment. They take as much time as each caller needs, provide thorough and personalized attention, and keep all calls confidential.

The CIS also provides live on-line assistance to users of NCI Web sites through LiveHelp, an instant messaging service that is available from 9 a.m. to 10 p.m. EST, Monday through Friday. Through LiveHelp, information specialists provide answers to questions about cancer and help in navigating Cancer.gov, the NCI's Web site.

CIS staffers can discuss concerns about cancer (including ways to prevent cancer, symptoms and risks, diagnosis, current treatments, and research studies), provide written materials from the NCI, and make referrals to clinical trials and cancer-related services such as treatment centers, mammography facilities, or other cancer organizations.

Through its Partnership Program, the CIS collaborates with established national, state, and regional organizations to reach minority and medically underserved audiences with cancer information. Partnership Program staff provide assistance to organizations developing programs that focus on breast and cervical cancer, clinical trials, tobacco control, and cancer awareness for special populations. To reach those in need, the CIS helps bring cancer information to people who do not traditionally seek health information or who may have trouble doing so because of educational, financial, cultural, or language barriers.

The CIS plays an important role in research by studying the most effective ways to communicate with people about healthy lifestyles; health risks; and options for preventing, diagnosing, and treating cancer. The ability to conduct health communications research is a unique aspect of the CIS. Results from these research studies can be applied to improving the way the CIS communicates about cancer and can help other programs communicate more effectively. For contact information, see Appendix I.

Cancer Legal Resource Center An organization that provides information on cancer-related legal issues. A joint program of Loyola Law School and the Western Law Center for Disability Rights, the center offers outreach to cancer support groups, cancer survivors, and caregivers. It also provides speakers for outreach programs at hospitals, community centers, cancer organizations, and for businesses.

The center also matches patients with volunteer attorneys and other professionals who can furnish additional legal information. It trains law students to appreciate and understand the legal needs of people battling cancer and cancer survivors. The organization works with major cancer centers in Los Angeles but accepts calls from the greater Los Angeles area, Orange County, and outside California. For contact information, see Appendix I.

Cancer Liaison Program A division of the U.S. Food and Drug Administration (FDA) that works directly with cancer patients and advocacy programs. It provides information and education on the FDA drug-approval process and cancer clinical trials as well as access to investigational drugs when participation in a clinical trial is not possible. For contact information, see Appendix I.

CancerMail CancerMail is a service of the NATIONAL CANCER INSTITUTE (NCI) that provides comprehensive cancer information summaries and other related information via e-mail. To obtain a contents list, consumers can send an e-mail to cancermail@cips.nci.nih.gov with the word *help* in the body of the message. CancerMail responds by sending a contents list via e-mail. Instructions for ordering documents through e-mail are also provided.

CancerNet A Web site providing cancer information from the NATIONAL CANCER INSTITUTE (NCI) that offers a wide range of cancer information, including details on treatment options, clinical trials, reduction of cancer risk, and coping with cancer. Information on support groups, financial assistance, and educational materials are also available. CancerNet can be found at http://cancernet.nci.nih.gov.

Cancer Research Foundation of America (CRFA) A nonprofit group that seeks to prevent cancer by funding research and providing educational materials on early detection and nutrition. The group focuses on cancers that can be prevented through lifestyle changes or early detection followed by prompt treatment.

When CRFA was established in 1988, cancer prevention was not regarded as a major strategy in the war against cancer. Instead, scientists focused on discovering new cancer treatments rather than thinking about ways to prevent disease.

Today, prevention research is recognized as essential to the fight against cancer. Now that scientists better understand how tumors develop, they are learning ways that people can reduce their cancer risks. Since its inception, the foundation has provided funding to more than 200 scientists at more than 100 leading academic institutions across the country. For contact information, see Appendix I.

Cancer Research Institute (CRI) A nonprofit organization that funds research projects and scientists across the country. The institute was founded in 1953 to foster the science of cancer immunology, which is based on the idea that the body's immune system can be mobilized against cancer. For more than five decades the institute has been a sustaining force in cancer and immunology research, supporting more than 2,500 scientists and clinicians at leading universities and research centers worldwide. All such funding decisions are made by its Scientific Advisory Council, consisting of 63 of the world's leading immunologists, including four Nobel Laureates, 24 members of the National Academy of Sciences, and 23 members of the Academy of Cancer Immunology. For contact information, see Appendix I.

Cancer Survivors Network A telephone- and Internet-based service for cancer survivors, their families, caregivers, and friends. The telephone component (1-877-333-HOPE) provides survivors

and families access to prerecorded discussions. The Web-based component offers live on-line chat sessions, virtual support groups, prerecorded talk shows, and personal stories. Cancer Survivors Network is supported by the AMERICAN CANCER SOCIETY. For contact information, see Appendix I.

cancerTrials A Web site sponsored by the NATIONAL CANCER INSTITUTE (NCI) that provides information and news about cancer research. The primary mission of cancerTrials is to help people consider clinical trials as an option when making cancer care decisions. The site can be accessed at http://cancertrials.nci.nih.gov.

Cancervive A Los Angeles nonprofit organization founded in 1985 by childhood cancer survivor Susan Nessium. The organization is dedicated to providing support, public education, and advocacy to those who have experienced cancer and to help survivors of cancer to reclaim their life. For contact information, see Appendix I.

carboplatin (Paraplatin) A type of platinum drug that belongs to the ALKYLATING AGENT group, administered intravenously to treat OVARIAN CANCER, ENDOMETRIAL CANCER, and CERVICAL CANCER. Carboplatin works by interfering with and then destroying cancer cells.

Common side effects include decreased white blood cell and platelet counts, brittle hair, altered kidney function, and birth defects (if a woman becomes pregnant while taking this drug). Less commonly, the drug may cause nausea and vomiting, mild DIARRHEA, loss of appetite, CONSTIPATION, or taste changes.

carboplatin, doxorubicin, and Cytoxan (CDC) A combination of the CHEMOTHERAPY drugs CARBOPLATIN, doxorubicin (ADRIAMYCIN), and cyclophosphamide (CYTOXAN) sometimes used to treat OVARIAN CANCER.

carcinoembryonic antigen (CEA) A substance sometimes found at an increased level in the blood, other body fluids, or tissues and that may suggest the presence of colon cancer. In some instances it may be elevated in patients with OVARIAN CANCER. CEA is considered to be a TUMOR MARKER or biomarker—a substance sometimes found in high levels in the body that may indicate the presence of a certain type of cancer. Other examples of tumor markers include CA 125 (ovarian cancer), CA 15-3 (breast cancer), and prostate-specific antigen (PSA) (prostate cancer).

carcinoma   Cancer that begins in the skin or in tissues that line or cover internal organs. Carcinomas are the most common category of gynecological tumors. Common types of gynecological carcinomas include squamous cell carcinoma, ADENOCARCINOMA, and malignant melanoma.

Adenocarcinoma   This type of carcinoma is found in tissues that excrete a substance, such as mucus or hormones. Most endometrial and OVARIAN CANCERS are adenocarcinomas, as are some cervical and VAGINAL CANCERS.

Squamous cell carcinoma   Squamous cells are flat cells that usually can be found on surfaces on the outside of the body. Environmental effects (sunlight) or HUMAN PAPILLOMAVIRUS trigger most squamous cell growth. This is the most common type of cancer that affects the vulva, vagina, and cervix. Squamous cell cancer is generally slow to develop and grow and often responds well to cancer treatment.

Malignant melanoma   This is an aggressive type of carcinoma that can affect the vulva or vagina. It begins in the melanocyte, a type of cell in the skin and mucous membranes that produces melanin (pigment).

carcinoma in situ   A precancer that is confined to its original position, usually considered to be the earliest stage of cancer (or stage 0). Surgical removal of carcinoma in situ is usually a cure.

carotenoid   A substance, found in yellow and orange fruits and vegetables and in dark green, leafy vegetables, that may reduce the risk of development of cancer. The most widespread pigments in the natural world, carotenoids play an important role in the colorful appearance of many plants and animals, including red peppers, tomatoes, paprika, flamingos, canaries, ladybugs, and salmon.

The color-producing properties of carotenoids are so powerful that many manufactured products, such as soft drinks, use carotenoids as coloring (although in such low concentrations that they do not produce much nutritional benefit). The most common individual carotenoid found naturally is BETA-CAROTENE, a yellow-orange pigment that lends its color to carrots, sweet potatoes, and other fruits and vegetables. Beta-carotene is a provitamin A carotenoid, that is, a type of carotenoid that the body can easily convert into vitamin A. In recent years, studies have linked a variety of carotenoids with the prevention of several different kinds of cancer.

Beta-carotene pills, lutein pills, and other carotenoids can be found at health food stores and supermarkets alongside other supplements. However, experts caution that scientists still do not totally understand how carotenoids work as preventative agents. Although studies indicate that a diet rich in fruits and vegetables may help prevent a wide variety of cancers, scientists do not know precisely how carotenoids reduce cancer risk and how they may interact with other agents. In addition, studies on the effects of carotenoids in supplement form, especially of beta-carotene, have also produced ambiguous results.

See also DIET.

Centers for Disease Control and Prevention (CDC) Division of Cancer Prevention and Control (DCPC)   A department of the federal government that conducts, supports, and promotes efforts to prevent cancer and to increase early detection of cancer. The Division of Cancer Prevention and Control (DCPC) works with partners in the government, private, and nonprofit sectors to develop, implement, and promote effective cancer prevention and control practices nationwide.

In addition to Centers for Disease Control (CDC) activities in monitoring cancer risk factors and use of cancer preventive services, the DCPC specifically supports systems for monitoring cancer incidence and mortality rates through funding and technical assistance. Data from these systems serve a critical role in identifying and monitoring cancer trends, gaps, disparities, barriers, and successes; developing, guiding, and evaluating cancer prevention and control activities; and prioritizing allocation of resources.

In addition, the DCPC helps translate basic research into public health practices, interventions, and health-delivery services and then promotes, implements, and evaluates their use. The DCPC conducts and funds studies to identify problems, needs, and opportunities related to modifiable behavioral and other risk factors for cancer and to identify the feasibility and effectiveness of cancer prevention and control strategies. Results are used to plan or improve cancer prevention and control activities.

The DCPC also develops health communication campaigns, prepares and provides cancer prevention educational materials, and recommends priorities for health promotion, health education, and cancer-risk reduction activities both for health professionals and for the public.

The DCPC provides cancer-related Web sites, a public inquiries e-mail service (cancerinfo@cdc.gov), a toll-free phone number (1-888-842-6355), and a Web-based information system on selected cancer legislative issues. The division also provides support and technical assistance to improve education, training, and skills in the prevention, detection, and control of selected cancers. For contact information, see Appendix I.

cervical biopsy   A test in which tissue samples are removed from the cervix for examination, usually when a PAP TEST result indicates a problem or when an abnormal area is seen on the cervix during a routine PELVIC EXAMINATION. When a stain result shows only minor cell changes, a BIOPSY probably will not be recommended unless the patient is in a high-risk category.

As in a regular pelvic exam, a speculum is inserted into the vagina and opened so that the cervix is visible. After swabbing the cervix with iodine or a vinegar solution to remove the mucus and highlight abnormal areas, the doctor positions the colposcope (a small microscope to magnify the surface of the vagina and cervix) at the opening of the vagina.

If any abnormal tissue is found, a biopsy may be taken by using a small biopsy forceps. A COLPOSCOPY

is painless; the biopsy may cause a brief pinching feeling when the tissue sample is removed, followed by some cramping.

Abnormal results of the biopsy may indicate abnormal tissue development or cell growth in the cervix (cervical DYSPLASIA) or cancer. The biopsy also may find cervical erosion or CERVICAL POLYPS. If the colposcopic biopsy does not show why the Pap smear is abnormal, a more extensive biopsy may be suggested.

cervical cancer   Cancer caused by abnormal cellular changes in the cervix, the lower end of the uterus that extends into the vagina. Once malignant cervical cells penetrate deep beneath the surface of the cervix, they can enter the network of small blood and lymphatic vessels lining the cervix, where they can then spread to other parts of the body. Cervical cancer cells also can spread by growing larger and invading nearby structures such as the bladder, rectum, or other tissues near the uterus and vagina.

Cervical cancer is the third most common type of cancer of the female reproductive system, and the most common in younger women. It usually affects women between the ages of 35 and 55 and may be caused by the HUMAN PAPILLOMAVIRUS (HPV), which can be transmitted during sexual intercourse.

About 40 years ago, cervical cancer is one of the most common causes of cancer deaths of women worldwide, but the routine use of the PAP TEST in the United States has helped lower cervical cancer deaths by 70 percent to 80 percent since 1960s. Cervical cancer now constitutes less than 2 percent of all cancers of women in the United States. Approximately 15,000 women will be diagnosed with cervical cancer this year in the United States, and 3,900 women will die of it. In many developing countries (where the Pap smear is not a routine test), this form of cancer is very common.

Types of Cervical Cancer

About 85 percent of cervical cancers are squamous cell carcinomas, which develop in the scaly, flat cells on the outside of the cervix. Most other cervical cancers develop from gland cells (ADENOCARCINOMAS) or a combination of cell types (adenosquamous carcinomas).

Development of Cervical Cancer

Dysplasia   Cervical cancer is the only gynecological cancer that can be prevented by regular screening. Most authorities believe cervical cancer develops slowly and in stages, beginning with progressive changes in normal cells that may develop over several years. Experts believe that cervical DYSPLASIA, a precancerous condition marked by abnormal cell development within the cervix, is the first step in the slow progression of abnormal cellular changes leading to CARCINOMA IN SITU, the earliest stage of cancer. In actuality, only 30 percent to 50 percent of women who have dysplasia ultimately have cancer if the condition is untreated, but this percentage is high enough that experts usually advocate treating dysplasia as a precancerous condition. If dysplasia is diagnosed, a doctor performs a biopsy to identify malignant cells.

Risk Factors

There are a number of identifiable risks that are associated with the development of cervical cancer.

Sexual practices   The risk for cervical cancer appears to rise the earlier a woman has had her first sexual intercourse, and as the number of sexual partners increases. Women who were younger than age 18 when they started regular sexual intercourse have a greater chance of development of cervical cancer. Having multiple partners (or having sex with a partner who has had many partners) is also a risk factor because cervical cancer is almost always caused by the sexually transmitted virus known as human papillomavirus. HPV can cause genital warts, some types of which are more likely to lead to the development of cervical cancer than others. Even if a woman has had only one sexual partner, if that man had many other sexual partners, he is at high risk for transmitting HPV to a partner. This risk in turns raises her risk for development of cervical cancer.

Most women who are infected with HPV never have visible warts and do not know they have the virus. Fortunately, in the great majority of cases, this viral infection produces no problems and does not result in cancer. There is some evidence that women who have these warts who have inherited certain types of the human leukocyte antigen may be at higher risk for development of invasive cervi-

cal cancer or its precursor lesion. Moreover, if a woman has had a sexually transmitted disease such as chlamydia, gonorrhea, herpes, or syphilis, she has a higher risk of also having an HPV infection.

Pap tests   Failure to have regular Papanicolaov (Pap) tests increases the risk of cervical cancer, because it eliminates the opportunity for early diagnosis.

Smoking   SMOKING or using tobacco products increases the risk of development of either a preinvasive abnormality or invasive cervical cancer. Tobacco by-products can be found in cervical cells.

Vitamin deficiency   Insufficient intake of vitamins A and C is associated with a higher risk of cervical cancer development.

Weak immune system   A weak IMMUNE SYSTEM is associated with cervical cancer. Because the immune system helps the body fight illness, women who are human immunodeficiency virus–(HIV)-positive or who have had an organ transplant have a greater risk of development of cervical cancer.

DES daughters   If a woman's mother used the drug DIETHYLSTILBESTROL (DES) when she was pregnant, the woman has a greater risk of development of cervical or VAGINAL CANCER in adulthood.

Socioeconomic status   Women in lower-income groups also have a higher risk of development of cervical cancer, perhaps because of lack of access to good health care and Pap tests.

Race   African-American women are at higher risk, but whether this is related to race or to lower access to Pap testing is not known. If a woman does not have a regular examination with a Pap test, it is more likely that a preinvasive abnormality will develop into cancer.

Age   Women age 60 and older are at greater risk for cervical cancer than are women in other age groups because these older women are less willing or able to seek medical care for early screening. One reason that many of these women are not screened for cervical cancer is that they often do not view themselves as being at risk.

Symptoms

Women who have precancerous lesions in the cervix usually have no symptoms; symptoms do not appear until the cells become malignant and begin to invade deeper parts of the cervix or other pelvic organs. That is why is it is so important that a woman's doctor regularly screen for it.

If cells do become malignant, symptoms may include spotting between menstrual periods, excessive bloody or foul-smelling discharge, or bleeding between periods or after sex. Pain and symptoms may not occur until the late stages of the disease. As the cancer becomes more advanced, a woman may experience pelvic pain, heavy vaginal bleeding, or swelling in a single leg.

Diagnosis: Pap Tests

A routine Pap test can detect cervical cancer early. A health-care provider uses a Pap test to obtain cells in order to identify any progressive cellular changes under a microscope. Because the Pap test can accurately and inexpensively detect up to 90 percent of cervical cancers even before symptoms develop, the number of deaths of cervical cancer has plummeted by more than 70 to 80 percent since the tests were introduced. If all women had Pap tests on a regular basis, deaths of this cancer could be eliminated. However, almost 40 percent of American women are not tested regularly.

The Pap test is simple and relatively painless and can be done in a doctor's office or a health clinic by an obstetrician-gynecologist, a family practitioner, or a nurse practitioner. The best time for a woman to have a Pap test is 10 to 20 days after her period.

During the procedure, a doctor uses a speculum to examine the upper part of the vagina and the cervix. A small sample of cells are then collected from the outer part of the cervix and vagina with a wooden scraper or a small brush, rubbed on a glass slide or placed in a liquid vial, and sent for analysis to a medical lab; results are reported within a few days.

Results are reported as abnormal in 5 percent to 10 percent of Pap smears performed each year on women in the United States. Abnormal cell types include:

- *Atypical squamous cells of undetermined significance (ASCUS).* Squamous cells are the thin flat cells that form the surface of the cervix.
- *Low-grade squamous intraepithelial lesion (LSIL).* This lesion indicates early changes in the size,

shape, and number of cells. The word *lesion* refers to an area of abnormal tissue; *intraepithelial* means that the abnormal cells are present only in the surface layer of cells.

- *High-grade squamous intraepithelial lesion (HSIL).* A high-grade lesion indicates a large number of precancerous cells that appear very different from normal cells.

Both ASCUS and LSIL are considered mild abnormalities. HSIL is more serious and has a higher likelihood of progression to invasive cancer. Experts agree that women who have HSIL cells on their Pap test result should have COLPOSCOPY, using a magnifying instrument to view the tissue surrounding the vagina and cervix to check for any abnormalities. Schiller's test may also be performed. For this test, the doctor coats the cervix with an iodine solution; healthy cells turn brown and abnormal cells turn white or yellow. Both of these procedures can be done in a doctor's office. Women who have HSIL may also need a BIOPSY.

However, there is no agreement among doctors about how to manage women who show ASCUS or LSIL cells. Most doctors either perform immediate colposcopy and, if necessary, biopsy, as for women with high-grade lesions. Since cells that have low-grade changes in many women tend to revert to normal spontaneously, other doctors choose to wait and repeat the Pap smear every four to six months, performing colposcopy if the abnormality is still present.

The NATIONAL CANCER INSTITUTE (NCI) is conducting a study (the ASCUS/LSIL Triage Study) to help doctors determine how best to manage these two abnormal cell types in women. So far, results show that it is helpful for women with ASCUS cells also to be tested for HPV to determine whether the abnormalities require immediate attention. The study found that women who have ASCUS cells who tested positive for HPV had precancer, or rarely, cancer. A negative HPV test result provided strong reassurance that precancer or cancer was not present.

If the Pap test result abnormality is unclear or minor, the doctor may repeat the test to ensure accuracy.

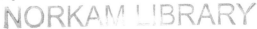

Pap test guidelines Because most cervical pre-cancers grow slowly, having Pap testing every two to three years detects almost all cervical precancers and cancers while they can be removed or treated successfully. The American Cancer Society issued new guidelines in November of 2002 addressing when and how often women should have early detection tests for cervical cancer and precancer. The new guidelines recommend:

- Cervical cancer screening should begin about three years after a woman begins having sex, but no later than age 21.
- Cervical screening should be done every year with regular Pap tests, or every two years using liquid-based Pap tests.
- At or after age 30, women who have had three normal test results in a row may be screened every two to three years. But a doctor may suggest having the test more often if a woman has certain risk factors such as human immunodeficiency virus infection or a weakened immune system.
- Women 70 years of age and older who have had three or more normal Pap test results and no abnormal results in the last 10 years may choose to stop cervical cancer screening.
- Screening after a total hysterectomy (with removal of the cervix) is not necessary unless the surgery was done as a treatment for cervical cancer or precancer.
- Women who have had a HYSTERECTOMY without removal of the cervix should continue cervical cancer screening at least until age 70.

HPV screening There is also a promising new test for human papillomavirus that has not yet been approved for screening by the U.S. Food and Drug Administration. This test eventually may be useful in detecting early cervical cancer in women older than 30 years of age. If the test is approved, it may be added to the guidelines.

Diagnosis: Further Tests

If the doctor or nurse notices something suspicious in the pelvic exam or if the Pap test finding is abnormal, the following tests can help the doctor determine whether the woman has cervical cancer.

Biopsy If a growth, sore, or other suspicious area is seen on the cervix during a pelvic examination or if a Pap test result shows an abnormality or cancer, the doctor performs a biopsy by removing a tissue sample for examination under a microscope. A diagnosis of cancer cannot be made without a tissue biopsy. The tissue sample is usually removed during colposcopy, in which a viewing tube with a magnifying lens is used to examine the cervix and choose the best biopsy site.

There are two different types of biopsy for this procedure—punch biopsy and ENDOCERVICAL CURETTAGE. In a punch biopsy, a tiny piece of the cervix is removed. In endocervical curettage, tissue that cannot be seen with the colposcope is scraped from the canal of the cervix.

Neither type of biopsy causes much pain or bleeding; both used together usually provide enough tissue to allow a pathologist to make a diagnosis.

Conization If the diagnosis with colposcopy is not clear, the doctor may perform a CONE BIOPSY, in which a larger piece of tissue deeper in the cervix is removed. When a cone biopsy is performed using a wire and electricity it is called a LOOP ELECTROSURGICAL EXCISION PROCEDURE (LEEP). The advantage of this procedure is that it can often be performed in the doctor's office after injection of an anesthetic into the cervix. After conization, the tissue is then sent to a pathologist for analysis.

Endometrial biopsy If the doctor cannot determine whether abnormal cells exist in the cervix or in the uterine lining (endometrium), the doctor may perform an endometrial biopsy. In this procedure, the doctor scrapes cells from the endometrium to determine whether the cancer is superficial (preinvasive) or invasive. This is important because treatment methods for preinvasive and invasive cancers are quite different.

Staging Cervical Cancer

If a woman has cervical cancer the doctor needs to determine its exact size and location in a process called staging. Staging begins with a physical examination of the pelvis and a variety of tests, including blood and urine tests, computed tomography (CT) scan, barium enema, and bone and liver scans, may be performed. Other tests may include the following:

Proctosigmoidoscopy   In this procedure, a doctor examines the rectum and the bottom part of the large intestine with a specialized instrument (sigmoidoscope) to see whether the tumor has spread to those areas.

CT, magnetic resonance imaging (MRI), and ultrasound scans   A doctor may order a scan to determine whether cancer has spread to the lymph nodes or to other internal organs such as the liver or lungs.

Cystoscopy   In this procedure, a doctor looks at the inside of the bladder with a specialized instrument (cystoscope) to see whether the tumor has spread to the bladder.

Intravenous pyelogram   This X-ray study of the kidneys, ureters, and bladder may not be needed if a CT has been performed.

The most commonly used staging system for cervical cancer is a system developed by the INTERNATIONAL FEDERATION OF GYNECOLOGY AND OBSTETRICS. In this system, numbers from 0 (the least serious or earliest stage) to IV (the most serious or advanced stage) represent the different stages of the cancer.

Stage 0: The tumor is still superficial and growing in the skin of the cervix; this is also called CARCINOMA IN SITU.

Stage I: The cancer has grown deeper into the cervix but has not spread to other pelvic organs and is still confined to the cervix.

Stage IA1: Cancers are less than three millimeters deep and less than seven millimeters wide.

Stage IA2: Cancers are between three and five millimeters deep and yet still less than seven millimeters wide.

Stage IB1: Cancers can be seen with the naked eye or are deeper than five millimeters or wider than seven millimeters. These cancers must be less than four centimeters and still found only in the cervix.

Stage IB2: Cancers are still found only in the cervix but are larger than four centimeters.

Stage II: Cancer is found near the cervix but not outside the pelvis.

Stage IIA: Cancer extends to the upper vagina without spreading into the tissues deeper than the vagina.

Stage IIB: Cancer has spread to the tissues surrounding the vagina and cervix, but not yet to the wall of the pelvis.

Stage III: Cancer has spread to the vagina or to the wall of the pelvis.

Stage IIIA: Cancer has spread to the lower vagina.

Stage IIIB: Cancers have spread to the soft tissues surrounding the vagina and cervix all the way to the wall of the pelvis or cause blockage of one or both kidneys.

Stage IV: Stage IV cancer has spread to other parts of the body such as the bladder, rectum, or lungs.

Treatment

Treatment of cervical cancer patients depends on how advanced the disease has become and how aggressive the cancer is (the tumor grade).

Early cancer   If a woman has lesions that have not invaded the normal cells of the cervix, treatments may be relatively easy and may not require hysterectomy. Instead, treatments for these women may include cryotherapy, laser therapy, and excision. Sometimes these procedures are also used to diagnose the cause of an abnormal Pap test result and to treat the problem at the same time. Occasionally, very early lesions are watched carefully without treatment because more than half the time they fade away spontaneously.

Invasive cancer   The treatment of invasive cancer depends on the extent of the tumor. If the tumor is small and confined to the cervix, a woman may be treated with either surgery or RADIATION THERAPY. When tumors are large or have spread to nearby tissues or lymph nodes, more intensive therapy, including radiation therapy and CHEMOTHERAPY, is needed.

Excision   Excision can be performed either with a knife or scalpel (conization) or with a loop excision. In an excision, the lesion is surgically removed; in cryotherapy the cells are frozen; in laser therapy the cells are burned. Some women may decide to have a hysterectomy, although this is not usually necessary unless abnormal cells that cannot be safely treated by cryotherapy, laser therapy, or excision exist inside the opening of the cervix.

Surgery   A variety of surgical procedures are used to treat cervical cancer, including LEEP, hysterectomy, cryosurgery, and pelvic exenteration.

Preinvasive lesions may only require a LEEP and can be performed in a doctor's office with local anesthesia. With an electrically charged wire loop, the doctor removes the outer part of the cervix where the abnormal tissue is. This tissue can then be examined under a microscope to make sure there is no cancer. In many cases, women are cured after one LEEP procedure. Since recurrence is possible, it is important that a woman continue to have Pap smears after a LEEP. Most women are able to return to full activity a day or so after a LEEP procedure. This procedure is used to treat stage IA1 cancers when a woman wants to stay fertile. However, LEEP may have a small increased risk of recurrence and therefore a lower chance of cure.

Hysterectomy involves the removal of the uterus through the abdomen or the vagina in a major surgical procedure that requires at least an overnight stay in a hospital. This is the standard treatment for stage IA1 invasive cancers, but there is rarely a reason to perform a hysterectomy for preinvasive lesions.

Advanced cervical cancer is treated with a radical hysterectomy, which involves the surgical removal of the uterus, the upper part of the vagina, and the ligaments and connective tissues that hold the uterus in place. Nearby LYMPH NODES are also removed (LYMPHADENECTOMY). Removing the lymph nodes within the abdominal area can confirm whether microscopic cancer cells have spread to those lymph nodes and into the ligaments that hold the uterus in place. This type of surgery is used to treat stage IA2, IB1, IB2, and IIA cancers. It is not necessary to remove the ovaries in a radical hysterectomy. After a radical hysterectomy, a woman no longer has menstrual periods and she cannot carry a child; however, she can have in-vitro fertilization with a surrogate mother carrying her baby to term. Radical hysterectomy requires several days in the hospital and several weeks of recovery time afterward. For patients who have this procedure, the cure rate for cervical cancer is 85 percent to 95 percent. This type of surgery should be performed only by a gynecologic oncologist.

The vaginal radical trachelectomy is still considered to be experimental. It is similar to a radical hysterectomy, but only the cervix is removed and the rest of the uterus is saved so the woman can still have children.

Larger and more extensive operations have more risks and are associated with more complications but, stage for stage, have a higher cure rate. Vaginal hysterectomies have shorter recovery times but may be difficult for obese women or when other gynecologic disorders are present (such as ovarian tumors).

Another technique for preinvasive lesions is cryosurgery, a procedure in which the doctor freezes and kills the abnormal cells on the cervix by placing a silver probe cooled with liquid nitrogen against the cervix, killing the outer layer of abnormal cells. This procedure is also performed in the doctor's office and usually anesthesia is not necessary. The use of cryosurgery has declined in the United States since the advent of LEEP.

For locally recurrent cervical cancer, a surgeon performs a pelvic exenteration, removing the bladder, connective tissues, urethra, and rectum, along with the tissues and organs removed in a radical hysterectomy.

Radiation therapy If the patient has early-stage cervical cancer, radiation can be used instead of surgery. Radiation therapy is also very effective in treating advanced cervical cancer that has not spread beyond the pelvic region. Radiation therapy is as effective as radical hysterectomy for treating small cervical cancers. When cancers are larger, however, radiation therapy is the preferred method.

Patients who are treated with radiation therapy often receive low-dose chemotherapy at the same time; the combination can make the radiation kill cancer cells more effectively. For early-stage or smaller cancers, radiation is as effective as surgery. Radiation is also used for larger tumors and advanced stage cancers.

Although radiation therapy usually causes few or no immediate problems, it can irritate the rectum and vagina. Delayed damage to the bladder and rectum may occur, and the ovaries usually stop functioning.

For external radiotherapy for cervical cancer, patients do not need to stay overnight in the hospital. In most cases, external radiation therapy does not permanently change the appearance of a woman's skin. It is very similar to having a chest X-ray, except that it lasts a few minutes and is usually repeated daily over four to five weeks. This type of radiation does not hurt and many women continue to carry on a normal life during external radiation. At the end of treatment, extra radiation, called a boost, may be directed at the area where the tumor started.

Side effects of radiation therapy appear a few days after treatment begins; they include diarrhea and more frequent or burning urination. Medication can help control these symptoms. Premenopausal women who have radiation no longer have menstrual periods and may experience hot flashes and other menopausal symptoms. Radiation can also have some long-term side effects. Radiation affects the normal tissues around the cervix, so that, rarely, a woman may have a hole in the bladder or rectum, chronic DIARRHEA, blood in the urine or stools, or blocked intestines. If the vagina should become narrow or shortened, making sex difficult or painful, a doctor can prescribe vaginal dilators after radiation to help prevent the condition.

Brachytherapy For cervical cancer, external radiation is usually followed by implant therapy (brachytherapy). For this type of internal radiation, the patient may have to stay in the hospital for two or three days. Patients also can receive alternative implant therapy (also called high-dose-rate brachytherapy) on an outpatient basis weekly for several weeks. In these treatments, a radioactive device is inserted inside the vagina and against the cervix to kill the abnormal cells. The device is left in place for a short time to send a high dose of radiation directly to the tumor itself. The implant is removed before the patient goes home, and her body does not remain radioactive after the treatment is finished.

In intracavitary brachytherapy, the radioactive "seeds" are placed in the vagina. In interstitial brachytherapy, radiation can be given by placing needles with radioactive material around the tumor.

Combination treatment Experts recommend that women who have large or metastatic cervical cancer receive a combination of radiation therapy

and chemotherapy. When these treatments are given together (known as radiosensization), the chemotherapy drugs boosts the action of the radiation. Some doctors prefer to use neoadjuvant therapy, in which chemotherapy is administered before radiation therapy in order to shrink the size of the tumor. This approach is still considered experimental.

Chemotherapy The National Cancer Institute recommends that doctors strongly consider administering chemotherapy simultaneously with radiation therapy for invasive cervical cancer. Five major studies showed that chemotherapy that includes the drug CISPLATIN, when given at the same time as radiation therapy, prolongs survival duration in women who have this disease. When used by itself, chemotherapy is not very effective against cervical cancer; more typically, it is combined with radiation therapy to increase the effectiveness of the radiation and to reduce the chance of cancer spreading to other parts of the body. When the therapies are used together, chemoradiation may be the only treatment for cervical cancer or be a supplemental treatment after surgery. Chemotherapy can also be used to treat patients whose disease has spread to multiple organs and who are not candidates for local treatments.

Chemotherapy for cervical cancer usually involves a combination of drugs given by intravenous injection, including cisplatin (Platinol), topotecon (Hycontin) CARBOPLATIN (Paraplatin), paclitaxel (Taxol), cyclophosphamide (CYTOXAN), ifosfamide (Ifex), and FLUOROURACIL (5-FU) (Adrucil, Efudex). For women whose cancer remains after treatment with radiation therapy or surgery, the use of chemotherapy is meant to slow or temporarily shrink the cancer. Chemotherapy rarely completely kills cervical cancer.

The side effects a patient may experience depend on the kind of drug, the amount, or combination of drugs she is taking. Common side effects of chemotherapy include nausea and vomiting, hair loss, mouth sores, diarrhea, and fatigue. Infections are potentially serious complications of chemotherapy. Infections occur because chemotherapy decreases the number of white blood cells, which fight infection. Any fever during the course of chemotherapy should be immediately reported to the doctor. If untreated, infections may lead to death.

Prevention

Women who smoke can lower their risk of cervical cancer development by quitting smoking. Other than not smoking, there is no definite way to prevent cervical cancer, so doctors recommend women have regular pelvic examinations and an annual Pap test. This way, the cancer can be detected at an early stage before it has spread.

Pap test   The Pap test can find an abnormality in the cervix long before it turns into an actual cancer. This simple, painless screening test is the most powerful tool in preventing cervical cancer. (For details, see the discussion of Pap tests.) Although Pap tests are the best way to detect cervical cancer, a single test may miss up to 15 percent of abnormal cells; for that reason, women should have the test yearly.

Pelvic exams   PELVIC EXAMS are another way to find cervical cancer. In a pelvic exam, the doctor checks the uterus, vagina, ovaries, fallopian tubes, bladder, and rectum for abnormalities. If a woman has risk factors, she should follow her doctor's or nurse's advice about when to have checkups.

HPV vaccine   Scientists have achieved exciting results using an HPV vaccine with cervical cancer, leading some experts to hope that the disease may someday be cured. They also hope it may help prevent many cases of the more rare VAGINAL CANCER, which is also linked to HPV. Although most types of cancer are caused primarily by genetic mutations and environmental factors, virtually all cases of cervical cancer and many cases of vaginal cancer are caused by HPV.

In a recent study, the HPV vaccine prevented HPV infection in every woman who had injections. Although it remains unclear how long the protection will last, researchers hope a vaccine could be available by 2007.

A vaccine for cervical cancer is urgently sought because the disease is still widespread in developing countries. In the United States, where Pap smears are widely used to screen for this cancer, it still develops in about 15,000 women annually and kills about 3,900.

The new HPV vaccine is aimed at the viral strain type 16, responsible for about half of all cervical cancers, and was tested on women between ages 16 and 23 in an 18-month study led by Merck & Co. and the University of Washington. (Merck developed the vaccine and funded the research.)

Of 768 women who had vaccine injections, none showed type 16 HPV infection or precancerous tissue. Of 765 who took placebo injections, 41 were infected with persistent HPV infections, and nine had precancerous tissue. Women who were vaccinated produced up to almost 60 times the amount of virus-fighting antibodies as unvaccinated women who were infected with HPV.

However, because cervical cancer is caused by many different strains of HPV, it is not clear whether the disease can ever be wiped out completely. In addition, scientists do not know whether the antibodies persist for more than five years, an important problem in planning for lifetime protection. Still, scientists hope that a vaccine targeting multiple viral strains encompassing the vast share of cases can be available fairly quickly. Such a vaccine could also stop other problems caused by the virus, including genital warts in both men and women and rare forms of penile, anal, vaginal, and oral cancers. The vaccine could also be administered to men to prevent them from infecting their partners.

cervical conization   See CONE BIOPSY.

cervical intraepithelial neoplasia   See DYSPLASIA.

cervical polyp   A fragile growth hanging from a stalk that projects outward into the canal of the cervix and can cause bleeding after sex; it may occur together with an endometrial polyp, which can lead to infertility. Cervical polyps are relatively common, especially among women older than age 20 who have had children. Typically, polyps are benign and easily removed; they rarely regrow.

Doctors do not fully understand what causes these polyps, which are often the result of an infection. They may be associated with chronic inflammation, an abnormal response to higher levels of ESTROGEN, or congestion of cervical blood vessels in the cervix. Most of the time polyps occur alone, but occasionally two or three are found together. They are rare before the onset of menstrual periods.

Symptoms

Signs of a cervical polyp include abnormal vaginal bleeding after sex or douching, between periods, or after menopause. A polyp also may cause an abnormally heavy period or white or yellow mucus discharge.

Diagnosis

A pelvic exam and a cervical BIOPSY can reveal mildly atypical cells and signs of infection.

Treatment

A doctor can remove the polyp during a simple outpatient procedure; often, gentle twisting of a cervical polyp is enough to remove it. Because many polyps are infected, an antibiotic may be administered after the removal. Although most cervical polyps are benign, the tissue should be sent to a pathologist to be sure; some CERVICAL CANCERS may first appear as a polyp.

CF A combination of the CHEMOTHERAPY drugs CISPLATIN and FLUOROURACIL (5-FU), sometimes used to treat GESTATIONAL TROPHOBLASTIC TUMOR.

CFL A combination of the CHEMOTHERAPY drugs CISPLATIN, FLUOROURACIL (5-FU), and LEUCOVORIN CALCIUM sometimes used to treat GESTATIONAL TROPHOBLASTIC DISEASE.

CHAD A combination of the CHEMOTHERAPY drugs cyclophosphamide (CYTOXAN), HEXAMETHYLMELAMINE, doxorubicin (ADRIAMYCIN), and CISPLATIN, sometimes used to treat OVARIAN CANCER.

CHEMOcare A program and Web site sponsored by the Scott Hamilton Cancer Alliance for Research Education and Survivorship (CARES) initiative, designed to provide the latest information about CHEMOTHERAPY to patients and their family.

The site contains information about having chemotherapy, managing side effects, and living well during treatment. For contact information, see Appendix I.

chemotherapy The use of toxic drugs to control cancer by interfering with the growth or production of malignant cells.

History

Chemotherapy agents were discovered by accident in the course of research related to chemical warfare. In experiments after World War I and during World War II, a large number of soldiers were mistakenly exposed to mustard gas. Doctors discovered these soldiers subsequently had unusually low white blood cell counts. Scientists soon realized that a drug that damaged rapidly growing white blood cells might also damage rapidly growing malignant cells. During the 1940s several patients who had lymphoma were thus injected with mustard gas, and experienced a remarkable (albeit temporary) improvement.

How It Works

Chemotherapy drugs interfere with the ability of cancer cells throughout the body to divide and reproduce. Whereas normal cells typically divide in very controlled ways, malignant cells grow and reproduce in a rapid, haphazard way. Chemotherapy drugs are taken up by rapidly dividing cells—which in addition to cancerous cells include some healthy cells that normally divide quickly, such as those in the lining of the mouth, the BONE MARROW, the hair follicles, and the digestive system. However, whereas healthy cells can repair the damage caused by chemotherapy, cancer cells cannot—and so they eventually die.

Chemotherapy drugs damage cancer cells in different ways. If a combination of drugs is used, each drug is chosen for its specific effects. Chemotherapy must be carefully planned so that it destroys more and more of the cancer cells during the course of treatment but does not destroy the normal cells and tissues. In some types of cancer, chemotherapy can destroy all the cancer cells and cure the disease.

Chemotherapy and Cervical Cancer

Chemotherapy for CERVICAL CANCER usually involves a combination of drugs given by intravenous injection. CISPLATIN (Platinol), CARBOPLATIN (Paraplatin), topotecan (Hycontin), paclitaxel (Taxol), cyclophosphamide (CYTOXAN), ifosfamide (Ifex), and FLUOROURACIL (5-FU, Adrucil, Efudex) are some of the drugs used to treat cervical cancer.

Chemotherapy and Endometrial Cancer

Common ENDOMETRIAL CANCER chemotherapy drugs include cisplatin (Platinol or carboplatin) doxorubicin (Adriamycin) and paclitaxel (Taxol).

Chemotherapy and Ovarian Cancer

Drugs used to treat OVARIAN CANCER include 9-aminocamptothecin (9-AC), among others.

Chemotherapy and Vaginal Cancer

There is no standard chemotherapy for the treatment of VAGINAL CANCER.

Chemotherapy and Vulval Cancer

Preinvasive vulva cancer may be treated with fluorouracil (5-FU) cream. Cisplatin is the most commonly used drug for advanced vulval cancer.

Adjuvant therapy To reduce the chance of cancer recurrence, chemotherapy may be given after surgery to remove the cancer, or after RADIATION THERAPY, to destroy any remaining cancer cells that are too small to see. In advanced cancer, if a cure is not possible, chemotherapy is given to shrink and control the cancer in order to extend life and improve its quality.

Neoadjuvant therapy When a cancer cannot be removed easily during an operation, chemotherapy can be given before surgery to shrink it and make it easier to remove. Chemotherapy can also be used in this way before radiation therapy.

How It Is Given

Chemotherapy may be given in different ways, depending on the type of cancer and the particular chemotherapy drugs used. They can be given in pill or liquid form by mouth, on the skin as a lotion, intravenously (IV), intramuscularly, subcutaneously (under the skin), intraarterially (into the artery), intrathecally (into the central nervous system through the cerebrospinal fluid), intrapleurally (into the chest cavity), intraperitoneally (into the abdomen), intravesically (into the bladder), or intralesionally (into the tumor itself).

Chemotherapy also can be given by IV lines through catheters, ports, and pumps. A catheter is a soft, thin flexible tube that is placed into a large vein, where it remains throughout treatment. Patients who need many IV treatments often have a catheter to avoid frequent needles. Drugs can be given and blood samples can be drawn through the same catheter. A catheter placed in a large vein in the chest is called a central venous catheter. A peripherally inserted central catheter is inserted into a vein in the arm. Catheters such as an intrathecal (delivering drugs into the spinal fluid) or intracavitary (placed in the abdomen, pelvis, or chest) also can be placed in an artery or other locations in the body. Drugs administered in this way tend to remain in the location in which they are given and do not affect cells in other parts of the body.

Sometimes the catheter is attached to a port—a small round plastic or metal disk placed under the skin, which is also used throughout treatment.

A pump (either external or internal) is used to control the rate at which the drug enters a catheter or port. Catheters, ports, and pumps cause no pain if they are properly placed, although a patient is aware of them.

Frequency

How often and how long a patient receives chemotherapy depend on the type of cancer, the treatment goals, the specific drugs, and the patient's body's response to treatment. Chemotherapy is often given in cycles of treatment periods with rest periods in between, to give the body a chance to produce healthy new cells and regain strength.

Chemotherapy on the Job

Most people can continue working while receiving chemotherapy, although they may need to change their work schedule if the drugs make them feel tired or sick. Federal and state laws require employers to let patients work a flexible schedule to meet treatment needs. Social workers and the staff of congressional or state representatives can provide information about state and federal laws that guarantee patient protections.

Side Effects

Different chemotherapy drugs cause a variety of side effects that may vary from person to person and treatment to treatment. Almost all side effects are short term and gradually end once the treatment has stopped. The main areas of the body that may be affected by chemotherapy are those where normal cells rapidly divide and grow, such as the lining of the mouth, digestive system, skin, hair, and bone marrow.

However, sometimes chemotherapy can cause permanent changes or damage to the heart, lungs, nerves, kidneys, reproductive organs, or other organs. Certain types of chemotherapy may have delayed effects (such as the occurrence of a second type of cancer) that do not appear until many years later. Patients need to balance their concerns about permanent effects with the immediate threat of cancer.

Great progress has been made in preventing and treating some of chemotherapy's common as well as rare severe side effects. Many new drugs and treatment methods destroy cancer more effectively while doing less harm to the body's healthy cells.

FATIGUE, infection, and unusual bleeding are all very common side effects because chemotherapy lowers the number of blood cells produced by the bone marrow—white blood cells that are essential for fighting infections, red blood cells that carry oxygen, and platelets that help clot blood and prevent bleeding.

Fatigue Fatigue is a very common side effect of chemotherapy that patients report is quite different from normal tiredness. Fatigue caused by chemotherapy can appear suddenly and may be experienced as lack of energy, weakness, and complete inability to work or think. Moreover, it seems unrelated to activity and does not improve with rest. It has been described as a total lack of energy that makes patients feel worn out and drained.

Fatigue associated with chemotherapy is related to low blood cell counts, stress, depression, poor appetite, lack of exercise, and many other factors. Chemotherapy can interfere with the bone marrow's ability to make red blood cells, which carry oxygen to all parts of the body. When there are too few red blood cells, body tissues do not receive enough oxygen to do their work and patients may become tired and lethargic. Because the amount of oxygen being carried around the body is lower, patients also may become breathless. These are all symptoms of anemia (a lack of hemoglobin in the blood). People who have anemia may also feel dizzy and light-headed and have aching muscles and joints. The tiredness fades away gradually once the chemotherapy has ended, but some people find that they still feel tired a year or more afterward.

ONCOLOGISTS order regular blood tests to measure hemoglobin during chemotherapy, and a blood transfusion can be given if the hemoglobin level falls too low. The extra red cells in the blood transfusion very quickly pick up the oxygen from the lungs and take it around the body; patients then feel more energetic, and the breathlessness improves. Some studies have also suggested that maintaining a moderate level of physical exercise (such as walking) can help prevent fatigue.

Nausea/vomiting Although many patients fear the nausea and vomiting that have historically been reported as a side effect of chemotherapy, in fact drugs used today have made these side effects far less common.

Because of very effective antinausea medications, many women do not become sick at all during their treatment, and if they do become sick, sickness is quite mild. It is particularly important that patients closely follow their physicians' guidelines regarding antinausea medication. This medication is usually given together with IV chemotherapy; patients generally should then take additional antinausea medication at home *before nausea begins*. Once nausea starts, controlling it is far more difficult. Low doses of steroids can be helpful in reducing nausea and vomiting.

Antinausea medications that are highly effective include lorazepam (Ativan), prochlorperazine (Compazine), promethazine (Anergan), metoclopramide (Reglan), dexamethasone (DECADRON), ondansetron (Zofran), Emend, and granisetron (Kytril).

Chemotherapy drugs cause nausea and vomiting because they tend to irritate the stomach lining, thereby stimulating nerves in the vomiting center in the brain. Certain chemotherapy medications are more likely to cause nausea and vomiting, including the following:

- Carboplatin
- Carmustine
- Cisplatin
- Cyclophosphamide

- Cytarabine
- Dacarbazine
- Dactinomycin
- Doxorubicin
- Etoposide
- Lomustine
- Mechlorethamine
- Melphalan
- Methotrexate
- Plicamycin
- Procarbazine
- Streptozocin

The reaction to chemotherapy varies from person to person and from drug to drug. If patients are going to feel sick, the symptoms usually begin a few minutes to several hours after chemotherapy, depending on the drugs given. The sickness may last for a few hours or for several days. Some people never vomit or feel nauseated. Others feel mildly nauseated most of the time; some become severely nauseated for a limited time during or after a treatment. Certain risk factors that influence severity of nausea include previous experience with motion sickness, age, alcohol use, and bad prior experiences with nausea and vomiting.

To prevent problems, women should

- Avoid big meals so the stomach will not feel too full. Eating small meals throughout the day is better than eating a few large meals.
- Drink liquids at least an hour before or after mealtime, instead of with meals.
- Eat and drink slowly.
- Avoid sweet, fried, or fatty foods.
- Eat foods cold or at room temperature to avoid strong smells. (Many patients swear by cold white foods, such as cold chicken or ice cream.)
- Chew food well for easier digestion.
- Drink cool, clear, unsweetened fruit juices, such as apple or grape juice. Avoid carbonated beverages, which can burn sensitive throats.
- Suck on ice cubes.

- Try to avoid bothersome odors such as cooking smells, smoke, or perfume.
- Prepare and freeze meals in advance.
- Rest in a chair after eating, but avoid lying flat for at least two hours after a meal.
- Breathe deeply and slowly during bouts of nausea.
- Use relaxation techniques.
- Avoid eating for at least a few hours before treatment if nausea usually occurs during chemotherapy.

Appetite loss/weight loss Patients who are receiving chemotherapy may lose their appetite and lose weight as a result of nausea and vomiting, and the drugs can also directly affect appetite by affecting the body's metabolism. In severe cases, loss of appetite can lead to CACHEXIA, a form of malnutrition. In general, appetite returns a few weeks after chemotherapy is completed. If loss of appetite is severe, doctors can prescribe medications that may improve the condition.

Bone marrow suppression Chemotherapy damages the blood cell–producing tissues of the bone marrow, triggering a condition called bone marrow suppression. While chemotherapy targets rapidly-dividing cancerous cells, it also affects normal rapidly-dividing cells in the body, such as those produced in bone marrow tissue. Until the bone marrow recovers from the damage, the patient has abnormally low numbers of white blood cells, red blood cells, and platelets. For this reason, the patient's blood is monitored weekly during chemotherapy.

Normally, blood cells are constantly replaced as they wear out (white blood cells last about six hours, platelets last about 10 days, and red blood cells last about four months). When chemotherapy is given, however, worn-out cells are not replaced, so blood counts begin to drop. Blood cell counts do not drop as soon as chemotherapy is given however, because the drugs do not affect cells circulating in the blood. Instead, new blood cells are temporarily prevented from forming in the marrow. The type of chemotherapy drug and the strength of the dosage influence the ways blood cells are affected.

In general, white blood cells and platelets drop to their lowest level within one or two weeks after a dose of chemotherapy. Because red blood cells last longer, their levels drop later. The side effects that result from low levels of various types of blood cells peak when the blood counts are lowest.

Low white blood cell count Because white blood cells fight infection, when a person's white cell count drops during chemotherapy, he or she becomes more vulnerable to infection. Neutrophils are the most common subtype of white blood cells; they are an important defense against infection. The normal range of neutrophils is between 2,500 and 6,000 cells per cubic millimeter; a patient who has a neutrophil count of 1,000 or less is considered to be at risk for infection, and a count of less than 500 is considered to be severely low. Because the risk of infection is great, chemotherapy treatments are delayed if a person has a very low white blood count.

When counts are low during chemotherapy, an infection can begin in almost any part of the body, including the mouth, skin, lungs, urinary tract, rectum, or reproductive tract. Fever is an important first sign of infection; for this reason, patients are usually told to call their doctor or nurse when they have a fever of 100.5°F or higher. Other signs of infection include sore throat, cough or shortness of breath, nasal congestion, shaking chills, burning during urination, and redness or swelling of the skin.

If patients contract an infection when their white blood cell level is very low, they may need antibiotics administered directly into the bloodstream. Sometimes, drugs called hematopoietic growth factors can help the bone marrow make more white blood cells. Growth factors are sometimes given after chemotherapy treatment to stimulate the bone marrow to produce new white cells quickly, thereby reducing the risk of infection. There are several naturally occurring growth factors, which are also called colony-stimulating factors. Scientists have recently discovered how to produce these in the lab, and growth factors are now available as drugs. The two growth factors that boost production of white blood cells are granulocyte-macrophage colony-stimulating factor (sargramostim [Leukine]) and GRANULOCYTE COLONY-STIMULATING FACTOR (filgrastim [Neupogen]).

Most infections a cancer patient may have originate from the bacteria normally found on the skin and in the intestines and genital tract. In some cases, the cause of an infection may not be known. When the white count is lower than normal, patients can try to prevent infections by taking the following steps:

- Washing hands often during the day, especially before meals or using the bathroom
- Cleaning the rectal area gently but thoroughly after each bowel movement
- Avoiding people who have communicable diseases (colds, flu, measles, or chickenpox)
- Avoiding crowds
- Avoiding people who have recently received immunizations, such as vaccines for polio, measles, mumps, and rubella (German measles)
- Preventing nicks when using scissors, needles, or knives. Substitution of an electric shaver for a razor can prevent breaks or cuts
- Using a soft toothbrush that will not cut gums
- Taking a warm (not hot) bath, shower, or sponge bath every day
- Cleaning cuts and scrapes immediately with warm water, soap, and an antiseptic

Low red blood count A person who does not have enough red blood cells is anemic. Normally, blood has between 4.0 and 6.0 million red blood cells per cubic millimeter. Another measurement used is the hematocrit—the percentage of total blood volume occupied by red blood cells. A normal hematocrit range is between 36 percent and 42 percent.

Patients who have ANEMIA feel tired, dizzy, and irritable and experience headaches, shortness of breath, and rapid breathing. Anemia caused by chemotherapy is temporary, but sometimes blood transfusions are needed until the bone marrow can begin producing red blood cells again. Alternatively, doctors may prescribe ERYTHROPOIETIN (Procrit, Aranesp), a naturally occurring growth factor that boosts production of red blood cells in the bone marrow. Erythropoietin is usually administered three times a week until the hematocrit rises to normal level.

Low platelet count Anticancer drugs can also compromise the bone marrow's ability to make platelets, the blood cells that help stop bleeding by making blood clot. Low platelet count (called *thrombocytopenia*) may cause a patient to bruise readily, bleed longer than usual after a minor cut, have bleeding gums or nose bleeds, and experience severe internal bleeding. Low platelet counts are temporary, but they can cause serious blood loss if an injury occurs. If counts are very low, a platelet transfusion can be given. Transfused platelets are short-lived, but a platelet growth factor can be administered as a drug to patients who have severe thrombocytopenia.

Patients should report to their doctor any symptoms of unexpected bruising, small red spots under the skin, reddish or pinkish urine, black or bloody bowel movements, or bleeding from gums or nose.

Diarrhea/constipation Up to 75 percent of people who receive chemotherapy may experience diarrhea because of the damage to rapidly dividing cells in the lining of the digestive system. The amount and duration of diarrhea depend in part on the type, dosage, and duration of drugs the patient receives. Some of the chemotherapy drugs that cause diarrhea are 5-fluorouracil, methotrexate, docetaxel and actinomycin D.

Although many patients may think of diarrhea as just an annoyance, in severe cases it can be life threatening if accompanied by dehydration, malnutrition, or electrolyte imbalance. In severe cases, the doctor may prescribe an antidiarrheal medicine. In addition, patients with diarrhea should

- Eat smaller amounts of food, but eat more often.
- Avoid high-fiber foods, such as whole grain breads and cereals, raw vegetables, beans, nuts, seeds, popcorn, and fresh and dried fruit.
- Eat low-fiber foods, such as white bread, white rice, noodles, creamed cereals, ripe bananas, canned or cooked fruit without skins, yogurt, eggs, mashed or baked potatoes without skin, pureed vegetables, chicken or turkey without skin, and fish.
- Avoid coffee, tea, alcohol, sweets, and fried, greasy, or highly spiced foods.
- Avoid milk and milk products.
- Eat more potassium-rich foods (bananas, oranges, potatoes, and peach and apricot nectars).

- Drink plenty of fluids to replace those lost through diarrhea. Mild clear liquids such as apple juice, water, weak tea, or clear broth are best.

Some chemotherapy drugs (such as vinblastine or vincristine) also can cause constipation, as can other drugs the patient may be taking at the same time (especially narcotic pain medications). Some patients become constipated because they are less active or less well nourished than usual. Dehydration, decreased fluid intake, and depression all can cause constipation. Patients can drink warm or hot fluids to help loosen the bowels and eat high-fiber foods (such as whole wheat bread or fresh fruit). Exercise—even just walking around the block—can also help, as can a more structured exercise program.

Mouth sores Good oral care is important during cancer treatment, because chemotherapy drugs can cause STOMATITIS and ESOPHAGITIS—sores in the mouth and throat. In addition to being painful and affecting the appetite, these sores can become infected by the germs in the mouth. Because infections can be hard to fight during chemotherapy and can lead to serious problems, it is important to take every possible step to prevent them.

Sores in the throat and mouth usually occur about five to 10 days after treatment and clear up within three to four weeks. Patients who have not been eating well since beginning chemotherapy are more likely to have mouth sores. Mouth sores usually begin with a pale, dry lining of the mouth, followed by inflamed gums, mouth, and throat. The tongue may begin to swell, and swallowing and eating may become painful and difficult.

If possible, patients should see a dentist before starting chemotherapy to have teeth cleaned and to take care of any problems, such as cavities, abscesses, gum disease, or poorly fitting dentures. Because chemotherapy can make a patient more likely to have cavities, a dentist may suggest using a fluoride rinse or gel each day to help prevent decay. Cleaning the teeth regularly and gently with a soft toothbrush helps to keep the mouth clean. If the mouth is very sore, gels, creams, or pastes can be used to paint over the ulcers to reduce soreness.

Chemotherapy also can alter a person's sense of taste. This sensation can affect appetite and nutrition. Food may seem more salty, bitter, or metallic. The patient may experience a sudden dislike of tomato products, beef, pork, or sweet foods. Typically, normal taste resumes after chemotherapy treatment ends.

Hair loss   Hair loss is one of the most common, and worrisome, side effects of chemotherapy. Although a few drugs used to treat cancer do not cause hair loss (or cause slight hair loss), most do cause partial or complete hair loss for a time. Chemotherapy affects the rapidly dividing cells of the hair follicles, making hair brittle so that it may break off near the scalp or spontaneously release. This usually occurs two to three weeks after the first chemotherapy treatment, although rarely it can start within a few days.

The amount of hair lost depends on the type of drug or combination of drugs used, the dosage given, and the person's individual reaction to the drug. Body hair may be lost as well, and some drugs even trigger loss of the eyelashes and eyebrows. Hair lost as a result of chemotherapy almost always regrows once treatment is over.

Patients who lose their hair during chemotherapy need to take special care of their scalp and any remaining hair. Patients should use mild shampoos, soft hairbrushes, and low heat when drying hair.

Once hair loss occurs, patients should use a sunscreen, sunblock, or hat to protect the scalp from the sun. Unlike some other side effects of chemotherapy, hair loss is not life threatening, but it can have a psychological impact on a person's life. Hair loss can cause depression, loss of self-esteem, and even grief reactions.

Skin/nail changes   Some drugs can affect the skin, making it drier or slightly discolored. These changes may be worsened by swimming, especially in chlorinated water. The drugs may also make skin more sensitive to sunlight during and after treatment. Nails may grow more slowly, and white lines may appear. Nails also may become more brittle and flaky.

Nerves   Some chemotherapy drugs can affect the nerves in the hands and feet, causing tingling, numbness, or a sensation of pins and needles known as peripheral neuropathy. In most cases this feeling gradually fades away after chemotherapy ends, but in severe ones nerves may be permanently damaged.

Nervous system   Some drugs can directly affect the central nervous system (the brain and spinal cord), causing feelings of anxiety and restlessness, dizziness, sleeplessness, headaches, or concentration and memory problems. Other drugs can lead to a loss of the ability to hear high-pitched sound or cause a continuous noise in the ears known as tinnitus.

Chemotherapy also can affect the cranial nerves—which are involved with movement and sensation of the head, face, and neck, and with vision—or the peripheral nerves, which are important in touch and movement.

Vaccinations   Patients who are having chemotherapy should not have live-virus vaccines, including those for polio, measles, rubella (German measles), measles, mumps, and rubella (MMR), bacille Calmette-Guérin (BCG) (tuberculosis), and yellow fever. Vaccines with killed viruses such as diphtheria, tetanus, flu, hepatitis A and B, rabies, cholera, and typhoid should not cause problems to chemotherapy patients.

Radiation recall   Some people who have had radiation therapy develop a skin problem during chemotherapy known as radiation recall during or shortly after certain anticancer drugs are given. In this condition, the skin over an area that has received radiation turns red and may blister and peel. This reaction may last hours or even days.

Kidney/bladder problems   When breakdown products from some anticancer drugs are excreted through the kidneys, they can irritate the bladder or cause temporary or permanent damage to the bladder or kidneys. Some anticancer drugs turn the urine orange, red, green, or yellow or give it a strong or medicinelike odor for 24 to 72 hours, although these changes are harmless. Symptoms of kidney damage include headache, lower back pain, weakness, nausea, vomiting, fatigue, high blood pressure, change in urination pattern, urgent need to urinate, and swelling. Patients who have had kidney problems are at higher risk for development of more problems during chemotherapy, especially if the drugs include high-dose methotrexate, ifosfamide, or streptozocin. Patients should always drink plenty of fluids to ensure good urine flow and help prevent problems.

Flu symptoms Symptoms of the flu may bother some patients a few hours to a few days after chemotherapy, especially if they are receiving BIOLOGICAL THERAPY at the same time. Aching muscles and joints, headache, fatigue, nausea, slight fever (less than 100°F), chills, and poor appetite may last one to three days. An infection or the cancer itself can also cause these symptoms.

Liver damage Chemotherapy drugs are broken down by the liver, which occasionally can become damaged during treatment. However, this problem is temporary and usually improves once treatment is stopped. Symptoms of liver damage include jaundice (yellowed skin and eyes), fatigue, and pain in the lower right ribs or right upper abdomen.

Older patients and those who have had hepatitis are more likely to have liver problems after chemotherapy, especially if they are taking drugs such as methotrexate, cytosine arabinoside (ara-C), high-dose cisplatin or cyclophosphamide (Cytoxan), vincristine, vinblastine, or doxorubicin (Adriamycin).

Heart problems About 10 percent of patients experience heart damage caused by certain chemotherapy drugs—especially daunorubicin and doxorubicin (Adriamycin). Symptoms of heart damage may include dry cough, ankle swelling, shortness of breath, puffiness, and erratic heartbeats. Patients at higher risk for heart damage include those with previous heart problems, high blood pressure, or prior radiation to the chest and patients who smoke. Because of the small risk of heart damage, assessments are made before and during chemotherapy to check for problems.

Fluid retention The body may retain fluid during chemotherapy. This may be due to hormonal changes from therapy, the drugs themselves, or the cancer. Patients may need to avoid table salt and foods that contain a lot of salt. If the problem is severe, a doctor may prescribe a diuretic to help rid the body of excess fluids.

Infertility Chemotherapy treatments may cause temporary or permanent infertility. The drugs can destroy both healthy and unhealthy cells, damaging the reproductive system. Risks vary by individual treatment regimens, and alkylating and platinum-based agents carry the greatest risk to the reproductive system. Data on the prevalence and duration of infertility are not yet available for most types of chemotherapy.

Long-term problems Although most side effects of chemotherapy end once treatment ends, some patients experience long-term problems related to their treatment for cancer. These long-term effects depend on the type of drugs used and whether other treatments (such as radiation therapy) were given.

Some drugs can permanently damage internal organs such as the heart or reproductive system. Changes in the nervous system can appear months or years after chemotherapy has stopped and may involve fatigue, sleepiness, memory problems, personality changes, shortened attention span, reduced intelligence quotient (IQ), or seizures. Long-term effects of nerve damage may include numbness, tingling, or prickling sensations.

Finally, it is also possible that some types of chemotherapy can lead to the development of a second type of cancer, including Hodgkin's disease and non-Hodgkin's lymphoma, leukemia, and a few types of solid tumors.

Cost The cost of chemotherapy varies with the types and dosages of drugs used, the duration and frequency of administration, and location of treatment (at home, in an office, or in a hospital). Most health insurance policies cover at least part of the cost of many kinds of chemotherapy. There are also organizations that will help with the cost of chemotherapy and with transportation costs. Nurses and social workers have information about these organizations. In some states, Medicaid (which makes health-care services available for people with financial need) may help pay for certain treatments.

Chemotherapy Foundation A public foundation, established in 1968, dedicated to the control, cure, and prevention of cancer through innovative medical therapies including chemotherapy, chemo-immunotherapy, chemohormonal therapy, chemo-prevention, and biotechnologies. The foundation is also dedicated to the education of physicians, patients, and the public through educational literature. The foundation currently sponsors selected basic and clinical research initiatives at six major

New York metropolitan medical centers. For contact information, see Appendix I.

CHEX-UP A combination of the CHEMOTHERAPY drugs cyclophosphamide (CYTOXAN), HEXAMETHYLMELAMINE, FLUOROURACIL (5-FU), and CISPLATIN sometimes used to treat OVARIAN CANCER.

choriocarcinoma A rare cancer in which cancer cells grow in uterine tissues after conception, also called GESTATIONAL TROPHOBLASTIC DISEASE, gestational trophoblastic neoplasia, gestational trophoblastic tumor, or molar pregnancy. This highly malignant type of cancer responds to CHEMOTHERAPY.

cigarettes See SMOKING.

cisplatin (Platinol) A platinum compound and ALKYLATING AGENT given intravenously to treat OVARIAN CANCER and CERVICAL CANCER. Cisplatin works by disrupting the growth of cancer cells.

More common side effects include nausea and vomiting; kidney damage; taste changes; pins and needles feeling in hands or feet; lowered levels of magnesium, potassium, and calcium; and decreased white blood cell and platelet counts. Other less common side effects may include FATIGUE, APPETITE LOSS, thinning of hair, and DIARRHEA.

clear cell adenocarcinoma A type of curable cancer that occurs in glandular tissue and that has been linked to the anti-miscarriage drug DIETHYLSTILBESTROL (DES). This synthetic hormone was prescribed to pregnant women between 1940 and 1971—about 4 million women in the United States alone.

Before 1971, clear cell adenocarcinoma of the vagina or cervix was a rare disease, diagnosed primarily in women over age 70. In 1971, however, doctors documented several cases of this cancer in young women whose mothers had taken DES during pregnancy. This discovery led the U.S. Food and Drug Administration (FDA) in 1971 to ban the use of DES during pregnancy.

Researchers have estimated that approximately one in 1,000 daughters of women who took DES (DES daughters) are at risk of developing the cancer, although this number may turn out to be higher as the daughters age. Fortunately, more than 80 percent of the women who have had clear cell adenocarcinoma recover.

So far, clear cell adenocarcinoma has been found in DES daughters between the ages of seven and 48. It is important for DES daughters and their physicians to be aware that there is no specific age after which the risk for this type of clear cell cancer is over. Today, the upper age limit for the development of the cancer is unknown.

Symptoms

Symptoms of adenocarcinoma in the vagina or cervix include bleeding or discharge not related to menstrual periods, difficult or painful urination, painful intercourse, pelvic pain, CONSTIPATION, or a mass that can be felt. Even if a woman has had a HYSTERECTOMY, she still has a chance of developing adenocarcinoma in the vagina.

Diagnosis

DES daughters should have a gynecological exam once a year, including a thorough pelvic examination with careful visual examination, a cervical Pap test, a vaginal Pap test taken from all four sides of the vagina (4-quadrant), and a manual inspection of the vagina. The recommended pelvic exam for a DES daughter is different from a routine women's exam (in the routine exam, the Pap smear is taken only from the cervix). In the DES exam, a separate Pap smear is taken from the surfaces of the upper vagina as well.

Treatment

The most common treatment is surgery—a radical hysterectomy (removal of uterus, fallopian tubes, and one or both ovaries), VAGINECTOMY (removal of all or part of the vagina), and LYMPHADENECTOMY (removal of surrounding LYMPH NODES). A vaginectomy is necessary only if diagnosis includes VAGINAL CANCER. Internal and external radiation may also be used to treat the cancer, alone or in conjunction with surgery.

clear cell carcinoma A rare type of tumor of the female genital tract in which the inside of the cells appears clear when seen under a microscope.

clear margin   An area of tissue surrounding a tumor that is free of cancer cells. During cancer surgery, the surgeon tries to remove the tumor and a wide margin of healthy tissue. If no cancer cells are found near the edges of the sample, it is said to have clear margins. After surgery, if the excised tissue is found by the lab to have cancer cells near the margin of healthy tissue, often the surgeon operates again in an attempt to remove a wider margin of healthy tissue around the original tumor.

clinical cancer centers   Cancer centers sponsored by the NATIONAL CANCER INSTITUTE that conduct programs in clinical and laboratory research and may also have programs in other areas such as basic research or prevention, control, and population-based research. The centers focus on both laboratory research and clinical research within the same institutional framework, which is a distinguishing characteristic of many clinical cancer centers. For contact information for individual clinical cancer centers, see Appendix II.

clinical trials   A research study designed to answer specific questions about vaccines, new drugs, or new ways of using known treatments, including whether they are both safe and effective. Carefully conducted clinical trials are the fastest and safest way to find treatments that work.

For all types of trials, the participant works with a research team that includes doctors, nurses, and social workers, who check the health of subjects at the beginning of the trial, give specific instructions for participation, and monitor participants carefully during and after the trial. Some clinical trials involve more tests and doctor visits than the participant would normally have for cancer.

To help someone decide whether or not to participate, scientists explain the study and provide an informed consent document that discusses the study's purpose, duration, required procedures, and key contacts. Risks and potential benefits are explained carefully and clearly, and then the participant decides whether or not to sign the document. Informed consent is not a contract—it is a means to ensure the participant understands all the pros and cons of the trial. The participant may withdraw from the trial at any time.

Well-designed clinical trials can help patients play an active role in their own health care, gain access to new treatments that are not widely available, obtain free expert medical care at leading hospitals, and help others by contributing to medical research.

Of course, there are risks in clinical trials. The treatment may have unpleasant, serious, or even life-threatening, side effects. It may not be effective for the participant. The protocol may require more time and effort than standard treatment, including trips to the study site, hospital stays, or complex dosage requirements.

However, the ethical and legal codes that govern medical practice also apply to clinical trials. Most clinical research is also regulated by the U.S. government, with built-in safeguards to protect participants. The trial follows a carefully controlled study plan that details what researchers will do. As a clinical trial progresses, researchers report the results of the trial at scientific meetings, to medical journals, and to various government agencies.

Types of Clinical Trials

There are a variety of types of clinical trials:

Screening trials test the best way to detect certain diseases or health conditions.
Prevention trials look for better ways to prevent disease in people who have never had the disease or to prevent recurrence of a disease. These means may include medicines, vitamins, vaccines, minerals, or lifestyle changes.
Diagnostic trials are conducted to find better tests or procedures for diagnosing a particular disease or condition.
Treatment trials test new treatments, new combinations of drugs, or new approaches to surgery or radiation therapy.
Quality of life trials (or "supportive care" trials) explore ways to improve comfort and the quality of life of individuals who have a chronic illness.

Phases of Clinical Trials

Clinical trials occur in four phases: PHASE I TRIALS test a new drug or treatment in a small group; PHASE II TRIALS expand the study to a larger group of people; PHASE III TRIALS expand the study to an even larger group of people; and PHASE IV TRIALS take place after the drug or treatment has been licensed and marketed.

Expanded Access Protocol

Most investigational new drugs are given during controlled clinical trials that assess their safety and efficacy. Sometimes patients do not qualify for these trials because of other health problems, age, or other factors. To help patients who may benefit from the drug but do not qualify for the trials, regulations allow manufacturers of investigational new drugs to apply for an expanded access protocol.

This allows people who have a life-threatening or serious disease to obtain a research drug. It also generates additional safety information about the drug. Expanded access protocols can be used only if scientists are actively studying the new treatment in well-controlled studies or all studies have been completed. There must be evidence that the drug may be an effective treatment for patients like those to be treated under the protocol. The drug cannot expose patients to unreasonable risks given the severity of the disease to be treated. Expanded access protocols are generally managed by the drug company, with the investigational treatment administered at a doctor's office or hospital.

See also Appendix III.

Coalition of National Cancer Cooperative Groups

The nation's premier network of cancer clinical trials specialists. Members include CANCER CENTERS, academic medical centers, community hospitals, physician practices, and patient advocate groups who represent the interests of more than 17,000 cancer investigators, hundreds of patient advocates, and thousands of patients around the world.

The coalition was created to address serious issues that affect cooperative groups, such as following regulatory requirements, competing for federal funding, working under the managed care system, and improving the clinical trials experience of patients and doctors. The coalition offers a variety of programs and information for doctors, payers, patient advocate groups, and patients, designed to improve the entire clinical trials process. For contact information, see Appendix I.

coenzyme Q10 (ubiquinone, ubidecarenone)

A compound produced naturally in the body that helps cells produce energy needed for cell growth and maintenance. Coenzyme Q10 is found in most body tissues, especially in the heart, liver, kidneys, and pancreas; the lowest amounts are found in the lungs. It is also an ANTIOXIDANT (a substance that protects cells from harmful chemicals called FREE RADICALS).

Studies of cancer patients have shown that coenzyme Q10 decreases the harmful effects on the heart of the CHEMOTHERAPY drug doxorubicin. However, no report of a randomized clinical trial of coenzyme Q10 as a treatment for cancer itself has been published in a peer-reviewed scientific journal.

Coenzyme Q10 was first identified in 1957, but scientists did not consider its use as a potential cancer drug until 1961, when a deficiency of the enzyme was noted in the blood of cancer patients.

Animal studies have found that coenzyme Q10 stimulated the IMMUNE SYSTEM and increased resistance to disease. In part because of this, researchers have theorized that coenzyme Q10 may be useful as an adjuvant therapy for cancer.

No serious side effects of the use of coenzyme Q10 have been reported. Some patients using coenzyme Q10 have experienced mild insomnia, higher levels of liver enzymes, rashes, nausea, and upper abdominal pain. Other reported side effects have included dizziness, visual sensitivity to light, irritability, headache, heartburn, and FATIGUE.

Patients should discuss with their health-care provider possible interactions between coenzyme Q10 and prescription drugs they may be taking. Certain drugs, such as those that are used to lower cholesterol or blood sugar levels, may also reduce the effects of coenzyme Q10. Coenzyme Q10 may also alter the body's response to warfarin (a drug that prevents blood clotting) and insulin.

Coenzyme Q10 is used by the body as an antioxidant, which protects cells from free radicals, the highly reactive chemicals that can damage them. Some conventional cancer therapies, such as chemotherapy and RADIATION THERAPY, are designed to kill cancer cells in part by triggering the formation of free radicals. Researchers are studying whether combining coenzyme Q10 with conventional therapies helps or hinders the fight against cancer.

Several companies distribute coenzyme Q10 as a dietary supplement, which is regulated as a food, not a drug. This means that evaluation and approval by the U.S. Food and Drug Administration are not required before marketing, unless specific health claims are made about the supplement. Because dietary supplements are not formally reviewed for manufacturing consistency, there may be variations in the composition of the supplement from one batch to another.

cognitive dysfunction   Difficulty in thinking ability that may include memory loss, distractibility, problems in performing multiple tasks at the same time, and trouble with arithmetic and language skills. All these impairments have been linked to administration of CHEMOTHERAPY. Problems related to cognitive functioning may range in severity, intensity, and duration.

Cognitive impairments may be subtle and unnoticed, but they may also cause a devastating collection of symptoms. The central nervous system, including the brain, is particularly vulnerable to many cancer treatments. Studies estimate that 18 percent of patients who receive standard-dose chemotherapy experience cognitive dysfunction; the percentage is even higher among those who receive high-dose chemotherapy.

Other cancer treatments also may affect a woman's ability to think clearly. Among the treatments for hormonally sensitive cancers such as OVARIAN CANCER are surgical or medication manipulations that reduce the level of circulating sex HORMONES. This effect causes a cognitive dysfunction that appears to be directly related to the reduction in sex hormone levels.

In addition, many medications used to manage medical complications—especially the immunosuppressive agents used in BONE MARROW TRANSPLANTS, antibiotics, steroids, and drugs used to manage pain or nausea—may cause cognitive impairment.

The symptoms of mild cognitive impairment are often referred to as chemo brain or mental fatigue; they include vulnerability in complex information handling, susceptibility to distraction, and exhaustion with tasks requiring mental energy. "Chemo brain" represents a lack of clear thought; examples include forgetting phone numbers and repeating questions.

A more extreme form of cognitive impairment more common in advanced illness is delirium. The symptoms of delirium include disordered attention and thinking commonly associated with lack of coordination in executing activities, disturbed sleep–wake cycle, disorganized thinking and speech, altered perceptions, and changes in mood. Unlike dementia, delirium usually appears suddenly, comes and goes, and generally affects only short-term memory.

cold knife cone biopsy   See CONE BIOPSY.

colony-stimulating factor (CSF, or hematopoietic growth factor)   A substance that encourages BONE MARROW stem cells to divide and develop into white blood cells, platelets, and red blood cells. Doctors use CSFs to help patients who are undergoing cancer treatment boost their blood counts.

Because CHEMOTHERAPY drugs can damage the body's ability to make white blood cells, red blood cells, and platelets, patients who receive these drugs have a higher risk of development of infections, become anemic, and bleed more readily. By using CSFs to stimulate blood cell production, doctors can increase the dosages of anticancer drugs without increasing the risk of infection or the need for transfusion with blood products. As a result, researchers have found CSFs particularly useful when combined with high-dose chemotherapy.

CSFs that are used in cancer therapy include the following:

- *GRANULOCYTE COLONY-STIMULATING FACTOR (G-CSF) (filgrastim) and granulocyte-macrophage colony-stimulating factor (GM-CSF) (sargramostim).* This increases the number of white blood cells, thereby reducing the risk of infection in patients who are receiving chemotherapy. They can also stimulate the production of stem cells in preparation for stem cell or BONE MARROW TRANSPLANTS.

- *ERYTHROPOIETIN.* This increases the number of red blood cells and reduces the need for red blood cell transfusions for patients receiving chemotherapy

- *Oprelvekin.* This reduces the need for platelet transfusions of chemotherapy patients.

colposcopy   A procedure in which a lighted magnifying instrument (colposcope) is used to examine the vagina and cervix to identify precancerous or abnormal areas. If abnormal areas are identified, small pieces of tissue are then removed for further analysis. The colposcope can magnify the area 10 to 40 times; some devices can also take photographs.

A colposcopy is ordered if a woman's PAP TEST result shows abnormal cell growth, or if the cervix, vagina, or vulva appears to be abnormal during a routine examination. The procedure may also be suggested for women who have genital warts and for daughters of women who used DIETHYLSTILBE-STROL (DES) during pregnancy.

The Procedure
A colposcopy is performed in a physician's office and is similar to a regular gynecologic exam. As a speculum holds the walls of the vagina open, the doctor places the colposcope at the opening of the vagina (not inside the vagina). The doctor looks inside the vagina to locate any potential abnormalities on the cervix or in the vagina. Abnormal areas can be identified by looking for a characteristic pattern made by malformed or dysfunctional blood vessels.

If there are any abnormal areas, the doctor performs a BIOPSY of the tissue during the colposcopy. When this is done, the doctor first numbs the area; numbing may cause a temporary pinch or cramp that usually ends within a few minutes. After the sample is removed, the doctor applies a solution to the area to stop the bleeding. Biopsy results are usually available within a week or two.

If the tissue sample suggests there is an area of abnormal growth (DYSPLASIA) or a precancerous condition, and if the entire abnormal area can be seen, the doctor can destroy the tissue by using one of several procedures: high heat (diathermy), extreme cold (cryosurgery), or lasers. Another procedure, called a LOOP ELECTROSURGICAL EXCISION PROCEDURE (LEEP), removes tissue by using low-voltage high-frequency radio waves. If any of the abnormal tissue is within the cervical canal, it may require a CONE BIOPSY or conization (removal of a conical section of the cervix for inspection).

Aftercare
It is normal to notice a dark fluid or some spotting for a few days after a colposcopy or biopsy. Because of the risk of infection, patients should not use tampons, douche, or have sex for at least a week after the procedure.

combined modality therapy   Use of two or more types of treatments to supplement each other. For instance, surgery, radiation, CHEMOTHERAPY, hormonal therapy, or immunotherapy may be used alternatively or together for maximal effectiveness.

Compazine (prochlorperazine)   A relatively inexpensive drug that is administered either intravenously or orally to help control the episodes of nausea and vomiting that occur more than 48 hours after administration of CHEMOTHER-APY. This drug belongs to a general class of drugs called phenothiazines. It works by blocking messages to the part of the brain that controls nausea and vomiting.

This drug can cause sleepiness, dry mouth, constipation, blurred vision, restlessness, weight gain, or increased heart rate. Rarely, it may cause jaundice, sensitivity to light, rash, or hives.

See also ANTINAUSEA MEDICATION.

complementary and alternative medicine (CAM)
A broad group of healing philosophies, approaches, and products (also referred to as integrative medicine) that are not presently considered to be part of conventional medicine. *Complementary treatment* is therapy used in addition to conventional approaches; *alternative* indicates that a treatment is used *instead of* conventional medicine. Conventional treatments are those that are widely accepted and practiced by the mainstream medical community.

Although there is scientific evidence of the effectiveness and safety of some CAM therapies, in general many of these therapies have not been scientifically tested. As CAM therapies are proved safe and effective through rigorous studies, they are adopted into conventional health care. Though grouped together, complementary and alternative medicines are different.

Complementary medicine is used together with conventional medicine. An example of complementary therapy is the use of aromatherapy to help lessen a patient's discomfort after surgery. Alternative medicine is used in place of conventional medicine—for example, use of a specific diet to treat cancer instead of undergoing surgery, RADIATION THERAPY, or CHEMOTHERAPY that has been recommended by a conventional health-care practitioner.

The National Center for Complementary and Alternative Medicine has classified CAM therapies into five groups:

- Alternative medical systems (for example, homeopathic medicine and traditional Chinese medicine)
- Mind-body interventions, such as visualization or relaxation
- Manipulative and body-based methods such as chiropractic therapy and massage
- Biologically based therapies such as vitamins and herbal products
- Energy therapies such as qi gong and therapeutic touch

Research indicates that the use of CAM therapies is increasing. A large-scale study published in the November 11, 1998, issue of the *Journal of the American Medical Association* found that CAM use among the general public increased from 34 percent in 1990 to 42 percent in 1997. Several surveys of CAM use by cancer patients have been conducted with small numbers of patients. A large study of CAM use in patients with different types of cancer was published in the July 2000 issue of the *Journal of Clinical Oncology*. That study found that 83 percent of 453 cancer patients had used at least one CAM therapy as part of their cancer treatment. The study included CAM therapies such as special diets, psychotherapy, spiritual practices, and vitamin supplements. When psychotherapy and spiritual practices were excluded, 69 percent of patients had had at least one CAM therapy in their cancer treatment.

Cancer patients who are considering complementary or alternative therapy should discuss this decision with their doctor, because some complementary and alternative therapies may interfere with standard treatment or may be harmful when used with conventional approaches. It is also a good idea to become informed about the therapy, including whether the results of scientific studies support the claims that are made for it.

Unlike conventional treatments for cancer, complementary and alternative therapies are often not covered by insurance companies.

comprehensive cancer center A type of cancer institution sponsored by the NATIONAL CANCER INSTITUTE (NCI) that conducts programs in all areas of research—basic research, clinical research, and prevention and control research—as well as in community outreach and education.

In 1990, there were 19 comprehensive cancer centers across the United States; today more than 40 cancer centers meet the NCI criteria for comprehensive status.

Each type of CANCER CENTER has special characteristics and capabilities for organizing new programs of research. To be recognized by the NCI as a comprehensive cancer center, an institution must pass rigorous peer review and must perform research in three major areas: basic research; clinical research; and cancer prevention, control, and population-based research. It must also have a strong body of interactive research that bridges these research areas.

In addition, a comprehensive cancer center must provide outreach, education, and information directed toward and accessible to both health care professionals and the lay community.

All NCI-designated cancer centers are reevaluated each time their grant comes up for renewal (generally every three to five years). For contact information on individual comprehensive cancer centers, see Appendix II.

cone biopsy A diagnostic and treatment procedure used to remove a cone-shaped section of tissue containing abnormal cells from the cervix. It is also known as cervical conization or cold knife cone biopsy. A cone biopsy is performed if the results of a CERVICAL BIOPSY indicates a precancerous condition in the cervix. (The cervix is the small cylindrical organ at the lower part of the uterus, which separates the uterus from the vagina.) A cone biopsy also may be performed if there is an abnormal PAP TEST finding.

The Procedure

During the procedure, the patient lies on the table with her legs raised in stirrups, similar to the position when having a Pap test. The patient is given general anesthesia, and the vagina is held open with a speculum as the doctor uses a scalpel or laser to remove a cone-shaped piece of the cervix containing the area with abnormal cells. The resulting crater is repaired by stitching flaps of tissue over the wound. Alternatively, the wound may be left open, and heat or freezing be used to stop bleeding.

Once the tissue has been removed, it is examined under a microscope for signs of cancer. If cancer is present, other tests are required, and surgery is performed to remove the cervix and uterus (HYSTERECTOMY).

If the abnormal cells are precancerous, a laser can be used to destroy them. Cone biopsy with a "cold knife" or a LEEP are the standard treatments for removing abnormal cells in the cervix. Cold knife cone biopsy is generally used only for specific situations (for example, if a biopsy did not remove all the abnormal cells, the cold knife cone procedure allows the physician to remove what is left). This procedure provides a larger sample than can be obtained by a cervical punch biopsy.

After the test, the patient may feel some cramping or discomfort for about a week. Women should not have sex, use tampons, or douche until after a follow-up appointment a week or more after the procedure.

Risks

Because cone biopsies carry risks such as bleeding and problems with subsequent pregnancies, they have been replaced with newer technologies except in a few circumstances. There is a slight risk of bleeding and infection after surgery. Cervical scarring may result from the procedure, occasionally causing painful menstrual periods or making evaluation of an abnormal Pap smear result. Having multiple cone biopsies may cause problems with a later pregnancy or may make conception more difficult if it damages the cervix and disrupts normal mucus production. It can also cause an incompetent cervix, which may open prematurely during pregnancy.

conization   See CONE BIOPSY.

constipation   The passage of hard, infrequent, dry stools, which is usually painful. Constipation affects a large proportion of women who have cancer and are undergoing CHEMOTHERAPY. Narcotic pain medications can also lead to constipation, as can decreased fluid intake, poor diet, lack of exercise, and depression.

Treatment

Patients can drink warm or hot fluids to help loosen the bowels, eat high-fiber foods (such as whole wheat bread or fresh fruit), and get some exercise. Simply going for a walk can help, as can a more structured exercise program.

core biopsy   Removal (with a large needle) of a piece of tissue to be sent to the lab for microscopic analysis.
See also BIOPSY.

Corporate Angel Network   The only charitable organization in the United States whose sole mission is to ease the emotional stress, physical discomfort, and financial burden of travel for cancer patients by arranging free flights to treatment centers, using the empty seats on corporate aircraft flying on routine business.

Based in White Plains, New York, in an office donated by the Westchester County Airport, 50 part-time volunteers and five paid staff work with patients, physicians, corporations, flight departments, and leading treatment facilities to arrange approximately 1,200 flights a year. Eligibility to participate in the program is open to all cancer patients, bone marrow donors, and bone marrow recipients who can walk and who do not need medical support while traveling.

Eligibility is not based on financial need, and patients may travel as often as necessary. Because of the cooperation of 500 of America's top corporations, including more than half of the top 100 in the Fortune 500, Corporate Angel Network has coordinated more than 14,000 flights since its founding in 1981. For contact information, see Appendix I.

CP   A combination of the CHEMOTHERAPY drugs cyclophosphamide (CYTOXAN) and CISPLATIN (Platinol) sometimes used to treat OVARIAN CANCER.

cyclophosphamide See CYTOXAN.

cyst A fluid-filled sac found in the body that is often benign. Cysts have a distinct appearance in computed tomography (CT) scans and ultrasounds; identifying cysts accurately is important because treatment of cystic tumors differs from that of solid tumors.

cytokines A class of proteins produced by cells of the immune system that help to regulate the immune response. Cytokines can also be produced in the laboratory by recombinant DNA technology and administered to influence immune responses.

cytotoxic drugs Drugs that can cause the death of cancer cells. The term usually refers to drugs used in CHEMOTHERAPY treatments.

cytotoxic T cells White blood cells that can directly destroy specific cells. T cells can be separated from other blood cells, grown in the laboratory, and then administered to a patient to destroy tumor cells. Certain CYTOKINES can also be used to help form cytotoxic T cells in a patient's body.

Cytoxan (cyclophosphamide) An alkylating agent, used to treat several types of cancer including OVARIAN CANCER, that works by disrupting the growth of cancer cells.

Side Effects
Side effects include nausea and vomiting, HAIR LOSS, appetite loss, mouth or lip sores, DIARRHEA, decreased sperm production, and decreased white blood cell count. Less common side effects include presence of blood in the urine, acne, FATIGUE, and decreased platelet count. Rarely, heart problems may occur at high dosages.

dactinomycin (Cosmegen) A type of CHEMO-THERAPY drug sometimes used to treat GESTATIONAL TROPHOBLASTIC DISEASE. Given by intravenous injection, the drug may cause side effects such as nausea and vomiting and HAIR LOSS. Less common side effects include BONE MARROW depression, mouth sores, acne, DIARRHEA, fever, FATIGUE, APPETITE LOSS, or skin rash.

danazol A commonly prescribed synthetic version of the male HORMONE androgen used to treat endometriosis that may raise the risk of OVARIAN CANCER, according to preliminary findings presented by the University of Pittsburgh Graduate School of Public Health.

Previous studies have found that women who have endometriosis are already at a 50 percent increased risk for ovarian cancer, and treating them with danazol appears to increase the risk further. This new result, even though it is preliminary, may factor into the equation when clinicians and their patients who have endometriosis are deciding on the best treatment.

Although the number of women studied was small, researchers believed that the results warrant further studies on a larger scale. Additional research studies are planned at the University of Pittsburgh to investigate further the link between androgens and ovarian cancer.

D&C The abbreviation for *dilation and curettage,* a procedure used to dilate the cervix and scrape out the lining and contents of the uterus. Doctors may perform a D&C to diagnose or treat the cause of abnormal bleeding (such as in early uterine or CERVICAL CANCER). This fairly minor surgical procedure may be performed in the hospital or clinic with general or local anesthesia. Rarely, a woman may need an emergency D&C that is performed if she experiences heavy bleeding that cannot be stopped with tablet treatment. However, a D&C is usually used to make a diagnosis and is not used in treating bleeding problems.

The Procedure
The cervical canal is widened (dilated) by using a metal rod; the doctor then inserts a curette (a metal loop on the end of a long thin handle) into the uterus and scrapes away the inner layer of the uterus. Tissue is usually collected for examination.

Risks
A D&C has relatively few risks. It can ease bleeding and can be used to diagnose problems such as infection, cancer, infertility, and other disease. There is a slight risk of damage to the inner lining of the uterus, inability of a dilated cervix to return to normal size, puncture of the uterus, laceration of the cervix, or scarring.

After Surgery
It is normal to experience irregular bleeding in the days after the D&C, as well as pelvic cramps and back pain for a few days. Pain can usually be managed well with medication. Tampon use is not recommended for a few weeks and sexual intercourse is not recommended for a few days. The woman should contact her doctor if heavy bleeding with large clots, severe lower abdominal pain, bleeding, or high fever occurs. The patient may resume normal activities the same day.

Decadron (dexamethasone) An antinausea medication that is also a strong anti-inflammatory agent, used in combination with other medications to prevent nausea and vomiting after CHEMOTHER-APY treatments.

Side Effects

Side effects include depression, weight gain, increased appetite, sleep problems, skin bruising, mood changes, delayed wound healing, increased risk of infection, increased blood sugar level, and sodium or fluid retention. Less common side effects include bone fractures, sweating, DIARRHEA, nausea, headache, increased heart rate, fungal infections, and decrease in potassium levels. Rarely, the drug may cause cataracts, personality changes, blurring of vision, or stomach ulcer.

DES See DIETHYLSTILBESTROL.

dexamethasone See DECADRON.

diarrhea Passage of loose or watery stools at least three times a day that may or may not be painful. Often, it is accompanied by gas, bloating, and cramps. Diarrhea occurs in about 75 percent of CHEMOTHERAPY patients because the drugs damage the rapidly dividing cells in the gastrointestinal tract. The severity of diarrhea depends on the type and dosage of chemotherapy. Some drugs that cause diarrhea are 5-FLUOROURACIL, methotrexate, docetaxel, and actinomycin D. Diarrhea can be life threatening if it triggers dehydration, malnutrition, and electrolyte imbalances.

diet Some evidence suggests a link between diet and some types of cancer. For example, studies have shown that diets rich in vitamins and antioxidants and low in fat can be protective against cancer. Increased levels of vitamin C also appear to reduce the risk of cervical cancer. Weight control can help reduce the risk of endometrial and uterine cancers.

Several substances, including LYCOPENES (found in high levels in some fruits and vegetables, such as tomatoes, grapefruit, and watermelon), vitamin E, and the mineral selenium may also lower cancer risk. Current studies are assessing whether or not these substances actually reduce risk.

Dietary fat Some studies suggest that a diet high in animal fat (saturated fat) may increase the risk of cancer, and that a diet high in fruits and vegetables may decrease the risk.

Foods that are low in fat are usually lower in calories than high-fat foods as well. There are three types of dietary fats—saturated, monounsaturated, and polyunsaturated fats:

- *Saturated fats* are almost exclusively produced from animal products such as meat, milk, and cheese; they have been linked to an increased risk of cancer.
- *Monounsaturated fats* are found in olive oil and canola oil.
- *Polyunsaturated fats* are found in vegetable oils.

Although the latter two types of fat are less closely linked to disease, since overall fat intake is associated with cancer, limiting intake of all three kinds is a good idea. Dietitians generally recommend that tub margarine is a better choice than butter, since butter is rich in both saturated fat and cholesterol, and the hazards of saturated fats are better documented and appear to be more severe than those of the hydrogenated fats in margarine. (Most margarine is made from vegetable fat and has no cholesterol.)

The usual recommendation is that people get no more than 10 percent of daily calories from saturated fats, and that total fat intake not exceed 30 percent of the day's calories.

Dietary fat consumption can be reduced by limiting the intake of red meat, choosing low-fat or no-fat varieties of milk and cheese, removing the skin from chicken and turkey, choosing pretzels instead of potato chips, and decreasing or eliminating fried foods, butter, and margarine. Cooking with small amounts of olive oil instead of butter significantly cuts saturated-fat intake. Choosing soy foods is also a good idea. Soy foods are high in ISOFLAVONES, which block some hormonal activity in cells. Diets high in SOY PRODUCTS have been associated with lower rates of cancers.

Antioxidants ANTIOXIDANT substances seek out and destroy naturally occurring toxic molecules called FREE RADICALS. These molecules can cause extensive damage to the body's cells, which may then lead to cancer development. Antioxidants reduce the number of free radicals, prevent tissue damage, and, quite possibly, prevent cancer. The antioxidants that have generated the most interest and research to date are vitamin C, vitamin E, BETA-CAROTENE, and selenium.

Good sources of vitamin C include citrus fruits, kiwi, cantaloupe, strawberries, peppers, tomatoes, potatoes, mangos, and cruciferous vegetables. Vitamin E can be found in green leafy vegetables, wheat germ, whole grain products, nuts, seeds, and vegetable oil. Beta-carotene often (but not always) is identified by its yellow, orange, or deep green color; it occurs in carrots, cantaloupe, sweet potatoes, apricots, broccoli, spinach, and other green leafy vegetables. Selenium is found in seafood, meat, and grains.

Phytochemicals These plant chemicals contribute to the color and flavor of vegetables and when eaten may suppress cancer development. Phytochemicals that may help prevent cancer include the following:

- The antioxidant beta-carotene
- Lutein in spinach, kale, and other green leafy vegetables
- Limonen and phenols in citrus fruits
- Allyl sulfides in garlic and onions
- Sulforaphane
- Indoles
- Isothiocyanates in broccoli, cauliflower, and other cruciferous vegetables

Pesticides

Health experts recommend eating a variety of fruits and vegetables for a healthy diet. Most believe that eating the small amount of synthetic pesticides in produce is not harmful; eating a wide variety of foods can prevent consuming too much of any one additive.

Preparation

Whenever possible, consumers should choose foods that are in a form as close to their natural state as possible—for example, by eating whole wheat bread rather than refined flour breads, fresh fruits and vegetables instead of canned, whole grain cereals instead of cereals that are heavily sugared. Refined products, such as white

rice and white bread, have often had most of the nutritious part of the grain removed during processing. These products may then be enriched; that is, they have certain vitamins and minerals added to them during processing. Although "enriched" foods sound good, many valuable nutrients (such as fiber) removed during the refining process are never readded. In addition, many refined products add other undesirable ingredients, such as salt or fats.

diethylstilbestrol (DES) A hormone similar to ESTROGEN that was given to pregnant women during the 1950s to prevent miscarriage. If a woman's mother took DES during pregnancy, the woman has a greater chance of development of cervical or VAGINAL CANCER as an adult.

differentiation The stage of maturity of cells. Differentiated tumor cells resemble normal cells and tend to grow and spread at a slower rate than undifferentiated or poorly differentiated tumor cells, which lack the structure and function of normal cells and grow uncontrollably.

dilation and curettage See D&C.

diploid Characteristic of tumor cells having a normal amount of DNA. Cells that have an unusual amount of DNA are called ANEUPLOID. Most cancerous cells have an abnormal amount of DNA (either too much or too little). In general, the more DNA a cancer cell has, the more aggressive the cancer.

DMC A combination of the CHEMOTHERAPY drugs DACTINOMYCIN (Cosmegen), methotrexate, and cyclophosphamide (CYTOXAN) sometimes used to treat GESTATIONAL TROPHOBLASTIC DISEASE.

do not resuscitate order (DNR order) A legal directive by a physician that instructs hospital staff not to try to help a patient whose heart has stopped or who has stopped breathing. A patient can request a DNR order either by filling out an ADVANCE DIRECTIVE form or by telling the doctor that cardiopulmonary resuscitation should not be performed. DNR orders are accepted by doctors and hospitals in all states.

doxorubicin   See ADRIAMYCIN.

dysgerminoma   The most common type of GERM CELL TUMOR, accounting for half of all germ cell tumor cases. About 20 percent of cases are diagnosed during pregnancy; 80 percent occur in women younger than age 30. Between 3 percent and 5 percent of all malignant OVARIAN CANCER tumors are dysgerminomas. Typically, a dysgerminoma is a solid, firm, or fleshy tumor composed of malignant germ cells. It is highly sensitive to RADIATION THERAPY and CHEMOTHERAPY.

dysplasia   Disordered growth of cells. Slow, progressive changes in normal cells may develop over several years. Experts believe that cervical dysplasia, a precancerous condition marked by abnormal cell development on the surface of the cervix, is the first step in the slow progression of abnormal cellular changes leading to CARCINOMA IN SITU, the earliest stage of CERVICAL CANCER (cancer localized to the superficial layer of the cervix). Mild dysplasia is designated *CIN I; CIN II* indicates moderate to marked dysplasia, and *CIN III* includes everything from severe dysplasia to carcinoma in situ.

Risk Factors

Cervical dysplasia may occur at anytime after age 15, with the peak incidence between ages 25 and 35. However, less than 5 percent of all PAP TESTS conducted note cervical dysplasia. Increased risk is associated with the following:

- Multiple sexual partners
- Early onset of sexual activity (before age 18)
- Early childbearing (before age 16)

- Past medical history of DIETHYLSTILBESTROL (DES) exposure or sexually transmitted diseases, especially HUMAN PAPILLOMAVIRUS (genital warts), genital herpes, or human immunodeficiency virus (HIV) infection

Symptoms

There are usually no symptoms of these early cervical changes.

Diagnosis

A pelvic exam cannot usually reveal dysplasia. A Pap smear can reveal mild, moderate, marked, or severe dysplasia. A COLPOSCOPY reveals white areas or a mosaic pattern on the cervical surface; both are caused by changes in the surface capillaries. A colposcopy-directed biopsy can confirm dysplasia and the extent to which the cervix is involved. If dysplasia is found, an endocervical curettage should be performed to rule out spread to the cervical canal. A CONE BIOPSY may be necessary to rule out invasive cancer.

Treatment

The treatment depends on how advanced the dysplasia is, and may range from careful observation with repeat Pap smears every three to six months (for mild dysplasia, which may disappear spontaneously) to removal of abnormal tissue by either electrocauterization, cryosurgery, laser vaporization, or surgery. In any case, consistent follow-up is essential.

Thirty percent to 50 percent of women who have dysplasia ultimately have cancer if the condition is untreated; this percentage is high enough that experts usually advocate treating dysplasia as a precancerous condition. If dysplasia is diagnosed, a doctor performs a biopsy to identify malignant cells. With early identification, adequate evaluation treatment and consistent follow-up nearly all cervical dysplasia can be cured.

embryonal carcinoma An uncommon type of OVARIAN GERM CELL TUMOR that occurs in children and young adults, usually together with a YOLK SAC TUMOR. Typically, an embryonal carcinoma is a solid tumor characterized by bleeding and tissue death. This highly malignant type of tumor is resistant to RADIATION THERAPY but responds to combination CHEMOTHERAPY.

endocervical curettage The removal of tissue from the inside of the cervix by a spoon-shaped instrument called a curette.

endodermal sinus tumors See GERM CELL TUMOR; YOLK SAC TUMOR.

end-of-life care A general term referring to the medical and psychological care given in the terminal stages of cancer. ADVANCE DIRECTIVES, including a living will, durable power of attorney, and HEALTH-CARE PROXY, allow people to express their decisions about end-of-life care ahead of time. Advance directives provide a way for patients to let family, friends, and health-care professionals know what their wishes are, to prevent later confusion should they become unable to communicate.

endometrial cancer The most common type of cancer of the female reproductive system. It begins in the lining of the uterus (the endometrium). (Another type of cancer that affects the uterus is called UTERINE SARCOMA, a rare condition that forms in uterine muscle instead of the lining.)

Endometrial cancer is usually curable when detected early; 92 percent of women survive this type of cancer when it is detected in its early stages, and 64 percent of women survive endometrial cancer even when it has spread to other parts of the body. The five-year survival rate of women who have endometrial cancer is 73 percent for all women. It is the fourth most common cancer in women, after lung, breast, and colon cancer; more than 40,000 women are diagnosed with endometrial cancer in the United States each year. Most women who have endometrial cancer are between the ages of 55 and 70.

Different women experience endometrial cancer in different ways; even patients who have the same type of cancer in the same stage who have the same treatment may have different results. For unknown reasons, this type of cancer may be eradicated in some women and may return or spread in others.

If endometrial cancer does spread, it tends to spread first to pelvic organs and lymph nodes nearest the uterus. From there, it may move to the cervix, vagina, ovaries, lungs, or bones.

The endometrium may also be affected by a precancerous condition called ENDOMETRIAL HYPERPLASIA. This overgrowth of cells in the endometrial lining may become malignant if untreated. Women who have endometrial hyperplasia may also experience unusual vaginal bleeding.

Benign Endometrial Conditions
There are conditions that affect the uterine lining that are not malignant but can cause symptoms similar to those of endometrial cancer. One of these conditions is endometrial polyps, which can cause bleeding.

Fibroids are another benign condition that may affect the endometrium. Also called leiomyomas, these common benign tumors sometimes form in the endometrial muscle. Women who have FIBROID TUMORS may experience unusual bleeding from the vagina and a frequent urge to urinate. Fibroid tumors usually require no specific treatment.

Risk Factors

A number of risk factors create higher likelihood of development of endometrial cancer. Being aware of the factors that raise the risk for endometrial cancer is important, because many can be controlled or modified. For example, a woman may slightly lower her risk by exercising regularly, eating a healthy DIET, and keeping blood sugar and blood pressure under control. Factors that cannot be controlled, such as a woman's age or race, should be called to the attention of a doctor.

Age   Most women who develop endometrial cancer are older than age 50; a woman is at higher risk if she is postmenopausal and older than 50.

Endometrial hyperplasia   This condition is indicated by an increase in the number of normal cells lining the uterus and is linked to a higher risk of endometrial cancer.

Estrogen levels   Since the incidence of endometrial cancer may be related to hormonal changes, any condition that raises HORMONE (ESTROGEN) levels may increase risk. Estrogen replacement therapy, some ovarian tumors, obesity, bearing of few or no children, and late menopause are all associated with elevated hormone levels.

Because women who use ESTROGEN REPLACEMENT THERAPY without additional progesterone have a higher chance of endometrial cancer, women who have an intact uterus who needed estrogen replacement therapy in the past used a combination of estrogen and progesterone. This combination protects the uterus but increases the risk of breast cancer and heart disease. It is no longer recommended for most women.

Overweight women are diagnosed with endometrial cancer twice as often as do women who are not overweight. Most young women who have this type of cancer are obese; however, it is unusual to develop endometrial cancer before the age of 45.

Women who have never been pregnant also have a higher chance of developing endometrial cancer, perhaps because high levels of progestins are produced during pregnancy.

If a woman does not ovulate regularly during her reproductive years, this condition can upset the delicate balance between estrogenic hormones that encourage the development of cancer and the progestigenic hormones that protect against cancer.

Other cancers   Women who have had colon, rectal, or breast cancer have a higher probability of developing endometrial cancer.

Race   Caucasian women have a higher probability of developing endometrial cancer than do non-Caucasian women. For reasons that are not entirely clear, this type of cancer is approximately twice as common in Caucasians as it is in African Americans and other non-Caucasians.

Tamoxifen   This drug, often prescribed for women with breast cancer, has been linked to a higher risk of developing endometrial cancer in women who have taken it for five or more years. Although several studies have shown that tamoxifen can significantly increase a woman's risk of endometrial cancer, experts believe its ability to lower the incidence of breast cancer deaths outweighs the increased risk of endometrial cancer. A woman who has been receiving tamoxifen does not need routine X-rays or biopsies, but she should be examined by her gynecologist at least once a year, (or immediately if irregular uterine bleeding occurs).

High blood pressure   High blood pressure has been weakly associated with endometrial cancer.

Diabetes   Women who have diabetes have twice the risk of endometrial cancer of women who do not have diabetes. However, many women who have diabetes are overweight, and experts are not sure how much of the increased risk in women with diabetes is due to the diabetic condition and how much is due to overweight.

Hereditary nonpolyposis colorectal cancer (HNPCC or Lynch syndrome II)   This is the most common type of hereditary endometrial cancer syndrome, in which multiple family members have cancers that begin in the colon, uterus, small intestine, kidney system, or ovaries.

Symptoms

Possible signs of endometrial cancer include unusual vaginal discharge, blood, or pain in the pelvis. Because symptoms of endometrial cancer can also be caused by less serious problems, a woman should discuss them with her doctor.

When endometrial cancer develops, it is almost always linked with unexpected vaginal bleeding, and often in a postmenopausal woman. The vaginal bleeding may appear watery at first, with a small amount of blood; eventually, the bleeding may appear less watery and more bloody. Other symptoms include pain during urination, pain during sex, and pelvic pain.

Diagnosis

Currently, there are no screening tests for endometrial cancer that are recommended for routine health care other than yearly pelvic exams by a gynecologist or other primary care doctor.

To determine the cause of any symptoms, a doctor performs a careful physical exam to check for any lumps or changes in the shape of the uterus, feeling the vagina, uterus, ovaries, bladder, and rectum. The doctor may also perform one or more of the following tests.

Pap test A PAP TEST is performed during a pelvic exam. Using a wooden spatula or small brush, the doctor takes a sample of cells from the cervix and upper vagina and examines them for abnormalities. However, the Pap test is used primarily to detect CERVICAL CANCER; because cancer of the endometrium begins inside the uterus, it does not usually show up in a Pap test. The Pap test will not find most endometrial cancers. For this reason, the doctor may also perform an endometrial biopsy or D&C or similar test to remove pieces of the lining of the uterus.

Endometrial biopsy The only way to be sure of a diagnosis of endometrial cancer is to perform an endometrial biopsy. During the procedure, a doctor removes some tissue from the inner endometrial lining by inserting a thin plastic tube through the vagina and cervix, into the uterus, which usually causes a brief period of endometrial cramping. The tissue specimen is then examined under a microscope by a pathologist; a formal report is given to the doctor and patient within several days.

Although most endometrial cancers occur in postmenopausal women, some cases develop in younger women. In these premenopausal women, an endometrial BIOPSY should be ordered if menstrual periods are very heavy or irregular. Irregular bleeding may be due to lack of regular ovulation,

but it also can be caused by the development of cancerous or precancerous uterine changes.

Dilation and curettage If the cervical canal is very narrow or a sample of tissue cannot be obtained by an endometrial biopsy, the doctor may need to perform a D&C of the endometrial cavity. This procedure is usually performed in an operating room with the patient under general anesthesia. During a D&C, the opening of the cervix is stretched with a spoon-shaped instrument and the walls of the uterus are gently scraped to remove any growths. This tissue is then checked for cancer cells. Afterward, the woman may experience mild cramps and vaginal bleeding for a few days. In order to check for tumors, a lighted scope may be inserted into the endometrial cavity during the D&C (a procedure called hysteroscopy).

Staging

When a woman is diagnosed with endometrial cancer, her doctor needs to know the stage of the cancer. Staging is based on the size of the tumor, the number of lymph nodes involved, and spreading of cancer to other organs. The most common staging system for endometrial cancer is a system developed by the INTERNATIONAL FEDERATION OF GYNECOLOGY AND OBSTETRICS in which numerals from 0 (the earliest stage) to IV (the most advanced stage) represent the stages of the cancer.

Stage 0: Endometrial hyperplasia (abnormal cell growth)
Stage I: The cancer is only in the body of the uterus.
Stage IA: The cancer is only in the endometrium (uterine lining).
Stage IB: The cancer has spread less than halfway through the myometrium (uterine muscle).
Stage IC: The cancer has spread halfway through the myometrium.
Stage II: The cancer has spread from the uterus to the cervix.
Stage IIA: The cancer is in the body of the uterus and the endocervical glands.
Stage IIB: The cancer is in the body of the uterus and the cervical stroma.
Stage III: The cancer has spread outside the body of the uterus but has not left the pelvic area.

Stage IIIA: The cancer has spread to the serosa of the uterus, or the adnexa, or there are cancer cells in peritoneal fluid.

Stage IIIB: The cancer has spread to the vagina.

Stage IIIC: The cancer has spread to the lymph nodes near the uterus.

Stage IV: The cancer has spread to the mucosa of the bladder or the rectum, the lymph nodes in the groin, or other organs such as the lungs or the bones.

Stage IVA: The cancer has spread to the mucosa or inner lining of the rectum or bladder.

Stage IVB: The cancer has spread to the lymph nodes in the groin area and/or other organs such as the lungs or bones.

Treatment

The treatment choices for each woman depend on the size and location of the tumor, the results of lab tests, and the stage or extent of the disease. A doctor also considers the woman's age and general health when deciding on a treatment plan.

Women whose endometrial cancer recurs may be treated with chemotherapy or hormonal therapy, as well as radiation therapy. These treatments are frequently used to relieve pain, nausea, and abnormal bowel function.

Surgery Surgery is the most common treatment for cancer of the endometrium. After the diagnosis of a cancer, surgery should be performed relatively soon. Several different types of surgery can be performed to treat endometrial cancer: *simple abdominal* HYSTERECTOMY, *vaginal hysterectomy,* or *radical hysterectomy,* with *bilateral* SALPINGO-OOPHORECTOMY.

In a simple hysterectomy, the uterus (including the cervix) is removed during a one- to three-hour operation, typically followed by a three- or four-day hospital stay. An abdominal hysterectomy is performed through an abdominal incision. In a vaginal hysterectomy, the uterus is removed through the vagina. Samples of LYMPH NODES in the area are usually taken during surgery to determine whether they include cancerous cells. (The lymph nodes are small, bean-shaped structures found throughout the body that produce and store infection-fighting cells but may also contain cancer cells.)

A radical hysterectomy is performed when the cancer has spread to the cervix or the tissues next to the uterus; this operation is uncommonly used for endometrial cancer. In this surgery the entire uterus is removed along with the tissues beside the uterus and the upper part of the vagina beside the cervix. A radical hysterectomy is performed through an abdominal incision. Women who have a radical hysterectomy also have a sample of nearby lymph nodes taken at the same time.

More recently, some gynecologic oncologists have been performing endometrial cancer surgery laparoscopically. The advantage of this approach is that smaller incisions are used and the hospitalization and recovery period is shorter.

In a bilateral salpingo-oophorectomy, both fallopian tubes and the ovaries are removed. In nearly all cases of endometrial cancer, the fallopian tubes and ovaries are removed. It is important to remove the ovaries during surgery because they are an area where endometrial cancer may spread. Lymph nodes from the pelvic and lower aortic areas are often removed to look for spread of the cancer, since this is the most common route of spread.

After hysterectomy, additional treatment with radiation therapy and/or chemotherapy is required in some cases in which spread of disease outside the uterus has been found or is suspected.

Radiation therapy The goal of radiation therapy is to kill cancer cells by using X-rays. This treatment can shrink a tumor before surgery, treat a tumor without the need for surgery, or get rid of any remaining cancer cells after surgery. Radiation therapy can also be used if the cancer has spread to distant organs, such as the brain or bones, to reduce pain or other symptoms.

External radiation may be directed at the body by a machine or may originate from a very small container of radioactive material placed directly into or near the tumor (called internal radiation or brachytherapy). Some patients receive both kinds of radiation therapy.

If a patient is having external beam radiation therapy of the pelvic area for endometrial cancer, treatment is given in an outpatient department of a hospital or clinic five days a week for four to six weeks. At the end of treatment, an extra boost of radiation is sometimes directed at a smaller area where the tumor first developed.

The radiation oncologist may also choose to use internal radiation therapy administered at the doctor's office over the course of several weeks. In most cases, the internal radiation is placed either after the external radiation or when the vagina has healed after the surgery. In these situations the implant is placed against the skin at the top of the vagina. If the radiation oncologist chooses to use standard-dose delivery (low- or high-dose-rate brachytherapy), the implant is placed at the hospital. This implant is temporary, and when it is removed, no radioactivity is left in the body.

Chemotherapy Anticancer drugs are used when the cancer can no longer be treated with local treatments alone. Chemotherapy can also be administered after surgery for patients who have a high risk for distant spread. The goal of chemotherapy in this setting is to kill any cells that may have spread before the tumor was surgically removed.

Chemotherapy is given in cycles. A woman who has endometrial cancer will have chemotherapy treatment for a certain length of time and then have a rest period; then treatment will begin again. Common endometrial cancer chemotherapy drugs include CISPLATIN (Platinol or carboplatin), doxorbicin (ADRIAMYCIN), and paclitaxel (Taxol). Potential side effects depend on the kind of drug the patient is taking. Common side effects of chemotherapy include nausea and vomiting, hair loss, CONSTIPATION or DIARRHEA, and FATIGUE. Other serious side effects that may occur as a consequence of a decrease in blood cell counts include infection and bleeding.

Hormonal therapy In this treatment method, drugs are used to prevent malignant cells from the hormones they need to grow. Response to hormone therapy can be predicted by factors such as tumor grade, presence of progesterone receptors, and (if the cancer has recurred) interval from the first treatment to recurrence.

Hormonal therapy may be used as a treatment if surgery is not possible. It can help the uterus shed the endometrial lining along with precancerous changes. Sometimes, hormonal therapy may shrink or completely kill endometrial cancer.

Hormonal therapy is usually given by injection or in the form of a PROGESTIN tablet that is taken daily for a specific period. Several progestin drugs and regimens have been studied for the treatment of advanced or recurrent endometrial cancer. Research suggests that the response rate of endometrial adenocarcinomas to progestin therapy ranges from 10 percent to 50 percent. Well- and moderately differentiated tumors respond more often to progesterone therapy than do poorly differentiated carcinomas.

Endometrial cancers are known to be dependent on estrogen for growth; women who have high levels of estrogen are at risk for the development of endometrial cancer. Estrogen is produced in the ovaries and by converting other hormones into estrogen in the body. In postmenopausal women, the conversion of testosterone into estrogen in fat tissue by the aromatase enzyme is an important source of estrogen; experts believe that inhibiting this conversion may be an effective manner of treating endometrial cancers.

Several such agents that competitively inhibit or inactivate the enzymes needed for the conversion of testosterone to estrogen have been developed. Estrogen antagonist aromatase inhibitors (such as TAMOXIFEN) are being evaluated in endometrial cancer. Tamoxifen inhibits the growth of estrogen-receptor-positive breast cancers, and when used by patients with recurrent or advanced endometrial cancer, can result in occasional durable responses and a significant incidence of disease stabilization. The objective response rate to tamoxifen in several studies is between 20 percent and 60 percent, with occasional long-term survivors. Although tamoxifen may be of some benefit to the occasional patient who has advanced or recurrent endometrial cancer, patients who have not been cured by initial hormonal therapy with progestin are unlikely to respond to estrogen antagonists.

After Treatment

Many women who have endometrial cancer feel tired for a period after treatment is finished. Such fatigue can interfere with daily life. It is important for the doctor to check a woman's red blood count, since anemia may be the cause of the lack of energy of some patients. In some cases, a blood transfusion may be necessary, or medications that increase red blood cell count may be prescribed. Some people do not want to eat or exercise when they are tired. However, having an unhealthy diet and little exercise can make the situation worse.

Prevention

There are certain changes a woman can make in her lifestyle to lessen her risk of endometrial cancer. These include the following.

Diet Studies have shown that eating foods that contain less fat may help prevent endometrial cancer. Consuming a plant-based diet low in fat, high in fiber, and rich in whole grains, vegetables, fruit, and legumes (especially soy beans) may reduce the risk of endometrial cancer, according to recent studies. This type of diet may partly explain the lower rates of uterine cancer in Asian countries compared with those in the United States. As with breast and ovarian cancers, rates for endometrial cancer are lower in Japan, China, and other Asian countries than they are in the United States and Europe. Consumption of less fiber and SOY PROD-UCTS and more fat may explain the increase in uterine cancer found among Asians who have immigrated to the West.

In recent years, researchers have focused on possible dietary factors that may influence these differences—especially the possibility that dietary fat increases the risk of endometrial cancer. In one study, energy intake from fat but not from other sources was positively associated with endometrial cancer. Among women who consumed the most dietary fat, the risk was 1.6 times greater than that of those who consumed the least fat. However, women who consumed the most fiber from cereals, vegetables, and fruit had a 29 percent to 46 percent reduction in cancer risk compared to that of those who ate the least amount of fiber.

In addition, several groups of PHYTOESTROGEN-rich foods (such as legumes, tofu, and other soy products) were linked to a lower risk of endometrial cancer. Phytoestrogens are plant compounds that have effects similar to those of the hormone estrogen. Women who ate the highest amount of foods rich in these compounds had a 54 percent reduction in cancer risk, compared with those who consumed the least. Phytoestrogens compete with estrogen for cell-receptor binding sites. In doing so,

they help control the level of estrogen circulating in the blood. Phytoestrogens' "antiestrogen effect" may block the development of endometrial cancer by reducing hormonal activities that cause endometrial cells to proliferate uncontrollably.

In one study, women who had never been pregnant and who ate less than nine grams of soy products a day were at 4.52 times the estimated risk of endometrial cancer.

Other preventive factors include:

- *Pregnancy.* Childbirth may lower a woman's chance of having endometrial cancer.
- *Body weight.* For women who are obese, significant weight loss can significantly lower risk of endometrial cancer.
- *Birth control pills.* Taking birth control pills with estrogens and/or progestins during childbearing years can lower a woman's risk of both endometrial and ovarian cancer.
- *Estrogen replacement therapy.* Taking estrogen later in life, after the childbearing years, can significantly lower a woman's risk of having endometrial cancer. However, it causes a higher risk of breast cancer and heart disease and is no longer recommended for most women.

endometrial hyperplasia An increase in the number of cells in the lining of the uterus. Although this increase in cells is not a malignant condition, it may sometimes result in cancer. Heavy menstrual periods, bleeding between periods, and bleeding after menopause are common symptoms of hyperplasia. The disease is most common after age 40.

Unless the lining of the uterus sheds regularly, tissues and glands will build up and may later become a breeding ground for abnormal cells. Any woman of childbearing age who has missed more than two consecutive periods but is not pregnant needs to investigate the reason.

During adolescence and in the years before menopause, women may have many cycles without ovulation during which there is continuous unopposed ESTROGEN activity. Polycystic ovary syndrome is another condition in which women do not ovulate and have unopposed estrogen. Similarly, HORMONE REPLACEMENT THERAPY with estrogen without progesterone may lead to endometrial hyperplasia.

To prevent endometrial hyperplasia from developing into cancer, a woman's doctor may recommend surgery to remove the uterus (HYSTERECTOMY) or treatment with progesterone and regular follow-up exams.

Types

Some cases of hyperplasia are more advanced than others. *Mild hyperplasia,* known as *cystic glandular hyperplasia* or *cystic endometrial hyperplasia,* is characterized by an excess of tissue with normal endometrial cells. This kind of hyperplasia is always caused by too much estrogen and rarely develops into cancer.

When mild hyperplasia is not treated, it may lead to *adenomatous hyperplasia without atypical cells.* This benign condition refers to a buildup of glandular cells (the glandular endometrial cells are growing but are still noncancerous). This kind of hyperplasia rarely develops into cancer.

Atypical adenomatous hyperplasia (also called *severe hyperplasia* or *carcinoma in situ—CIS*) means that either a small area on the endometrium or the entire lining consists of cells that are abnormal. The cells seem to be more aggressive but may still be harmless. It still is not malignant, but more women with severe hyperplasia may go on to develop uterine cancer.

Risk Factors

Women who are 25 to 50 pounds overweight are three times as likely to develop hyperplasia; women who are more than 50 pounds overweight are nine times as likely to develop hyperplasia. Women at higher risk also include those who have always had irregular periods or who have diabetes. Other potential causes of excess estrogen include environmental toxins; certain herbs (such as ginseng); hormone-fed meats and poultry; certain cosmetics made from estrogen; and hormonal contraceptives that contain estrogen.

Diagnosis

This diagnosis can only be made by the pathologist who examines a sample of tissue removed from the thickened endometrium by a sampling procedure such as an endometrial biopsy or a D&C.

Treatment

In younger women particularly, severe hyperplasia can be reversed with HORMONAL THERAPY. Adding progesterone by taking a PROGESTIN or resuming ovulation (spontaneously or with medications) can eliminate hyperplasia. If this does not work, a D&C is the next logical step. A HYSTERECTOMY is not necessary unless the hyperplasia persists after the lining is removed. If severe hyperplasia persists and keeps redeveloping despite HRT and a repeat D&C, then a hysterectomy may be required.

endometrium The lining of the uterus.

See also ENDOMETRIAL CANCER; ENDOMETRIAL HYPERPLASIA; UTERINE CANCER; UTERINE SARCOMA.

endostatin A drug known as an ANGIOGENESIS INHIBITOR that was heralded in 1998 for its ability in animal research to starve a malignant tumor by drying up its source of blood. Angiogenesis inhibitors are drugs that kill cancer cells by interfering with their blood supply. Human tests of endostatin were launched in 1999 at the M. D. Anderson Cancer Center, the University of Wisconsin, and the Dana-Farber Cancer Center.

Endostatin can decrease blood flow to some tumors in patients and promote death in cancer and blood vessel cells. Researchers concluded the drug, even at different dosages, was both safe for and well tolerated by the 25 patients who received it. Patients used the drug for a median period of 69 days. In two patients, there was evidence of minor antitumor activity—several tumors were observed to shrink—but no long-term responses were seen.

environmental hormones Chemicals found in the environment that may mimic natural HORMONES. Natural hormones are chemicals that are produced by endocrine glands and travel through the bloodstream, helping to guide development, growth, reproduction, and behavior. Endocrine glands include the pituitary, thyroid, and adrenal glands.

Chemicals that interfere with the normal functioning of this complex system are known as endocrine disruptors. Disruption of the endocrine system can occur in various ways. For example, some chemicals may mimic a natural hormone, fooling the body into overresponding as though to an excess of the hormone. Other chemicals may block the effects of a hormone in parts of the body normally sensitive to it. Still others may directly stimulate or inhibit the endocrine system, leading to reproduction or underproduction of hormones. Some types of ENDOMETRIAL CANCER are exacerbated by overproduction of the hormone ESTROGEN.

epithelial ovarian carcinoma   Cancerous epithelial tumors that begin in the ovaries; about 85 percent of OVARIAN CANCERS are epithelial ovarian carcinomas.

Most epithelial ovarian tumors are benign and therefore do not spread, nor do they usually lead to serious illness. There are several types of benign epithelial tumors, including serous adenomas, mucinous adenomas, and Brenner tumors.

When viewed under the microscope, some ovarian epithelial tumors do not appear to be cancerous—these are called TUMORS OF LOW MALIGNANT POTENTIAL, or borderline tumors.

Epithelial ovarian carcinoma cells have several features that can be recognized under the microscope and are used to classify epithelial ovarian carcinomas into serous, mucinous, endometrioid, and clear cell types. Undifferentiated epithelial ovarian carcinomas do not resemble any of these four subtypes, and they tend to grow and spread more quickly.

In addition to their classification by cell type, epithelial ovarian carcinomas are also given a grade and a stage. The grade is on a scale of 1 to 3: grade 1 epithelial ovarian carcinomas more closely resemble normal tissue and tend to have a better prognosis; grade 3 carcinomas less closely resemble normal tissue and usually have a poorer outlook.

The tumor stage describes how far the tumor has spread from the site where it started in the ovary.

erythropoietin (Epogen, Aranesp, Procrit)   Produced in the adult kidney, this substance triggers the production of red blood cells and can reverse anemia in cancer patients who are receiving CHEMOTHERAPY.

esophagitis   Inflammation of the esophagus. It can be a direct result of taking CHEMOTHERAPY drugs for cancer and in such cases, generally develops between 5 and 14 days after chemotherapy. Esophagitis can lead to bleeding, painful ulcers, and infection. However, sores in the esophagus are usually temporary and heal completely once chemotherapy is finished.

Symptoms
Symptoms include chest pain or a burning feeling in the throat that can be heavy or sharp. Pain from esophagitis may be constant or intermittent. Problems include worsening of existing chest pain when swallowing or a feeling of food sticking in the chest after swallowing. Less often, blood may appear in a patient's vomit or stools.

Prognosis
In most cases symptoms begin to improve within a week or two after the chemotherapy treatment, symptoms may not end completely for weeks.

estrogen   One of the hormones produced by the body. Estrogen is the HORMONE primarily responsible for directing endometrial cells to multiply or proliferate. Although proliferation is necessary during the "buildup" phase of the endometrium's cycle, the effects must be constrained by other hormones, such as progesterone.

If estrogen stimulation continues unchecked, it can cause ENDOMETRIAL HYPERPLASIA. This condition is a known risk factor for the later development of ENDOMETRIAL CANCER.

estrogen replacement therapy (ERT)   The use of ESTROGEN to replace that which a woman no longer produces herself because of natural or induced menopause. Once recommended for women without a uterus as a way of easing menopause symptoms, research released in 2004 found that women who took estrogen alone after menopause had a significantly increased risk of stroke and possibly a higher risk of dementia too, according to the National Institutes of Health. The NIH decided to stop the estrogen-only study a year before its planned completion because enough data had been collected to assess overall risks and benefits.

The government ended early the last major study of estrogen because of the health risks, noting that estrogen alone is not as bad as combining it with the hormone PROGESTIN—officials advise, however, that estrogen still is too risky for long-term use.

Estrogen alone did not increase the risk of breast cancer, a surprise to researchers because the estrogen-progestin combination had increased that risk by 26 percent.

For a long time, doctors had thought that using estrogen (alone or together with progestin) would keep women healthier after menopause by reducing heart attacks and keeping the brain sharp. However, millions of women abandoned the estrogen-progestin combination in 2002, when a major federal study concluded that those pills raised the risk of breast cancer, strokes and heart attacks. At that time, the scientists were not sure whether estrogen alone was as risky. (Only women who have undergone a hysterectomy can even consider taking estrogen alone; in other women, progestin use with estrogen is crucial to protect against uterine cancer.)

Then, in March 2004, the NIH shut down its study of estrogen-only use as well, telling the 11,000 women enrolled to quit their pills, essentially ending hope that estrogen alone would have some usefulness that the hormone combination did not. The women in the study were healthy 50- to 79-year-olds who took either estrogen or a dummy pill for nearly seven years. The study's primary purpose was to see if estrogen could prevent heart disease after menopause.

In stopping the study, the government revealed that estrogen alone increased the risk of a stroke as much as combination estrogen-progestin does. For every 10,000 women, those taking hormones suffer eight more strokes per year than nonhormone users. At the same time, estrogen alone had no effect on heart disease. (In contrast, the estrogen-progestin combination increases heart attack risk by 29 percent.)

Neither type of hormone therapy seems good for women's brains. Preliminary data from a related study of women 65 and older suggest those taking estrogen alone were more likely to suffer some degree of dementia than those taking a placebo. Likewise, scientists announced in 2003 that the estrogen-progestin combination doubled the risk of Alzheimer's and other forms of dementia.

Benefits

Estrogen (and estrogen-progestin) decrease the risk of a hip fracture from bone-thinning osteoporosis, although only women who cannot take one of the nation's many other osteoporosis treatments should consider estrogen for that use, according to the government.

European Organisation for Research and Treatment of Cancer (EORTC) An international nonprofit group that conducts, coordinates, and stimulates laboratory and clinical research in Europe to improve the management of cancer. Because comprehensive research in this field is often beyond the means of individual European laboratories and hospitals, the organization allows multidisciplinary, multinational efforts of basic research scientists and clinicians of the European continent.

The ultimate goals of the EORTC are to improve the standard of cancer treatment in Europe through the development of new drugs and innovative approaches and to test more effective treatments with drugs, surgery, and RADIATION THERAPY.

The organization was founded as an international organization under Belgian law in 1962 by eminent oncologists working in the main cancer research institutes of the European Union (EU) countries and Switzerland. Named Groupe Européen de Chimiothérapie Anticancéreuse, it became the European Organisation for Research and Treatment of Cancer in 1968. For contact information, see Appendix I.

Exceptional Cancer Patients A nonprofit organization dedicated to promoting a comprehensive integrative philosophy of the importance of the mind–body connection in health care for cancer patients and others who have chronic illnesses.

Exceptional Cancer Patients was founded in 1978 by Bernie Siegel, M.D., and successfully operated for many years; it was acquired in 1999 by the

Mind-Body Wellness Center in order to build upon and advance the organization and its principles. Today it is owned and operated by Meadville Medical Center and MMC Health Systems, Inc., to offer comprehensive, integrative "whole person" programs in a traditional medical setting.

The center provides resources, comprehensive professional training programs, and interdisciplinary retreats to help people facing the challenges of cancer discover their inner healing resources. These programs are based upon the science of mind–body–spirit medicine. For contact information, see Appendix I.

excisional biopsy   A type of BIOPSY in which the surgeon removes all of a lump or suspicious area plus an area of healthy tissue around the edges. This technique is more aggressive than an *incisional biopsy*, in which the surgeon simply cuts out a sample of a lump or suspicious area. In either case, a pathologist then examines the tissue under a microscope to check for cancer cells.

exercise   Exercise in general is extremely beneficial to overall health; it also can help prevent certain types of cancer, including ENDOMETRIAL CANCER. Exercise helps the body function properly so that all food and fiber are used optimally, builds lean muscle, and burns calories. A sedentary lifestyle contributes to obesity, which is a risk factor for many cancers.

The amount of exercise that is sufficient is controversial, however. Although some studies recommend that even only 30 minutes of moderate exercise a day—not even at one time—is enough, other studies indicate the benefit may result only from vigorous exercise. Most scientists believe that a brisk walk of 30 to 40 minutes on most days of the week is probably the minimal level that people should be trying to achieve.

The AMERICAN CANCER SOCIETY is also putting a new emphasis on exercise as a way to reduce the risk of cancer, and of surviving the disease once it is diagnosed. Studies suggest that weight control, through proper nutrition and physical activity, independently reduces risk. Although studies have not found that cancer risk falls if people lose weight, experts suspect risk would fall because studies do show a lower cancer risk among people who are not overweight.

The society's minimal recommendation for cancer prevention in adults is at least 30 minutes of moderate activity, such as a brisk walk, five days a week. In addition, 45 minutes or more of moderate-to-vigorous activity, five or more days a week, may further reduce cancer risk. Vigorous activity can range from jogging to martial arts, basketball, or masonry work. The guidelines also call for children and adolescents to perform at least 60 minutes a day of moderate-to-vigorous physical activity, five days a week, to create lifetime habits that will keep them in shape as they get older.

fallopian tube cancer   The rarest of all types of female reproductive cancers, making up just 0.3 percent to 0.5 percent of all gynecologic cancers. Only 1,500 to 2,000 cases have been reported throughout the world. Fallopian tube cancer develops from cells inside the fallopian tubes (the twin tubes connecting the ovaries and the uterus). There are several forms of cancer that may start in this way. The most common is ADENOCARCINOMA; more rare types include LEIOMYOSARCOMA and TRANSITIONAL CELL CARCINOMA.

Most of the time, cancer that is found in the fallopian tubes did not originate there but spread from other sites in the body (usually an ovary or the endometrium). In fact, between about 80 percent and 90 percent of cancers involving the tube have spread from the ovary, uterus, endometrium, appendix, or colon. It is often difficult for a surgeon to determine definitely whether an adenocarcinoma has originated in the fallopian tube or the ovary, because the cells from these neighboring organs appear so similar. Fallopian tube cancer is so rare that even a major cancer center may see no more than a few cases over many years.

Cause

Very little is known about the origins of cancer of the fallopian tube. These cancers typically appear in middle-aged women who have had children, and often after menopause. Some experts suspect there may be a genetic factor involved.

Risk Factors

Because fallopian tube cancer is so rare, scientists have not been able to determine any specific environmental or lifestyle factors that increase the risk of this malignancy. Currently, researchers are trying to find out whether there is some inherited tendency to have the illness. In particular, there is some evi-dence that women who have inherited a mutation in the *BRCA1* gene (a gene connected with an OVARIAN CANCER–BREAST CANCER LINK) also have an increased risk of development of fallopian tube cancer.

Symptoms

There may not be any symptoms early in the disease. When fallopian tube cells become malignant, the resulting tumor slowly grows, eventually distending the inner passageway of the fallopian tube and causing pelvic pain. Over time, the tumor can also invade the wall of the fallopian tube, penetrate the tube's outer surface, and spread throughout the pelvis and abdomen. When symptoms do appear, they may include the following:

- Vague abdominal discomfort
- Watery, clear, or blood-tinged discharge from the vagina
- Abdominal pressure or cramping
- Lump or mass in the abdomen
- Increased abdominal swelling without weight gain elsewhere
- Abdominal swelling that does not recede with diet or exercise
- Feelings of pressure on the bowel or bladder
- Sensation that the bowel or bladder cannot be completely emptied

Diagnosis

Cancer of the fallopian tubes is not easy to diagnose because of the lack of symptoms early in the disease. The diagnosis of fallopian tube cancer is rarely suspected until the condition is discovered during surgery in another ailment.

If this type of cancer is suspected, the doctor conducts an internal pelvic examination to determine the shape, size, and position of the pelvic organs. Blood tests and an ultrasound of the pelvis may be ordered.

Staging

As in all cancers, once the tumor is removed the doctor determines the stage to plan treatment. Fallopian tube cancer staging is as follows:

Stage 0: This represents an in situ cancer that is only minimally aggressive and has not spread beyond the fallopian tubes.

Stage I: Growth of the tumor is limited to the fallopian tubes.

Stage II: The tumor involves one or both fallopian tubes and has spread to the pelvis.

Stage III: The tumor involves one or both fallopian tubes and has spread outside the pelvis.

Stage IV: The tumor involves one or both fallopian tubes with distant metastases.

Treatment

Almost always, aggressive surgery entails a HYS-TERECTOMY and removal of both tubes and both ovaries, together with a selection of abdominal and pelvic lymph glands. Patients in the advanced stages of the disease are normally also given CHEMOTHERAPY (typically paclitaxel [Taxol]) and CISPLATIN) or RADIATION THERAPY.

However, if the disease is diagnosed early, is limited to one fallopian tube, and occurs in a young woman who wants to retain fertility, the surgeon may simply remove the fallopian tube and ovary on the affected side (a SALPINGO-OOPHORECTOMY), as well as the omentum (fatty tissue beneath the bottom of the stomach and including part of the bowel) and LYMPH NODES in the pelvis.

Prognosis

The prognosis for recovery depends on the stage of the disease at the time of diagnosis. The earlier stages of this illness carry a very good prognosis, but statistics are limited because the condition is rare. If the cancer is growing only along the inside passageway of the tube, 91 percent of patients survive for at least five years after diagnosis. However, if the cancer has penetrated below the lining and involves the wall of the fallopian tube, the five-year survival rate drops to 53 percent. For tumors

that have spread entirely through the wall to involve the tube's outer surface, the five-year survival rate is less than 25 percent.

Prevention

Because experts know very little about the risk factors for fallopian tube cancer, there is no way to prevent it. Eventually, scientists hope to develop screening blood tests that can identify women who are at higher-than-average risk of development of fallopian tube cancer or ovarian cancer, either by identifying *BRCA1* mutations or by measuring levels of a tumor marker called CA 125 in the blood.

fat, dietary Some studies suggest that a DIET high in animal fat (saturated fat) may increase the risk of cancer, and that a diet high in fruits and vegetables may decrease the risk.

Although the results of these studies are inconclusive regarding cancer risk, a diet low in animal fat may have other health benefits. For example, soy foods, a good source of nonanimal-fat protein, are high in ISOFLAVONES, which block some hormonal activity in cells. Diets that include high intake of soy products have been associated with lower rates of cancers.

There are three types of dietary fats—saturated, monounsaturated, and polyunsaturated fats:

- *Saturated fats* are almost exclusively derived from animal products such as meat, milk, and cheese and have been linked to an increased risk of cancer.

- *Monounsaturated fats* are found in olive oil and canola oil.

- *Polyunsaturated fats* are found in vegetable oils.

Although the latter two types of fat are less closely linked to disease, since overall fat intake is associated with cancer, limiting use of all three kinds is a good idea. Dietitians generally recommend use of tub margarine as a better choice than butter, since butter is rich in both saturated fat and cholesterol, and the hazards of saturated fats are better documented and appear to be more severe than the risks associated with the hydrogenated fats in margarine (most margarine is made from vegetable fat and has no cholesterol). The usual recommendation is that people derive no more than 10 percent of daily calories from saturated fats and that total fat intake not exceed 30 percent of the day's calories.

Dietary fat use can be reduced by limiting one's intake of red meat, choosing low-fat or no-fat varieties of milk and cheese, removing the skin from chicken and turkey, eating pretzels instead of potato chips, and decreasing or eliminating fried foods, butter, and margarine. Cooking with small amounts of olive oil instead of butter significantly cuts saturated-fat intake.

fatigue The most common side effect experienced by cancer patients, usually as a result of surgery, RADIATION THERAPY, CHEMOTHERAPY, or BIOLOGICAL THERAPY. Although it occurs most frequently in those who are undergoing treatment, overwhelming fatigue may continue after treatment.

Although scientists are not sure of its exact cause, some researchers believe fatigue may be caused by the waste products produced as a tumor shrinks or may be related to the energy the body needs to fight cancer. Others believe fatigue may be related to interruptions in the signals sent through the nervous system. A low blood count (anemia) as a result of chemotherapy, sleep disturbances, stress, depression, poor DIET, infection, and other medication side effects can all contribute to this exhaustion.

Symptoms

The symptoms of cancer-related fatigue are different from normal feelings of being tired. Fatigue can begin suddenly and be all-consuming; naps may not help. Fatigue can be physically and emotionally draining on the patient as well as the family. General weakness may be accompanied by limb heaviness, decreased ability to concentrate, sleeplessness, and/or irritability.

Diagnosis

Patients who experience this type of extreme tiredness should consult a health-care provider, who can conduct a few simple tests, including a blood count to check for anemia or infection, and a physical examination.

Treatment

If symptoms are fatigue related, there are several ways patients can help manage those symptoms. It is important to eat healthy, appetite-stimulating foods. The complex carbohydrates found in pasta, fresh fruits, and whole grain breads provide long-term energy. Studies have shown that a moderate amount of exercise may actually help improve energy level.

Sleep is also important. Patients should go to bed at a regular time each day and follow a regular routine.

Fertile Hope A national nonprofit organization that addresses the reproductive needs of cancer patients and survivors. The group provides education, financial help, research, and support.

Fertile Hope programs and services include supporting research, increasing awareness of fertility risks among patients; and providing credible, accurate educational resources. Fertile Hope also provides financial assistance for patients whose medical treatments threaten reproductive function and offers support to help patients cope with the physical and emotional issues associated with infertility, fertility preservation, assisted reproduction, family planning, genetic counseling, pregnancy, adoption, and other related issues. For contact information, see Appendix I.

fertility drugs Drugs given to women to help them became pregnant. Whereas some controversial data associate ovulation stimulation drugs, such as gonadotropins, with a higher risk of OVARIAN CANCER, the overwhelming majority of studies have found no connection between fertility drugs and cancer.

Fertility drugs are the mainstay of treatment for infertility. Some women are unable to become pregnant because they do not secrete enough hormones at the right time during their menstrual cycle and, as a result, do not ovulate. Fertility drugs are given to such women to ensure not only that they ovulate, but that they ovulate at a particular time so that artificial insemination can be planned accurately for their most fertile period. If a woman is going to have several eggs retrieved for assisted reproductive technologies, fertility drugs may also be used to boost the number of eggs produced.

Some experts believe that the extra ovulations caused by fertility drugs promote cancer through the constant irritation of the ovary's surface. They believe that uninterrupted "incessant ovulations" during a woman's lifetime increase her probability of development of ovarian cancer. This theory may explain why events that interrupt the constant cycle of ovulations (pregnancy, breast-feeding, and oral contraceptive use) are associated with a decreased risk of ovarian cancer.

Another theory is that increased levels of certain hormones associated with ovulation (such as human chorionic gonadotropin) increase the risk of ovarian cancer. Fertility drugs can increase both the number of ovulations and the levels of hormones associated with ovulation.

The first study to suggest a direct link between fertility drugs and cancer was published in 1992 in the *American Journal of Epidemiology*. It found that women who used fertility drugs and never conceived had a higher risk of ovarian cancer. Interestingly, women who used fertility drugs and *did* conceive did not have a higher cancer risk. It is unclear whether the degree of cancer risk was linked to the fertility drugs.

Another study found that using the fertility drug clomiphene citrate for more than a year may increase the risk of development of ovarian tumors of low malignant potential. This type of tumor responds better to treatment than epithelial ovarian cancer, the most common type of ovarian cancer.

These studies and other recent research raise questions about whether infertile women who use fertility drugs and do not become pregnant and women who use certain fertility drugs for extended periods, may be at increased risk of ovarian cancer. These risks have not yet been proved.

Women who have taken fertility drugs and who are concerned about their risk of ovarian cancer should discuss their previous fertility drug treatment with a gynecologist. At this time, there are no screening tests that are consistently accurate enough to detect ovarian cancer at an early stage when there are no symptoms.

Although research to clarify this issue is under way, infertility experts advise that the careful use of gonadotropins is still reasonable, especially considering that pregnancy and breast-feeding reduce cancer risk. Most doctors do not advise taking any fertility drug for more than several months at a time, and certainly not for more than a total of six months to a year.

fibroid tumor The common name for a benign uterine leiomyoma—a lump of smooth muscle cells and fibrous connective tissue that develops within the wall of the uterus. Fibroids may appear alone or in clusters, ranging from less than an inch to more than eight inches, and may grow within the wall of the uterus or project into the interior cavity or outer surface of the uterus. In rare cases, they may grow on stalks projecting from the wall of the uterus.

Experts do not know what causes fibroids; most occur in women of reproductive age and tend to occur twice as often in black women as in white women. They are seldom seen in young girls, and they usually stabilize or fade away after menopause.

Fibroids are the most common pelvic tumor in women, and they almost never become malignant; nor do they increase a woman's risk for UTERINE CANCER.

Risk Factors

Experts have not definitely identified risk factors; a few small studies suggest that as a group, women who have had two children have half the risk of having fibroids of women who have never given birth. It is unclear whether giving birth protects a woman from fibroids development or whether fibroids contribute to infertility.

Symptoms

Most fibroids do not cause symptoms and do not require treatment other than observation. Some women may experience excessive or painful bleeding during menstruation, bleeding between periods, a feeling of fullness in the lower abdomen, pain during sex, low back pain, or frequent urination because the fibroid is pressing on the bladder. Rarely, a fibroid can block the fallopian tube, preventing fertilization and migration of the egg; after surgical removal of the fibroid, fertility is generally restored.

Diagnosis

Fibroids are usually discovered during a routine gynecologic examination or during prenatal care.

Treatment

Until very recently, HYSTERECTOMY was often recommended for an enlarging fibroid. However, more commonly today doctors believe that uterine fibroids may require no intervention—or, at most, limited treatment. Some women never exhibit any symptoms or have any problems associated with fibroids, in which case no treatment is necessary. Women who have occasional pelvic pain or discomfort may take a mild anti-inflammatory drug. More bothersome cases may require stronger drugs available by prescription.

financial issues Treating cancer can be very expensive, but health insurance plans usually cover much of the cost. Patients who belong to a health maintenance organization (HMO) or preferred provider organization (PPO) should become familiar with their provider choices and their financial responsibility if they receive care "out of network" from a doctor not covered by the health plan.

Cancer patients who do not have insurance should contact their local Social Security office to determine whether they qualify for supplemental security income (SSI) or SOCIAL SECURITY DISABILITY INSURANCE (SSDI). The medical requirements and disability determination process are the same for both programs. However, whereas eligibility for SSDI is based on employment history, SSI is based on financial need.

Free Hospital Care

Cancer patients without insurance can also receive care from hospitals who receive federal grants from Hill-Burton funds. These funds allow hospitals and nursing homes to provide low-cost or no-cost medical care. To receive a listing of hospitals or nursing homes participating in the Hill-Burton program, patients can call (800) 638-0742 or visit the Hill-Burton Web site (www.hrsa.gov/osp/dfcr/). (See also HILL-BURTON FREE HOSPITAL CARE.)

Prescription Drugs

Most major pharmaceutical companies have patient-assistance programs that offer a free three-month supply of medication to those who cannot afford their prescriptions. To obtain guidelines and a listing of participating companies, patients can call the Pharmaceutical Manufacturers' Association at (800) 762-4636. The medication request must be completed by a physician.

Free Air Transportation

Many nonprofit agencies offer free air transportation for patients who travel to treatment centers, relying on private pilots who donate their time and use of their own planes. Patients can obtain a list of these services at http://www.aircareall.org. In addition, major airlines sometimes offer reduced or no-cost travel through an assistance program.

Local Transportation

For local travel assistance to and from treatments, a hospital social worker may be able to provide van service or cab or bus vouchers. Some local AMERICAN CANCER SOCIETY offices run volunteer transportation programs or provide funds to reimburse travel expenses. Some communities offer MediVans for those who qualify as a result of illness or disability. Local nursing homes, park districts, or YMCAs also may offer van transportation to local hospitals. In addition, many communities offer seniors reduced-fare taxi service within the community.

Temporary Housing

Temporary housing is sometimes required by cancer patients who must travel for consultation or treatment or for families who visit hospitalized patients. The AMERICAN CANCER SOCIETY may be able to arrange a low-cost hotel room for those receiving treatment. In addition, many hospitals negotiate discount rates at local hotels or provide dormitory-style housing. The National Association of Hospitality Houses (800-542-9730) also provides referral information to anyone in need of lodging while undergoing treatment away from home.

Utilities

Assistance programs are offered by many gas, electric, water, and phone companies for cancer patients who may have problems in paying monthly bills. Many states have regulations that prohibit companies from turning off utilities; a doctor or social worker may need to write letters describing why the services are medically necessary. The regulations do not lessen a patient's responsibility for paying bills but may allow families more time to pay or lower monthly payments. In an emergency, local help lines and social service agencies may be able to provide one-time emergency help with utility bills.

Home Care/Respite

Some insurance plans offer coverage for home care ranging from skilled nursing to companionship. If companion care is not a covered benefit, patients can contact various agencies for assistance. Respite care allows the caregiver a few hours each week to take a break while someone watches over the patient. Many caregivers use this time to run errands, take care of personal health needs, or unwind.

Local respite caregivers can be located by calling the National Respite Locator at (800) 773-5433. The locator service can also provide a listing of qualifying conditions.

In addition, the National Federation of Interfaith Volunteer Caregivers, a not-for-profit group that oversees 400 regional offices, sends volunteers into the homes of people who need care, company, and supervision. They can be reached at (800) 350-7438.

Medical Supplies

The CANCER FUND OF AMERICA (800-578-5284) can provide nonprescription medical items such as nutritional supplements. Items available vary as the group receives products donated from companies. Patients or family members can call to be listed in their database for specific needs.

Food Programs

Meals on Wheels coordinates thousands of programs throughout the United States dedicated to delivering meals to those who are homebound. Some programs require a small donation; eligibility is determined by each program. For a local referral to Meals on Wheels, patients can contact the national office at (616) 530-0929.

Income Tax Deductions

Medical costs that are not covered by insurance policies can sometimes be deducted from annual income before taxes. Examples of tax-deductible expenses may include mileage for trips to and from medical appointments, out-of-pocket costs for treatment, prescription drugs or equipment, and

the cost of meals during lengthy medical visits. The local Internal Revenue Service office, tax consultants, or certified public accountants can determine medical costs that are tax deductible. Their telephone numbers are in the local telephone directory.

Medicaid

Medicaid is a jointly funded federal-state health insurance program for people who need financial assistance for medical expenses, coordinated by the Centers for Medicare & Medicaid Services (CMS) (formerly the Health Care Financing Administration). At a minimum, states must provide home care services to people who receive federal income assistance such as Social Security income and Aid to Families with Dependent Children. Medicaid coverage includes part-time nursing, home-care aide services, and medical supplies and equipment. Information about coverage is available from local state welfare offices, state health departments, state social service agencies, or the state Medicaid office.

Medicare

This federal health insurance program is administered by the CMS. Eligible individuals include those who are 65 or older, people of any age who have permanent kidney failure, and disabled people younger than age 65. Medicare may offer reimbursement for some home care services. Cancer patients who qualify for Medicare may also be eligible for coverage of HOSPICE services if they are accepted into a Medicare-certified hospice program. To receive information on eligibility, explanations of coverage, and related publications, call Medicare at 1-800-633-4227 (1-800-MEDICARE) or visit their Web site at: www.medicare.gov. Some publications are available in Spanish.

Patient Assistance Programs

The PATIENT ADVOCATE FOUNDATION is a national nonprofit organization that provides referrals to cancer patients and survivors concerning managed care, insurance, financial issues, job discrimination, and debt crisis matters. (For contact information, see Appendix I.)

Veterans' Benefits

Eligible veterans and their dependents may receive cancer treatment at a Veterans Administration

Medical Center. Treatment for service-connected conditions is provided, and treatment for other conditions may be available, depending on the veteran's financial need.

Viatical Settlement Companies

Viatical companies purchase a patient's life insurance policy at a discounted rate and provide money for patients to use as they choose. The seller, in turn, signs over the policy to the viatical company.

In general, any life insurance policy (group or individual) can be sold, but the rate of return and eligibility criteria vary among companies. However, patients should consider tax implications and the effect of a viatical settlement on assistance programs.

A free brochure, "Viatical Settlements: A Guide for People with Terminal Illnesses," is available at the Federal Trade Commission at (202) 326-2222. The National Viatical Association (202-347-7361) offers a listing of viatical companies.

Life Insurance Loans

LifeWise Family Financial Security, Inc., allows patients to take out a loan against their existing life insurance policy if their life expectancy is five years or less. There is no obligation to repay the loan, but the option is available, thereby creating a different option from selling an insurance policy to a viatical company. If a patient chooses not to repay the loan, the life insurance policy proceeds are the sole source of repayment. All surplus funds are remitted to the patient's family. LifeWise has counselors available to answer any questions and publishes *The Financial Resource Guide: A Comprehensive, Step-by-Step Reference for Individuals Facing Life-Threatening or Terminal Illnesses.* Advice from counselors and a copy of the guide are available by calling (800) 219-7385.

fine-needle aspiration The use of a thin, hollow needle to withdraw tissue from the body. A fine-needle aspiration (also called a needle-aspiration biopsy) is less expensive, is less painful, and carries less risk of infection than a surgical BIOPSY. Because of its safety, cost-effectiveness, and accuracy, it is often the first biopsy procedure of choice in evaluating a variety of different masses.

A core-needle biopsy is similar to needle aspiration, but it uses a wider needle in order to obtain a larger tissue sample. Fine-needle aspiration is less painful than core biopsy and therefore can be performed as an outpatient procedure and at periodic intervals for serial follow-up.

five-year survival rate The percentage of people who have cancer who are expected to survive five years or longer with the disease. Although the rates are based on the most recent information available, they may include data from patients treated several years earlier. Although still statistically valid, five-year survival rates may not reflect advances in cancer treatment, which often occur very quickly. They should not be seen as predictive in individual cases.

flow cytometry A procedure that measures cellular DNA that can be used to assess the aggressiveness of a malignant cell and the likelihood of cancer recurrence.

Once malignant cells are removed, a fluorescent dye is added to the cells and attaches itself to the DNA. A laser instrument called a flow cytometer measures the amount of DNA; excessive or insufficient DNA may indicate the risk of recurrence. This type of modern technology can provide an answer about likelihood of recurrence in just a few minutes.

fluorouracil (5-fluorouracil, commonly called 5-FU) An antimetabolite cancer drug that prevents cell growth at a short, specific time in its reproduction cycle by interfering with important enzyme reactions within the cell. This type of CHEMOTHERAPY is applied as a cream to treat precancerous vulval disease.

FORCE: Facing Our Risk of Cancer Empowered A nonprofit organization for women at high risk of OVARIAN CANCER or breast cancer due to their family history and genetic status, and for members of families who carry a *BRCA* gene mutation. The group provides women with information to determine whether they are at high risk for breast and ovarian cancer as a result of genetic predisposition, family history, or other factors and provides information about options for managing and living with these risk factors. FORCE also supports families facing these risks and represents the concerns of these high-risk members to the cancer advocacy community, the scientific and medical community, the legislative community, and the general public. In addition, they promote research related specifically to hereditary cancer. For contact information, see Appendix I.

free radicals   Highly charged destructive forms of oxygen generated by each cell in the body that destroy cellular membranes through the oxidation process. Free radicals can damage important cellular molecules such as DNA or lipids in other parts of the cell.

Because free radicals are essential to many reactions in the body (they are generated by the immune system to fend off microbes and help the digestive system break down food), they should not be entirely destroyed. It is only when their levels become too high that damage can occur.

Free radical damage can be offset by molecules called ANTIOXIDANTS, which neutralize free radicals, preventing them from damaging cells. Antioxidants include BETA-CAROTENE, selenium, and vitamins E and C. Although there are no guarantees of the effectiveness of the dietary supplements of antioxidants in preventing cell damage, many doctors recommend them to their patients.

frozen section   A technique in which a part of BIOPSY tissue is frozen immediately after removal, and a thin slice is then mounted on a microscope slide, enabling a pathologist to analyze it in just a few minutes for a diagnosis.

garlic The edible bulb of a plant in the lily family (*Allium* genus) that research suggests may effectively inhibit the cancer process. Studies reveal that the benefits of garlic are not limited to a specific species, to a particular tissue, or to a specific carcinogen. Of 37 observational studies in humans using garlic and related allyl sulfur components, 28 studies showed some cancer-preventive effect. However, all of the available information is from observational studies comparing cancer incidence in populations who eat or do not eat garlic, animal models, or observations of cells in culture. These findings have not yet been verified by clinical trials in humans.

Although the health benefits of garlic are frequently reported, eating too much can also have unpleasant effects, such as garlic odor on breath and skin, occasional allergic reactions, stomach disorders and diarrhea, decrease in protein and calcium levels, association with bronchial asthma, and contact dermatitis.

Because garlic preparations vary in concentration and in the number of active compounds they contain, quality control is important when considering the use of garlic as a cancer-fighting agent.

Several compounds are involved in garlic's possible anticancer effects. Garlic contains allyl sulfur and other compounds that slow or prevent growth of tumor cells. Allyl sulfur compounds, which occur naturally in garlic and onions, make cells vulnerable to the stress created by products of cell division. Because cancer cells divide very quickly, they generate more stressors than most normal cells. Thus, cancer cells are damaged by the presence of allyl sulfur compounds to a much greater extent than normal cells. However, the chemical characteristics of garlic are complicated, and the ultimate quality of garlic products depends on the manufacturing process.

Peeling garlic and processing garlic into oil or powder can increase the number and variety of active compounds. Peeling garlic releases an enzyme called allinase and starts a series of chemical reactions that produce diallyl disulfide (DADS). DADS is also formed when raw garlic is cut or crushed. However, if garlic is cooked immediately after peeling, the allinase is inactivated and the cancer-fighting benefit of DADS is lost. This is why scientists recommend waiting 15 minutes between peeling and cooking garlic to allow the allinase reaction to occur.

Processing garlic into powder or garlic oil releases other cancer-fighting agents; the inconsistent results of garlic research may be due, at least in part, to problems in standardizing all of the active compounds in garlic preparations. Some of the garlic compounds currently under investigation are allin (responsible for the typical garlic odor), alline (odorless compound), ajoene (naturally occurring disulfide), diallyl sulfide, diallyl disulfide, diallyl trisulfide, *S*-allylcysteine, organosulfur compounds, and allyl sulfur compounds.

genes The hereditary unit carrying characteristics from parent to child. Some genes appear to increase a woman's risk of development of different types of cancer.

germ cell ovarian cancer A type of OVARIAN CANCER that begins in the egg-producing cells within the body of the ovary. This type of cancer can occur in women of all ages, but most tumors are diagnosed during late adolescence. It is rare in comparison to EPITHELIAL OVARIAN CARCINOMA.

Germ cell ovarian cancer is the second largest group of ovarian cancers (about 20 percent). In children and adolescents, more than 60 percent of ovarian tumors are of germ cell origin, of which a third are malignant.

There are six main types of germ cell carcinomas; the three most common types are TERATOMAS, DYSGERMINOMAS, and YOLK SAC TUMORS. There are also many tumors that arise in the germ cells that are benign.

See also GERM CELL TUMOR.

germ cells Germ cells in females are the eggs (ova).
See also GERM CELL TUMOR.

germ cell tumor A type of OVARIAN CANCER. Germ cells are the cells that usually form in the ova (eggs). There are several subtypes of germ cell tumors, most of which are benign; some, however, are cancerous and may be life threatening. The most common germ cell tumors are TERATOMA, DYSGERMINOMA, YOLK SAC TUMOR, and CHORIOCARCINOMA. About 20 percent of ovarian cancers are malignant germ cell tumors.

Teratoma

The teratoma has a benign form (mature teratoma) and a cancerous form (immature teratoma). The mature teratoma is the most common ovarian germ cell tumor and usually affects women of reproductive age. It is often called a dermoid CYST because its lining resembles skin. These tumors or cysts also contain a variety of other benign tissues that may resemble adult respiratory passages, bone, nervous tissue, teeth, and other tissues. They can be surgically removed.

Immature teratomas usually occur in girls younger than age 18. Just like mature teratomas, these rare cancers may contain connective tissue, brain tissue, and tissue from respiratory passages. Tumors that are not very immature (grade 1 immature teratoma) and have not spread beyond the ovary are cured by surgical removal of the ovary. When they have spread beyond the ovary and/or much of the tumor has a very immature appearance (grade 2 or 3 immature teratomas), chemotherapy is recommended in addition to surgical removal of the ovary.

Dysgerminoma

Although dysgerminoma is the most common germ cell ovarian cancer, it represents only 2 percent of all ovarian cancers. It usually affects women in their teens and 20s. Although dysgerminomas are malignant, most do not grow or spread very rapidly. When they are limited to the ovary, more than 95 percent can be cured by surgical removal of the ovary without further treatment. Even when the tumor has spread farther, the combination of surgery and chemotherapy is effective in about 90 percent of cases.

Endodermal Sinus Tumor (Yolk Sac Tumor) and Choriocarcinoma

Endodermal sinus tumor and choriocarcinoma are very rare tumors that typically affect girls and young women and tend to grow and spread rapidly. However, they are usually sensitive to chemotherapy. Choriocarcinomas more commonly start in the placenta during pregnancy rather than in the ovary and are usually even more responsive to chemotherapy than ovarian choriocarcinomas.

gestational trophoblastic disease (GTD) A group of diseases that begin when abnormal cells grow in the uterus after a woman has conceived. GTD is always related to some aspect of pregnancy. After a sperm fertilizes an egg, several new tissues that normally would form the fetus and a placenta develop. In gestational trophoblastic disease (also known as molar pregnancy), the tissue originally destined to become the placenta instead forms a tumor that can become malignant and spread beyond the uterus. Usually there is no normal fetal tissue, but sometimes incomplete fetal tissues can develop in addition to the molar tissue. Most molar pregnancies (even those that spread) are benign, but a few are cancerous. However, almost all—even the cancerous type—are curable.

Most molar pregnancies are benign and confined to the uterus. If, on rare occasions, the mole becomes malignant, it is called a CHORIOCARCINOMA. Half of all choriocarcinomas form as the result of a molar pregnancy, but others can appear during a tubal pregnancy, an aborted pregnancy, a miscarriage, or a healthy pregnancy.

According to the AMERICAN CANCER SOCIETY, these moles occur in about one of 1,200 to 1,500 pregnancies in the United States. GTD accounts for less than 1 percent of gynecologic cancers.

Risk Factors

Choriocarcinoma and all other types of molar pregnancy are more common in women of Asian or African descent, although experts also believe some environmental conditions predispose women to this disease. In addition, most women at higher risk of molar pregnancy are older than age 40 or younger than age 20. Women who have had one mole are at risk of having another molar pregnancy, as are women who have blood type AB or B (as opposed O or A). Some studies suggest that a diet low in beta-carotene or vitamin A may increase a woman's risk of having GTD as well.

Symptoms

GTD can exaggerate symptoms of pregnancy or may mimic symptoms associated with miscarriage. Choriocarcinomas also can cause symptoms during or after pregnancy—even after a mole has been removed. The most common symptom is vaginal bleeding, especially between the sixth and 16th weeks of pregnancy or continuing for a long time after delivery. Occasionally, grapelike bits of tissue may pass vaginally.

Choriocarcinoma also may cause the following symptoms:

- Unusually rapid abdominal swelling during the first trimester of pregnancy
- Abnormal vomiting during pregnancy
- Fatigue that results from heavy bleeding
- Sudden severe abdominal pain
- Pelvic cramps
- Vaginal discharge
- Shortness of breath, cough, or blood in sputum

Diagnosis

GTD may be suspected because of symptoms that occur during or after pregnancy or because the uterus is unusually large early in pregnancy. In addition, high levels of human chorionic gonadotropin suggest GTD. A pelvic ultrasound can confirm a GTD diagnosis, and additional testing can determine whether the mole is malignant. Testing may include X-rays, computed tomography scans, or magnetic resonance imaging scans to view the chest, abdomen, pelvis, and brain, along with blood chemical tests and a complete blood count.

Treatment

Surgery is the treatment of choice for this rare type of gestational trophoblastic disease, with the evacuation of the uterine contents as the first step. If the mole is malignant, surgery may be followed by CHEMOTHERAPY. RADIATION THERAPY has not been shown to be very effective in treating GTD except in some unusual cases in which the cancer cells have spread to the brain. If radiation is used, it is generally given five days a week for four to six weeks.

Close follow-up with monitoring of blood tests for human chorionic gonadotropin (HCG) is necessary. If the HCG does not disappear, further treatment with chemotherapy may be needed.

With appropriate treatment, all moles are curable and nearly all cases of more aggressive molar tumors can be cured as well. Even 80 percent to 90 percent of tumors that have a poor prognosis can be cured with a combination of surgery and chemotherapy.

Prevention

The only foolproof way a woman can protect herself against GTD is by never becoming pregnant.

gestational trophoblastic neoplasia   See GESTATIONAL TROPHOBLASTIC DISEASE.

Gilda Radner Familial Ovarian Cancer Registry

An international registry of families in which two or more relatives have OVARIAN CANCER. In addition to ovarian cancer research, the registry offers a helpline, education, information, and peer support for women at high risk of ovarian cancer. The registry hopes to identify new genes associated with familial ovarian cancer, thereby improving genetic and psychosocial counseling for individuals and families. They also hope to identify lifestyle choices (oral contraceptive use, HORMONE REPLACEMENT THERAPY, number of pregnancies) that reduce ovarian cancer risk in women who may be more susceptible to the disease. The group's goals include improved detection of ovarian cancer, predictive testing for cancer predisposition, and ultimately, an understanding of means to prevent the disease in future generations. The group is currently collecting family histories, medical records, and tissue samples of ovarian cancer patients. For contact information, see Appendix I.

See also GILDA'S CLUBS.

Gilda's Clubs   Nonprofit locations where those who have any type of cancer and their families and friends can build social and emotional support as a supplement to medical care. Gilda's Clubs offer free support and networking groups, lectures, workshops, and social events in a nonresidential, homelike setting. Funding is solicited from private individuals, corporations, and foundations.

The Gilda's Club program is composed of the following elements, which are offered in every clubhouse:

• Support and networking groups, including Weekly Wellness Groups for those living with cancer, Family Groups for family members and friends, and monthly Networking Groups on specific forms of cancer or topics of common interest (such as cancer of young adults and living solo with cancer).

• Lectures and workshops: Typical lecture topics, which are selected on the basis of members' interests, include stress reduction, nutrition, talking to children about cancer, and managing pain. Major workshop areas include art and other forms of self-expression, meditation, exercise and yoga, and cooking.

• Social activities: A range of gatherings including potluck suppers with music, karaoke nights, joke fests, comedy nights, and major celebrations around special holidays are offered.

• Team convene: Two-hour sessions requested by a person with cancer or family member to create a network to provide support at the time of diagnosis and during any challenging situations that may follow. Sessions include all significant friends and family in a member's life, who join together to provide support for transportation, food preparation, child care, and so on.

• Family focus: A meeting is facilitated by a staff member designed to enlist all family members as a resource and help them learn together how to live with cancer. It seeks to identify and discuss family beliefs about cancer, critical family issues, and immediate practical problems as well as solutions.

Gilda's Clubs are named in memory of the comedian Gilda Radner, who died of ovarian cancer in 1989. Radner is best known for her work on NBC's *Saturday Night Live*. Her book, *It's Always Something,* describes her life with cancer. The clubs were founded by Joanna Bull, Gilda's therapist; Gene Wilder, Gilda's husband; and Joel Siegel. For contact information, see Appendix I.

grade   A measure of the extent of resemblance of a cancer to normal tissue of its same type and of the cancer's probable rate of growth.

grading   A diagnostic laboratory process that measures how aggressive or malignant cells taken from a tumor may be. The cancer cells are evaluated to determine by the extent to which they resemble normal cells—in other words, their degree of DIFFERENTIATION. The more normal the cell (that is, the more differentiated), the lower the grade and the less quickly the cancer cells are likely to spread—and the better the prognosis. Tumor grade often plays a role in treatment decisions.

granulocyte   A type of white blood cell that is produced in BONE MARROW, and which includes neutrophils, basophils, and eosinophils. These white blood cells fight infection by engulfing infecting organisms; their actions may contribute to inflammation and are responsible for allergic reactions.

granulocyte colony-stimulating factor (G-CSF) (filgrastim [Neupogen])   A natural chemical in the body that helps to control the production of white blood cells in the BONE MARROW. G-CSF is sometimes used as medication with or after chemotherapy, as a way of stimulating the production of white blood cells. This mechanism can help to decrease the risk of infection.

G-CSF was one of the first hematopoietic growth factors approved and is an important part of BIOLOGICAL THERAPY. G-CSF also may allow patients to tolerate stronger CHEMOTHERAPY regimens and may enhance the effectiveness of chemotherapy drugs.

gynecological cancer   See REPRODUCTIVE CANCER.

gynecological examination   An examination of a woman's breasts and internal reproductive organs. With the woman sitting and then lying down, the doctor inspects the breasts for irregularities, dimpling, tightened skin, lumps, or discharge. The LYMPH NODES under each arm are also checked for enlargement. The doctor also feels the neck and the thyroid gland for lumps and abnormalities, along with the area between the rib cage and pelvis. Although the woman may experience some discomfort when the doctor presses deeply, the examination should not be painful. To help identify abnormalities, the doctor may listen with a stethoscope for the activity of the intestine and for any abnormal noises made by the circulation.

During a pelvic examination, the woman lies on her back with her hips angled and knees bent while the doctor inspects the external genital area. The doctor notes the distribution of hair as well as any abnormalities, discoloration, discharge, or inflammation. This inspection may reveal hormonal problems, cancer, infections, injury, or physical abuse.

The doctor spreads the labia with gloved fingers to examine the opening of the vagina. Using a warmed, lubricated speculum, the doctor examines the deeper areas of the vagina and the cervix for signs of irritation or cancer and scrapes cells from the cervix's surface for a PAP TEST. A small bristle brush is used to obtain a sample of cells from the canal of the cervix, which are then placed on a glass slide, sprayed with a preservative, and sent to a laboratory, where they are examined under a microscope for signs of cervical cancer.

The Pap test can identify up to 85 percent of CERVICAL CANCERS, even in the earliest stages. The test is most accurate if the woman does not douche or use vaginal medications for at least 24 hours before the examination.

After removing the speculum, the doctor performs a two-handed examination, inserting the index and middle fingers of one gloved hand into the vagina and placing the fingers of the other hand on the lower abdomen above the pubic bone. Between the two hands, the uterus can usually be felt as a pear-shaped, smooth, firm structure, and its position, size, consistency, and degree of tenderness can be determined. Then the doctor attempts to feel the ovaries by moving the hand on the abdomen more to the side and exerting slightly more pressure. Because the ovaries are small and much more difficult to feel than the uterus, more pressure is required; the woman may find this part of the examination uncomfortable. The doctor determines how large the ovaries are and whether they are tender and checks for growths or tender areas within the vagina.

Finally, the doctor performs a rectovaginal examination by inserting the index finger into the vagina and the middle finger into the rectum. In this way, the back wall of the vagina can be examined for abnormal growths or thickness and the rectum can be examined for fissures, polyps, and lumps. A woman may be given a take-home kit to test for unseen blood in the stool.

Gynecologic Cancer Foundation   Nonprofit charitable organization established by the SOCIETY OF GYNECOLOGIC ONCOLOGISTS in 1991 to raise funds for programs benefiting women who have or are at risk for gynecologic cancer. The foundation's programs are designed to raise public awareness of ways to prevent, detect, and treat gynecologic cancers; to provide education; and to support gynecologic cancer research. For contact information, see Appendix I.

gynecologic oncologist   A cancer specialist expert in the treatment of cancer affecting the female reproductive system (ovaries, uterus, cervix, vulva, fallopian tubes, and vagina). Gynecologic ONCOLOGISTS must have five years of postgraduate training as obstetrician-gynecologists, after which they are given two to four years of structured training in all of the effective forms of treatment of gynecologic cancers (surgery, radiation therapy, chemotherapy and experimental treatments) as well as the biology and pathology of gynecologic cancer. They can be board certified through the Board of Obstetrics and Gynecology.

Gynecologic oncologists practice in a variety of settings, including teaching hospitals, CANCER CENTERS, and regional and local hospitals. A gynecologic oncologist can perform screening and the initial diagnosis of a gynecological cancer, through subsequent treatment with surgery and chemotherapy and palliative care, if necessary.

Recent studies suggest that women with OVARIAN CANCER who were treated by a gynecologic oncologist were more likely to receive the appropriate treatment than those treated by other doctors, and that women with advanced ovarian cancer lived significantly longer when treated by a gynecological oncologist. This is important because many women do not realize that their regular obstetrician-gynecologist is not trained to perform radical pelvic surgery for gynecologic cancer.

gynecologic oncology A field of medical specialization that involves the study and treatment of malignancies of the female reproductive tract, including those of the ovary, uterine lining, cervix, vulva, and vagina. Although these types of malignancies are often discussed as a group, there are many differences in cause, prevention, detection, treatment, and prognosis.

See also GYNECOLOGIC ONCOLOGIST; REPRODUCTIVE CANCER.

hair loss Known medically as alopecia, this is one of the most well-known side effects of CHEMOTHERAPY treatments often prescribed for cancer patients. The fast-growing hair follicle cells are affected by chemotherapy, causing brittle hair that breaks off at the scalp or is spontaneously released from the follicle. Although a few drugs used to treat cancer do not cause hair loss (or cause slight hair loss), most do cause partial or complete hair loss for a time.

The amount of hair lost depends on the type of drug or combination of drugs used, the dosage given, and the person's individual reaction to the drug. If hair loss is going to happen, it usually begins within a few weeks of the start of treatment, although rarely it can start within a few days. Body hair may be lost as well, and some drugs even trigger loss of the eyelashes and eyebrows; however, this loss is usually less severe, since growth is less active in these hair follicles than on the scalp.

Hair loss can profoundly affect a patient's quality of life and psychological well-being. In fact, alopecia can cause loss of self-confidence, depression, and grief reactions.

If patients do lose their hair as a result of chemotherapy, it regrows once treatment ends. However, the color or texture may be different, and hair often grows back quite curly, no matter how straight it was originally. Hair starts to grow again three to four months after hair loss.

health-care proxy A legal type of ADVANCE DIRECTIVE (also called a health-care power of attorney) that gives another person the authority to make decisions related to health care for a patient who has become unable to do so. Patients usually choose someone to be a proxy whom they trust to represent their preferences when they can no longer communicate their wishes.

A patient should be sure to ask whether this person is willing to serve as proxy, since an agent may have to exercise judgment in the event of a medical decision for which the patient's wishes are not known.

The health-care proxy is a legal document that should be signed, dated, witnessed, notarized, copied, distributed, and incorporated into the patient's medical record.

Patients may also want to appoint someone to manage their financial affairs if they cannot. This durable power of attorney for finances is a different legal document from the health-care proxy. Patients may choose different people to act as their health-care proxy and their agent in financial matters.

hereditary nonpolyposis colon cancer (HNPCC or Lynch syndrome II) A genetic colon cancer syndrome in which mutations in any one of a number of genes confers an increased lifetime risk of developing colorectal cancer and, in women, an increased risk of OVARIAN CANCER (12 percent) and ENDOMETRIAL CANCER (between 40 and 60 percent).

This syndrome caused by inherited gene mutations reduces the body's ability to repair damage to its DNA, leading to very high risks for colorectal cancer and endometrial cancer as well as a somewhat higher risk of ovarian cancer. The risk for ovarian cancer in HNPCC syndrome is much lower than for *BRCA1* or *BRCA2* gene defects. These gene mutations cause about 1 percent of all ovarian epithelial cancers.

Some individuals who have HNPCC do not have an affected parent; they have a new mutation of the gene. Once the mutation appears, however, the abnormal gene can be passed on to any children.

The vast majority of individuals who have HNPCC have cancer.

A clinical diagnosis of HNPCC is made when all of the following characteristics are present in a family:

- three or more relatives have colorectal cancer or other HNPCC-related cancer (including cancer of the endometrium, ovary, small bowel, ureter, or renal pelvis)
- cancer affects at least two successive generations
- one person with cancer is a first-degree relative of the other two
- at least one case of cancer is diagnosed in a relative under the age of 50
- a diagnosis of familial adenomatous polyposis (FAP) has been excluded
- the reported history of cancer has been verified by a pathology report

Alterations of one of five genes are now known to be responsible for most cases of HNPCC: *MSH2*, *MSH6*, and *PMS1* on chromosome 2, *MLH1* on chromosome 3, *MSH3* on chromosome 5, and *PMS2* on chromosome 7. *MLH1* and *MSH2* are the genes most commonly implicated.

The genes responsible for HNPCC are mismatch-repair genes, which correct "spelling errors" in DNA that happen during the cell division process. When these genes are altered, however, mismatches in the DNA remain. If mismatches accumulate in cell growth control genes such as TUMOR SUPPRESSOR GENES, this will eventually lead to uncontrolled and malignant cell growth. Both copies of a mismatch-repair gene must be altered before a person will develop cancer.

The first (germline) mutation is inherited from either the mother or the father and is therefore present in all cells of the body. Whether a person with a germline mutation will develop cancer—and where—depends on the cell type in which the second mutation occurs. For example, if the second mutation is in the ovary, then ovarian cancer may develop. The process of tumor development requires mutations in several growth control genes.

Loss of both copies of a particular mismatch-repair gene is just the first step in the process. What causes additional mutations is unknown but could be related to chemical, physical, or biological environmental exposures or chance errors in DNA replication.

Some people who inherit a germline mismatch-repair gene mutation never develop cancer because they never get the second mutation necessary to disturb the genetic function and trigger tumor formation. This can make cancer appear to skip generations in a family, when in reality the mutation still exists.

People with a mutation, regardless of whether they develop cancer, have a 50/50 chance of passing the mutation on to their children. Because the mismatch-repair genes responsible for HNPCC are not located on the sex chromosomes, mutations can be inherited from the mother or the father.

Other genes yet to be discovered also may cause HNPCC. Gene tests for HNPCC are available for certain people in families who have HNPCC; a family member who has HNPCC should be tested first.

Early diagnosis is important if the cancers are to be found early or prevented. When HNPCC is detected early, the chance of cure is much better. Exam guidelines for people at risk include a colonoscopy every one to three years starting at age 25, or five to 10 years before the age of earliest colorectal cancer diagnosis in family. Annual hemocult tests should begin when colonoscopy begins.

In addition to these guidelines, women should have a yearly pelvic exam with PAP TEST from age 18 (or younger if sexually active). A TRANSVAGINAL ULTRASOUND or endometrial screening with biopsy should begin at age 25 to 35 and continued yearly.

Positive HNPCC gene test finding   Women who have a positive HNPCC gene test result should have a colonoscopy every year along with following the other guidelines. In addition, other ways to prevent cancer, such as surgery, may be considered.

Negative HNPCC test finding   Women who have a negative HNPCC gene test result still require careful evaluation by a doctor and a genetic counselor to determine the best screening guidelines to follow, as the available gene test cannot detect all HNPCC-causing genes.

heredity and cancer   See GENES.

HER-2/neu gene A gene that supports the production of a protein (HER2/neu, or human epidermal growth factor receptor 2) that may help cancer cells reproduce. An OVARIAN CANCER patient who has multiple copies of the *HER-2/neu* gene may have a higher probability of recurrence.

HER-2 protein overexpression See *HER-2/NEU* GENE.

hexamethylmelamine A type of CHEMOTHERAPY drug sometimes used to treat OVARIAN CANCER.

Hill-Burton Free Hospital Care A program sponsored by the U.S. government in which certain medical facilities or hospitals must provide free or low-cost care to patients who meet certain low-income guidelines. Hill-Burton facilities also are responsible for providing emergency treatment and for treating all patients who live in the service area, regardless of race, color, national origin, creed, or Medicare or Medicaid status.

Each facility chooses the services it will provide at no or reduced cost. Services fully covered by third-party insurance or a government program such as Medicare or Medicaid are not eligible for Hill-Burton coverage. However, Hill-Burton may cover services not covered by the government programs.

Private pharmacy and private physician fees are not covered by this program, but services provided by doctors may be covered.

Hill-Burton facilities include hospitals, nursing homes, and clinics. To find local Hill-Burton facilities, patients can check the state-by-state directory listing at the Hill-Burton Web site (www.hrsa. gov/osp/dfcr). Although a facility may be listed in the directory, patients must call the facility to be certain that it has available funds and that the service desired is still covered. A patient interested in free care should apply at the admissions, business, or patient accounts office. Eligibility is based on a person's family size and income, calculated on actual income for the past 12 months (or last three months' income times 4, whichever is less). Patients may qualify if their income falls within the federal poverty guidelines, or if income is up to double (or triple for nursing home services) the poverty guidelines. Gross income includes interest and dividends

earned and child support payments, but not assets, food stamps, gifts, loans, or one-time insurance payments. (For self-employed people, income is determined after deductions for business expenses.)

Patients may apply for Hill-Burton assistance at any time before or after receiving care—even after a bill has been sent to a collection agency. If a hospital obtains a court judgment before the patient applies for Hill-Burton assistance, the solution must be worked out within the judicial system, but if patients applied for Hill-Burton before a judgment was rendered and they are found eligible, they receive Hill-Burton aid even if a judgment was given while waiting for a response to their application. The program is open to both citizens and noncitizens who have lived in the United States for at least three months.

Patients who believe they have been unfairly denied services or discriminated against should contact the Office for Civil Rights at 1-800-368-1019.

Hispanic/Latina women Cancer affects women of all racial and ethnic groups, but in unequal ways. Many of the differences in cancer incidence and mortality rates among racial and ethnic groups may be due to factors associated with social class rather than ethnicity. Socioeconomic status in particular appears to play a major role in the differences in cancer incidence and mortality rates, risk factors, and screening prevalence among racial and ethnic minorities. Moreover, studies have found that socioeconomic status more than race predicts the likelihood of a group's access to education, certain jobs, and health insurance, as well as income level and living conditions. All of these factors are associated with a person's chance of having and surviving cancer.

Of all ethnic groups, Hispanic Americans are the most likely to lack health insurance; only 43 percent of Hispanic Americans have employment-based health insurance, compared to 73 percent of whites. More often than any other group, Hispanic Americans have no regular source of health care. In addition, the low income of many Hispanic Americans as compared to that of other groups makes obtaining individual health insurance outside employer- or government-sponsored plans difficult. Even when they are eligible for

Medicaid or state-sponsored child health insurance programs, many Hispanic-American families fear that enrollment of family members in such plans could be used against them when they apply for citizenship.

Compared with Caucasian women, Hispanic-American women are three times as likely to lack health insurance, according to a 1999 study by the Commonwealth Fund. African-American and Asian-American women are twice as likely as Caucasian women to lack health insurance.

Cervical Cancer

Hispanics and Latina women have the highest incidence of cervical cancer among all racial groups in the United States (17.5 per 100,000, compared to 13.3 for African-American women, 11.7 for Asians and Pacific Islanders, 9.6 for Caucasians, and 7.7 for Native Americans and Alaskan Natives).

They have the second-highest death rate from cervical cancer (3.8 per 100,000, compared to 6.7 for African-American women and 2.8 for Caucasians).

hormonal therapy A type of treatment that prevents cancer cells from receiving the hormones they need to grow. Hormonal therapy may include the use of hormones, hormone analogs, and certain surgical techniques to treat cancer alone in combination with other hormones, or in combination with other methods of treatment.

Hormonal therapy is used to treat advanced ENDOMETRIAL CANCER, among other cancers, because this type of malignancy is usually dependent on hormones to grow and hormone therapy can be an effective way to alleviate symptoms and retard development of the disease. It may be used as a treatment if surgery is not possible or not needed. It may also be used in addition to local treatment, or as a means to ease symptoms by shrinking a painful tumor. Sometimes this type of therapy is used to prevent cancer recurrence after surgery or RADIATION THERAPY.

Hormones may often be used to treat precancerous changes of the uterus and may help the uterus shed the endometrial lining along with precancerous cells.

Several PROGESTIN drugs and regimens have been studied for the treatment of advanced or recurrent endometrial cancer. The response rate of endometrial ADENOCARCINOMAS to progestin therapy ranges from 10 percent to 50 percent in published studies. Factors that doctors look at to predict the response are tumor grade, presence of progesterone receptors, and interval from the first treatment to recurrence. Well- and moderately differentiated tumors respond more frequently to progesterone therapy than do poorly differentiated carcinomas. Hormonal therapy that includes progestins is a useful, relatively nontoxic method for the treatment of advanced endometrial adenocarcinomas. Between 20 and 30 percent of patients are likely to benefit from this treatment.

Estrogen antagonist aromatase inhibitors Endometrial cancers are known to be ESTROGEN dependent, and women who have high levels of estrogen are at risk for the development of endometrial cancer. In postmenopausal women, the conversion of testosterone into estrogen in fat tissue by the aromatase enzyme is an important source of estrogen; it is thought that inhibition of this conversion may be an effective manner of treating endometrial cancers. Several such agents that competitively inhibit or inactivate the enzymes needed for the conversion of testosterone to estrogen have been developed. To date, most studies have investigated the use of these agents in the treatment of breast cancer. These aromatase inhibitors are also being evaluated for their value in treating endometrial cancer. TAMOXIFEN is known to inhibit the growth of estrogen-receptor-positive breast cancers. The use of tamoxifen for recurrent or advanced endometrial cancer can result in occasional durable responses and a significant incidence of disease stabilization. The objective response rate to tamoxifen in several studies is 20 percent to 60 percent, with occasional long-term survivors. Although tamoxifen may occasionally be of some benefit to a patient who has advanced or recurrent endometrial cancer, patients for whom initial hormonal therapy with a progestational agent has failed are unlikely to have a durable response.

hormone replacement therapy (HRT) A type of therapy that combines ESTROGEN and PROGESTIN to provide women with the female HORMONES that decrease as they age. When the hormone estrogen is given alone, it is usually referred to as ESTROGEN REPLACEMENT THERAPY.

Estrogen is a female hormone that brings about changes in several organs in the body, whereas progesterone is a female hormone that specifically affects the uterus, preparing it each month for a pregnancy. During the transition to menopause, these hormone levels begin to fluctuate, causing some uncomfortable symptoms such as hot flashes, sweats, and disturbed sleep. Eventually, the ovaries completely stop producing estrogen and progesterone, and the woman's menstrual periods cease—she experiences menopause. Hormone therapy has been used in the past to relieve the short-term symptoms of menopause and to help prevent or alleviate a higher rate of bone loss.

There are some significant long-term risks, including an increased risk of some cancers. When estrogen is taken alone, it raises the risk of ENDOMETRIAL CANCER (cancer in the lining of the uterus). Adding progestin to estrogen can dramatically reduce this risk. Progestin is added to prevent the overgrowth (HYPERPLASIA) of cells in the lining of the uterus; therefore, women who have an intact uterus are generally given this combined therapy.

However, the National Institutes of Health's Women's Health Initiative (WHI) stopped a major clinical trial of HRT early, in 2002, as a result of the discovery of an increased risk of invasive breast cancer from HRT. The increased risk of breast cancer appeared after four years of hormone use. After 5.2 years, estrogen-plus-progestin use resulted in a 26 percent increase in the risk of breast cancer—or eight more breast cancers each year for every 10,000 women. Women who had used estrogen plus progestin before entering the study were more likely than others to have breast cancer, an indication that the therapy may have a cumulative effect.

Research released in 2004 also found that women who took estrogen alone after menopause had a significantly increased risk of stroke and possibly a higher risk of dementia too, according to the National Institutes of Health. For many years, doctors had thought that using estrogen (alone or together with progestin) would keep women healthier after menopause by reducing heart attacks and keeping the brain sharp.

As a result, the NIH decided to stop the last major estrogen-only study a year before its planned completion because sufficient data had been collected to assess overall risks and benefits. The government noted that estrogen alone does not have as many serious effects as when it is combined with progestin, but officials still advise that estrogen continues to be too risky for long-term use.

However, estrogen alone did not increase the risk of breast cancer, which was a surprise to researchers because the estrogen-progestin combination had increased that risk by 26 percent.

In stopping the study, the government revealed that estrogen alone increased the risk of a stroke as much as combination estrogen-progestin does. For every 10,000 women, those taking hormones suffer eight more strokes per year than nonhormone users. At the same time, estrogen alone had no effect on heart disease. (In contrast, the estrogen-progestin combination increases heart attack risk by 29 percent.)

Neither type of hormone therapy seems good for women's brains. Preliminary data from a related study of women 65 and older suggest those taking estrogen alone were more likely to suffer some degree of dementia than those taking a placebo. Likewise, scientists announced in 2003 that the estrogen-progestin combination doubled the risk of Alzheimer's and other forms of dementia. Estrogen (and estrogen-progestin) decrease the risk of a hip fracture from bone-thinning osteoporosis, although only women who cannot take one of the nation's many other osteoporosis treatments should consider estrogen for that use, according to the government.

Data from the Postmenopausal Estrogen/Progestin Interventions trial at the NCI indicate that about 25 percent of women who use combined HRT have an increase in breast density found on their mammograms, compared to about 8 percent of women who take estrogen alone. One study showed that stopping HRT for about two weeks before having a mammogram improved its readability, but more research is needed to confirm the usefulness of this approach.

Women who are still taking HRT should watch for dangerous symptoms, such as abnormal bleeding, breast lumps, shortness of breath, dizziness, severe headaches, or chest pain.

hormones   A chemical produced in the body that runs the activity of another organ or cell. Many hormones are believed to stimulate the growth of a variety of cancers.

hospice   A concept rather than a place, which focuses on a holistic model of services designed neither to hasten nor to postpone death, but rather to make a patient's final days as positive and symptom-free as possible. The concept of hospice is based on a philosophy of caring that respects and values the dignity and worth of each person. Although hospices care for people approaching death, they cherish and emphasize life by helping patients and their families live each day to the fullest. There are almost 3,000 hospice and palliative care organizations in the United States. Hospice services, which are most often provided to terminally ill patients living at home, can also be provided to a patient in a nursing home; the patient would receive visits from hospice nurses, home health aides, chaplains, social workers, and volunteers, in addition to other care and services provided by the nursing home.

A few hospice programs have their own facilities or have arrangements with freestanding hospice houses, hospitals, or inpatient residential centers to care for patients who cannot reside in a private residence. These patients may require an alternative place to live during this final phase of their life when they need extra care.

The modern American hospice movement began in 1974 when the Connecticut Hospice was established in New Haven. It was founded on a care model outlined by Dame Cicely Saunders, M.D., who opened the Saint Christopher's Hospice in 1967 in Sydenham, England. This center became the model for hospice care around the world.

How It Works

Hospice care usually starts as soon as a formal referral is made by the patient's doctor. Often a hospice program representative tries to visit the patient on the day the referral is made; in any case, care is ready to begin within a day or two of a referral.

Typically, a family member serves as the primary caregiver and, when appropriate, helps make decisions for the terminally ill individual. Hospice is a medical benefit covered by most insurance plans, enabling patients to live at home at the end of their life and receive care from an integrated hospice team of nurses, medical social workers, physical and occupational therapists, nutritionists, home aid workers, pastoral counselors, and trained volunteers.

Patients can continue to be treated by their own physician or by the hospice physician. If the hospice patient chooses to have the family doctor involved in the medical care, both the patient's physician and the hospice medical director may work together to coordinate the patient's medical care, especially when managing symptoms is difficult.

Members of the hospice staff make regular visits to assess the patient and provide additional care or other services and are on call 24 hours a day, seven days a week. Every hospice patient can take advantage of services offered by a registered nurse, social worker, home health aide, and chaplain. Typically, full-time registered nurses provide care to about 12 different families, and social workers usually handle about twice that number. If needed, home health aides who can provide personal care to the patient visit most often, but all visits are subject to the needs described in the care plan and to the condition of the patient during the course of the illness. The availability and frequency of spiritual care generally depend on the family's request.

In addition, hospice volunteers enhance quality of life and ease the burden of caregiving. Volunteers usually can provide different types of support to patients and their family, including running errands, preparing light meals, staying with a patient to give family members a break, lending emotional support and companionship, and helping out with light housekeeping.

Care Plan

The hospice team develops a care plan that meets the patient's individual needs for pain management and symptom control and outlines the medical and support services required such as nursing care, personal care (dressing, bathing), social services, physician visits, counseling, and homemaker services. It also identifies the medical equipment, tests, procedures, medication, and treatments necessary to provide high-quality comfort care.

While patients are at home, all necessary symptom-relieving medications are provided by hospice workers, along with any necessary special medical equipment. In emergencies, hospice workers take patients to a hospital or hospice inpatient unit designed to be as homelike as possible. Inpatient respite care is also available to provide a break for families.

Other Services

Besides medical aid, hospice workers help patients with practical support (such as shopping) and emotional support, including life closure, grief, and spiritual counseling. Depending on the hospice's resources, it may also provide other services such as art, touch, and music therapy.

Paying for Hospice

MEDICARE, private health insurance, and Medicaid (in 43 states) cover hospice care for patients who meet eligibility criteria. As with any health-care program, there may be copayments and deductibles that families pay to receive care, but many hospices also rely on community support for donations. Each hospice has its own policies about payment, but traditionally hospice offers services on the basis of need rather than the ability to pay.

Hospice care is available as a benefit under Medicare Part A, which is designed to give patients who have terminal illness and their families special support and services not otherwise covered by Medicare. Under the Medicare Hospice Benefit, beneficiaries choose to receive noncurative treatment and services for their terminal illness by waiving the standard Medicare benefits for treatment of a terminal illness. However, the beneficiary may continue to access standard Medicare benefits for treatment of conditions unrelated to the terminal illness. Medicare law states that to qualify for hospice care, a patient must have "a medical prognosis that life expectancy is six months or less if the illness runs its normal course." However, it is difficult to predict the length of time left to a cancer patient, and beneficiaries are not restricted to six months of coverage by hospice rules.

Finding a Program

Patients and families can obtain information about local hospices from health-care professionals, social workers, clergy, counselors, their local or state Office on Aging or senior centers, health-related Web sites, or the yellow pages. Alternatively, patients may contact the NATIONAL HOSPICE AND PALLIATIVE CARE ORGANIZATION, which represents most hospice programs in the United States.

See also HOSPICE EDUCATION INSTITUTE; HOSPICE FOUNDATION OF AMERICA; HOSPICELINK.

Hospice Education Institute An independent nonprofit organization, founded in 1985, that serves a wide range of individuals and organizations interested in improving and expanding HOSPICE and palliative care throughout the United States and around the world. The institute works to inform, educate, and support people who are seeking or providing care for the dying and the bereaved or those coping with loss or advanced illness.

The institute offers seminars, books, and pamphlets. It also offers a range of programs, plus HOSPICELINK, which maintains a directory of hospice programs; and a program offering small gifts to patients and families. For contact information, see Appendix I.

Hospice Foundation of America A nonprofit organization that promotes HOSPICE care and educates professionals and those they serve about care giving, terminal illness, loss, and bereavement. The foundation provides leadership in the development and application of hospice and its philosophy of care. Hospice Foundation, Inc., was chartered in 1982 as a way to help raise money for hospices operating in South Florida, before passage of the MEDICARE hospice benefit. In 1990, the foundation expanded its scope to a national level in order to provide leadership in the entire spectrum of end-of-life issues.

To reflect its national scope more accurately, in 1992 the foundation opened a Washington, D.C., office and in 1994 it changed its name to *Hospice Foundation of America.* For contact information, see Appendix I.

HOSPICELINK A service offered by the HOSPICE EDUCATION INSTITUTE that maintains a computerized directory of all hospice and palliative care programs in the United States. The toll-free telephone number (800-331-1620) provides referrals to hospice and palliative care programs as well as general information about the principles and practices of good hospice and palliative care. For contact information, see Appendix I.

hot flashes   A sensation of heat and flushing that occurs suddenly during perimenopause and during treatment with some medications. The cause of hot flashes in association with HORMONE THERAPY is not well understood, but they appear to be linked to sudden drop in hormone level and the effect of hormones on blood vessels.

There are different treatments for the hot flashes associated with hormone therapy. Medications include the blood pressure medicine clonidine (Catapres), the hormones megestrol acetate (Megace), and medroxyprogesterone acetate (Provera or Depo-Provera), the antidepressant venlafaxine, and DIETHYLSTILBESTROL. Limiting caffeine use and avoiding very warm temperatures and excessive exercise may also help minimize hot flashes.

human papillomavirus (HPV)   A virus that causes the common wart on hands and feet as well as warts in the genital area. Infection by human papillomavirus is one of the most important avoidable risk factors for CERVICAL CANCER. Women who are infected by HPV have a significantly higher risk of development of low- and high-grade cervical lesions than women who are not.

Types of HPV
HPVs are a group of more than 100 types of viruses called papillomaviruses because they can cause warts (papillomas). More than 30 types of HPV are transmitted through sexual contact, and about half of these have been linked to cancer. Different HPV types cause different types of warts in different parts of the body, and HPV infections cause symptoms in some but not all patients. Some types cause common warts on the hands and feet, lips, or tongue; certain other HPV types can infect the genitals and the anal area. For years HPV has been recognized as the major cause of cancer of the cervix, but it also has been associated with some cancers of the vulva and vagina, as well as with cancers of the

anus, penis, and middle throat (including the base of the tongue and the tonsils).

Low-risk infections   Most genital warts are caused by two sexually transmitted HPV types, HPV-6 and HPV-11, but these rarely develop into cancer and are called low-risk viruses. The warts may appear within weeks of sexual contact with an HPV-infected person or may appear years later, or not at all.

High-risk infections   Other sexually transmitted HPVs have been linked with genital cancers in women. These high-risk HPV types (HPV-16, HPV-18, HPV-31, HPV-33, HPV-35, and HPV-45) can cause growths that are usually flat and difficult to see and can lead to the development of cancer. A test for the viral DNA in the affected tissue can reveal the type of HPV that is present.

HPV and Cancer
In women, certain types of HPV infection can cause abnormal changes in the outermost layer of cells (epithelium) covering the cervix. These abnormal cells are called squamous intraepithelial lesions (SILs) (or DYSPLASIA or cervical intraepithelial neoplasia). Although they are not malignant, they can continue to change and turn into cancer later in life. SILs can be detected by a PAP TEST performed during a GYNECOLOGICAL EXAMINATION.

Many low-grade dysplasias fade away and become normal over a period of months or years. In these patients, the Pap test result may become normal, and the HPV is considered to be latent or possibly eliminated by the patient's immune system. It is believed that a latent infection can be reactivated years after initial exposure to HPV.

In patients who have cervical cancer, the HPV persists or is reactivated, and the SILs progress over many years, becoming increasingly abnormal and invading deeper and deeper levels of the epithelium. High-grade SILs include abnormal cells that extend through the full thickness of the epithelium, also known as CARCINOMA IN SITU—an early form of cervical cancer.

The mechanism by which HPV transforms a cell into a malignancy is probably controlled by two viral genes (*E6* and *E7*) in HPV-infected cells. The *E6* and *E7* proteins bind to and inactivate the host cell's TUMOR SUPPRESSOR GENE, leading to uncontrolled growth.

Risk Factors

Risk factors for HPV infection (and thus for cervical cancer) include initiation of sexual activity at an early age (before age 16), multiple sexual partners, sex with a partner who has had multiple partners, and unprotected sex at any age. Infection with a high-risk type of HPV such as HPV-16 increases the risk of development of the abnormal cells (SILs) caused by HPV into cancer. Smoking, use of oral contraceptives, infection with other sexually transmitted diseases or with the human immunodeficiency virus (HIV), or birth of many children may act together with HPV in some way to increase the probability that abnormal cells will lead to cancer.

Symptoms

When HPV infects the skin of the external genital organs and the anal area, the virus often causes raised bumpy warts that range from barely visible to several inches across.

Diagnosis

A patient whose Pap test finding is abnormal is referred for COLPOSCOPY (examination of the cervix and vagina with a magnifying instrument). The doctor takes BIOPSY specimens from abnormal areas, and the tissue is examined to determine the grade of the abnormality and detect the presence of cancer.

New tests that can directly identify the DNA from HPVs and identify the exact HPV type that is causing an infection are available. However, it is not clear how treatment would be affected by knowing the exact type of HPV. HPV testing and typing are not presently routinely recommended, and most health-care providers do not do this testing.

There is a promising new test for HPV now being developed, although it has not yet been approved by the U.S. Food and Drug Administration for use as a screening tool. If approved, this test eventually could be useful in detecting early cervical cancer in women older than 30 years of age.

Treatment

There is currently no cure for human papillomavirus infection, but the warts and abnormal cell growth caused by these viruses can be effectively destroyed, to prevent them from developing into cancer.

A high-grade SIL may be treated with a laser, LOOP ELECTROSURGICAL EXCISION PROCEDURE, cryosurgery, surgical excision (including CONE BIOPSY), or CHEMOTHERAPY. Genital warts may be treated with some of these same procedures.

hydatidiform mole   A tumorous growth of tissue that develops after a miscarriage or a full-term pregnancy. The growth most often develops from a fertilized egg as an independent abnormal growth or from placental or afterbirth tissue.

Although most hydatidiform moles are benign, 15 percent can become malignant and burrow into the wall of the uterus, where they can cause serious bleeding. Another 5 percent develop into fast-growing cancers called CHORIOCARCINOMAS. Some of these tumors spread very quickly outside the uterus to other parts of the body. Fortunately, cancer development from these moles is rare and highly curable.

In the United States, these growths occur in about one of every 1,500 pregnancies, and are nearly 10 times more common among Asian women. In fact, in Asia the incidence may be as high as 1 in 200. A hydatidiform mole (*hydatid* means "drop of water" and *mole* means "spot") is most likely to occur in younger and older women (especially after age 45) than in those between ages 20 and 40. About 1 percent to 2 percent of the time a woman who has had one molar pregnancy has a second one.

Symptoms

Hydatidiform moles often become apparent shortly after conception. Women who have a hydatidiform mole have a positive pregnancy test result and often believe they have a normal pregnancy for the first three or four months. However, in these cases the uterus grows abnormally fast. By the end of the third month (if not earlier) the woman experiences vaginal bleeding ranging from scant spotting to excessive bleeding. She may have hyperthyroidism (overproduction of thyroid hormones, which causes symptoms such as weight loss, increased appetite, and intolerance to heat). Sometimes, the grapelike cluster of cells itself is shed with the blood during this time. Other symptoms may include severe nausea and vomiting and high blood pressure. As the pregnancy progresses, the fetus does not move and there is no fetal heartbeat.

Symptoms of severe nausea and vomiting with vaginal bleeding indicate the need for immediate medical attention. Even benign hydatidiform moles can cause serious complications, including infections, bleeding, and toxemia of pregnancy.

Diagnosis

Previously, the physician might not have suspected a molar pregnancy until after the third month or later, when the absence of a fetal heartbeat together with bleeding and severe nausea and vomiting indicates something is wrong. With recent increase of early ultrasounds during pregnancy, however, moles are now diagnosed much earlier.

If a mole is observed on ultrasound, the physician then checks the level of human chorionic gonadotropin (hCG), a hormone that is normally produced by both a placenta and a mole. Abnormally high levels of hCG together with the symptoms of vaginal bleeding, lack of fetal heartbeat, and an unusually large uterus all indicate a molar pregnancy. An ultrasound of the uterus to make sure there is no living fetus confirms the diagnosis.

As the mole decays, small bits of the material may pass through the vagina. The diagnosis can be confirmed by examining this material under a microscope.

Treatment

It is extremely important to make sure that all of the mole is removed from the uterus, since the tissue is potentially cancerous, by performing a D&C.

Alternatively, a vacuum aspiration can be performed to remove it. In a procedure similar to a dilation and curettage, a woman is given an anesthetic, her cervix is dilated, and the contents of the uterus are gently suctioned out. After most of the mole has been removed, gentle scraping of the uterine lining is usually performed.

Only rarely is HYSTERECTOMY required. If the woman is older and does not want more children, the doctor may choose to remove the uterus instead of performing a vacuum aspiration because of the higher risk in this age group that a cancerous mole will recur.

Because of the cancer risk, the physician continues to monitor the patient for at least two months after the end of a molar pregnancy. The hCG level is measured to make sure the mole was completely removed. When removal is complete, the level returns to normal within eight weeks and remains normal. However, if a woman who has had a mole removed becomes pregnant soon thereafter, interpretation of a high hCG level becomes difficult because it could be caused by the pregnancy or by part of the mole that was not removed. This is why women who have had a mole removed are advised not to become pregnant for six months.

Malignant moles require CHEMOTHERAPY, usually including Methotrexate, DACTINOMYCIN, or a combination of these drugs. If the cancer has spread to other parts of the body, RADIATION THERAPY is added. Specific treatment depends on how advanced the cancer is.

The cure rate is virtually 100 percent for women whose disease is less advanced and about 85 percent for women whose disease has spread widely. Most women are still able to have children after treatment.

hyperplasia   Enlargement of an organ or tissue caused by an increase in the number of constituent cells.

See also ENDOMETRIAL HYPERPLASIA.

hysterectomy   An operation in which a woman's uterus is removed; sometimes the fallopian tubes, ovaries, and cervix are also removed at the same time. Hysterectomy is the second most common major surgery among women in the United States, after cesarean section delivery. Each year, more than 600,000 hysterectomies are done, and about a third of women in the United States have had a hysterectomy by age 60.

Cancers affecting the pelvic organs account for only about 10 percent of all hysterectomies. ENDOMETRIAL CANCER (cancer of the lining of the uterus), UTERINE SARCOMA, CERVICAL CANCER, OVARIAN CANCER, and FALLOPIAN TUBE CANCER often require hysterectomy. Depending on the type and extent of the cancer, other kinds of treatment such as radiation or HORMONAL THERAPY may be used as well.

There are several types of hysterectomy:

- *Complete or total hysterectomy.* This is the most common type of hysterectomy, in which both the cervix and the uterus are removed.

- *Partial or subtotal hysterectomy (supracervical hysterectomy).* This is a procedure in which the doctor removes the upper part of the uterus and leaves the cervix in place.

- *Radical hysterectomy.* This is removal of the uterus, cervix, upper part of the vagina, and supporting tissues. This is done in some cases of cancer.

A bilateral SALPINGO-OOPHORECTOMY is a procedure in which both ovaries and both fallopian tubes are removed at the same time as the uterus. If a woman's ovaries are removed before she reaches menopause, the sudden loss of her main source of female hormones causes her to enter menopause suddenly (surgical menopause). This condition can cause more severe symptoms than a natural menopause.

The uterus may be removed through an incision in either the abdomen (abdominal hysterectomy) or the vagina (vaginal hysterectomy). Sometimes an instrument called a laparoscope is used for a better view of the inside of the abdomen. The choice of surgical technique depends on the reason for the surgery. Abdominal hysterectomies are more common than vaginal hysterectomies and usually require a longer recovery time.

Side Effects

Some women suffer serious complications of hysterectomy, including reactions to anesthetics, pain, infection, bleeding, and fatigue. Sometimes other pelvic organs such as the bladder and bowel are injured during a hysterectomy. Hysterectomy is also linked to urinary incontinence, loss of ovarian function, and early menopause. Some women experience depression and sexual dysfunction after hysterectomy.

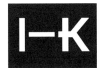

immune system A body system that plays a critical role in controlling cancerous cell development in addition to attacking and killing a range of foreign substances such as viruses and bacteria. The immune system attacks cancer cells not because they are foreign—they are not—but because the cells' biological function has gone awry so that it cannot respond to the body's normal methods of controlling cell growth and reproduction. As a result, the abnormal cells continue to grow, and their growth leads to cancer. This is why cancer is 100 times more likely to occur in people who take drugs that suppress the immune system (such as those who have had organ transplantation) than in people who have a normal immune system.

Most of the time, the body is protected against cancer by immune system cells, which can detect the appearance of tumor antigens on cancer cells; these antigens attract the attention of certain kinds of white blood cells that are responsible for destroying cancer cells.

An antigen is a foreign substance that the body's immune system recognizes and targets for destruction. Antigens are found on the surface of all cells; when a cell becomes cancerous, new antigens that the immune system does not recognize suddenly appear on the cell's surface. With luck, the immune system may regard these new "tumor antigens" as foreign and may be able to contain or destroy the cancer cells. Unfortunately, even a very healthy immune system cannot always destroy every cancer cell.

So far, tumor antigens have been identified in several types of cancer, including malignant melanoma, bone cancer, and some stomach cancers. People who have these cancers may have antibodies against the tumor antigens, but the antigens generally do not trigger a strong enough immune response to control the cancer. For some reason, the immune system's antibodies do not seem to be able to destroy the cancer; sometimes, they even seem to stimulate the tumor's growth.

Certain tumor antigens can be used to help diagnose cancer, however. Antigens released into the bloodstream by some cancers can be detected with blood tests; in this case, they are called tumor markers because their presence in the blood indicates that a tumor is growing. Scientists are trying to determine whether tumor markers can be used to screen healthy people for cancer. Because the tests are expensive and not very specific, their routine use is not recommended. On the other hand, tumor markers are quite valuable in both diagnosis and treatment of cancer. Blood tests can help determine whether a cancer treatment is effective, because after treatment if the tumor marker no longer appears in the blood, it is reasonable to assume that the cancerous cells are gone. If the marker disappears and later reappears, the doctor assumes the cancer has probably returned.

Alpha-fetoprotein (AFP) normally produced by fetal liver cells is also found in the blood of people with certain types of germ cell cancers.

Human chorionic gonadotropin (hCG) is a hormone produced during pregnancy that also appears in various types of cancer. Beta-hCG is a very sensitive tumor marker used to monitor the effects of treatment.

incisional biopsy A procedure in which a surgeon removes a sample of a lump or suspicious area, and a pathologist then examines the tissue under a microscope to check for cancer cells. This method is less aggressive than an *excisional biopsy*, in which the surgeon removes all of a lump or suspicious area, plus an area of healthy tissue around the edges.

Indian Health Service (IHS)   A program of the U.S. Department of Health and Human Services that provides hospital and ambulatory medical care as well as preventive and rehabilitative health-care services for Native Americans and Alaska Natives who are members of a federally recognized tribe.

The provision of health services to members of federally recognized tribes grew out of the government-to-government relationship between the federal government and Native American tribes. This relationship, established in 1787, is based on the Constitution and has been given form and substance by numerous treaties, laws, Supreme Court decisions, and Executive Orders. The IHS is the principal federal health-care provider and health advocate for Native Americans. Its goal is to raise the health status of about 1.5 million Native Americans and Alaska Natives, who are members of more than 557 federally recognized tribes in 35 states, to the highest possible level. For contact information, see Appendix I.

See also NATIVE AMERICAN/ALASKA-NATIVE WOMEN.

infertility and cancer   Cancer survivors typically have more problems conceiving a child than do women who have never had cancer. Birth rates among cancer survivors are only 40 percent to 85 percent those of the general population. Today, as millions of women of childbearing age are surviving cancer, the question of reproduction is arising as a paramount consideration in planning treatment, since both CHEMOTHERAPY and RADIATION THERAPY can harm egg and sperm cells.

The more closely radiation treatments are localized to a woman's reproductive organs, the higher the risk for infertility.

Cancer treatment may cause genetic damage to sperm cells exposed to chemotherapy or radiation therapy for up to two years after treatment; that is why experts recommend that women use birth control during this time. After two years, rates of

birth defects in children born after a woman's cancer treatment appear to be similar to those of the general population. No unusual cancer risk has been identified in the children of cancer survivors in families who carry genetic cancer syndromes such as the BRCA gene mutations.

infusion pump   A device that delivers a constant flow of CHEMOTHERAPY drugs or pain medication. Infusion pumps are especially useful for drugs that must not be administered too quickly.

Institutional Review Board   A group of scientists, doctors, and consumers who oversee the protocols for clinical trials. The review board is designed to protect patients who take part in studies and must review and approve the protocols for all clinical trials funded by the U.S. federal government. The board ensures that a study is well designed, does not involve undue risks, and includes safeguards for patients.

insurance coverage   The cost of treating cancer can be high, but health insurance plans usually cover much of the cost. Patients who belong to a health maintenance organization (HMO) or preferred provider organization (PPO) should become familiar with their provider choices and their financial responsibility if they receive care "out of network" from a doctor not covered by the health plan.

Testing Coverage

Most health insurance plans, including MEDICARE, cover PAP TESTS and others for patients over age 50.

Uninsured Patients

Cancer patients who do not have insurance should contact the local Social Security office to determine whether they qualify for Supplemental Security Income (SSI) or SOCIAL SECURITY DISABILITY INSURANCE (SSDI). The medical requirements and disability determination process are the same in both programs. However, whereas eligibility for SSDI is based on employment history, SSI eligibility is based on financial need.

Cancer patients who do not have insurance can also receive care from hospitals who receive federal grants from Hill-Burton Funds, which allow hospitals and nursing homes to provide low-cost or no-cost medical care. To receive a listing of hospitals or nursing homes that participate in the Hill-Burton program, patients can call (800) 638-0742.

See also FINANCIAL ISSUES.

Intercultural Cancer Council (ICC) A nonprofit group that promotes policies, programs, partnerships, and research to eliminate the unequal access to cancer care among racial and ethnic minorities and medically underserved populations in the United States and its associated territories.

The council believes that all Americans need equal access to cancer prevention, detection, diagnosis, treatment, rehabilitation, mental health, and long-term care services. In addition, it believes that minorities ought to have major roles in developing health policies and programs intended for their community. The council supports the development of culturally appropriate literature and new programs to promote educational efforts to counteract ignorance and overcome fears.

The council also tries to ensure that diverse populations are fully represented in clinical studies and research supported by public and private sector funds, which requires third-party coverage of patient-care costs associated with these trials, including maximum cooperation from managed-care systems.

International Cancer Alliance A nonprofit organization that provides cancer information to patients and doctors on a person-to-person basis. The organization has developed several unique patient-centered programs through an extensive process of collection, evaluation, and dissemination of information, putting the cancer patient in contact with top physicians and scientists around the world. This organization is operated by a network of people that includes scientists, clinicians, staff, and lay volunteers, many of whom are patients themselves. For contact information, see Appendix I.

International Federation of Gynecology and Obstetrics An international professional organization that developed the most commonly used staging system for many types of cancer. In this system, numerals from 0 (the least serious or earliest stage) to IV (the most serious or advanced stage) represent the different stages of a cancer.

International Union Against Cancer (IUAC) Nonprofit group devoted exclusively to all aspects of the worldwide fight against cancer. Its objectives are to advance scientific and medical knowledge in research, diagnosis, treatment, and prevention of cancer and to promote all other aspects of the campaign against cancer throughout the world. Particular emphasis is placed on professional and public education. IUAC is an independent association of more than 290 member organizations in about 85 countries. Members are voluntary cancer leagues and societies, cancer research and/or treatment centers, and, in some countries, ministries of health. For contact information, see Appendix I.

investigational new drug A drug allowed by the Food and Drug Administration to be used in clinical trials, but not yet approved for sale to the general public.

isoflavones Plant compounds found in SOY PRODUCTS and clover that may help prevent cancer. Isoflavones are also known as PHYTOESTROGENS because they are similar in chemical shape and properties to the human hormone ESTROGEN, though less potent.

Studies on the effects of isoflavones show complex and sometimes contradictory results. Effects depend in part on the number of estrogen receptors and the level of human estrogen in the body. In addition, isoflavones work differently in different parts of the body. Most significantly, isoflavones may mimic human estrogen—but they may also block human estrogen, and thus alter its effects. They are also believed to work differently in premenopausal women than they do in postmenopausal women.

Research suggests that eating soy products may decrease the risk of breast cancer, and perhaps of ENDOMETRIAL CANCER, in premenopausal women. Dietary isoflavones can affect menstrual cycle length, which is one of the risk factors for breast cancer. Some experts believe that Asian women have a lower risk for breast cancer because they have longer menstrual cycles and lower estrogen blood concentrations.

Animal studies also suggest that isoflavones are natural anticancer agents that are involved in regulating cell growth as well as cell death. On the other hand, there is little proof that soy intake decreases the risk of breast cancer in post-menopausal women.

Soy Products

There are many soy products on the market, including soy milk, soy nuts, tofu (soybean curd), and tempeh, but not all soy foods contain isoflavones. Soy foods that are made from soy protein concentrate may contain little or no isoflavone. Experts recommend that patients consume 30 to 50 mg of isoflavones each day to reduce risk of cancer. The following are estimated accounts of isoflavones in soy products:

- Soy milk: 30 mg isoflavones in eight ounces
- Soy nuts: 60 mg isoflavones in one-fourth cup
- Tempeh: 35 mg isoflavones in one-fourth cup
- Tofu: 35 mg isoflavones in one-half cup

Consumers should read labels to learn the actual amount of isoflavones in a given product.

Contraindications

Consumers should also understand that soy foods and isoflavone extracts (pills or tablets) are not the same. Although there is little danger of overdosage of soy foods, experts do not know the safe maximum dosage for isoflavone supplements.

High isoflavone intake (about 50 grams of soy protein per day) may help relieve hot flashes and night sweats in the short term (two years or less), according to the American College of Obstetricians. But although isoflavones are safe when eaten in normal dietary amounts, consumption of extraordinary amounts of soy and isoflavone supplements may interact with estrogen and may be harmful to women who have a history of estrogen-dependent breast cancer and possibly to other high-risk women as well.

2IT-BAD monoclonal antibody 170 A type of MONOCLONAL ANTIBODY used in cancer detection or therapy. Monoclonal antibodies are laboratory-produced substances that can locate and bind to cancer cells.

Japanese women See ASIAN WOMEN.

killer cell A type of white blood cell that attacks tumor cells and body cells that have been invaded by foreign substances.

Laetrile A purified form of the chemical amygdalin, a substance found in the pits of many fruits and in numerous plants, which some people have used as a cancer treatment. However, Laetrile has exhibited little anticancer activity in animal studies and no anticancer activity in human clinical trials. It is not approved for use in the United States.

Used as a poison in ancient Egypt, Laetrile was first used in Russia in 1845, and in the United States in the 1920s. Some people thought that the cyanide contained in Laetrile might fight cancer. In the 1970s, Laetrile gained popularity as an anticancer agent, and by 1978 more than 70,000 individuals in the United States were reported to have been treated with it.

laparoscopy A type of surgical procedure in which a small incision is made (usually in the navel) and through it a viewing tube (laparoscope) is inserted. The viewing tube has a small camera on the eyepiece, which allows a doctor to examine the reproductive organs on a video monitor connected to the tube. Other small incisions can be made to insert instruments to perform a variety of procedures. A laparoscopy can be done to diagnose conditions or to perform certain types of operations. It is less invasive than regular open abdominal surgery, which is called LAPAROTOMY.

Laparoscopy has been a popular diagnostic and treatment tool since the late 1980s, although the technique dates to 1901, when it was reportedly first used in a gynecologic procedure performed in Russia. Gynecologists were the first to use laparoscopy to diagnose and treat conditions of the uterus, fallopian tubes, and ovaries.

Laparoscopy plays a role in the diagnosis, staging, and treatment of a variety of cancers; however, the use of laparoscopy instead of open surgery for the complete removal of cancerous growths and surrounding tissues is controversial. Experts are not sure whether it is as effective as open surgery for complex operations. Laparoscopy is also being investigated as a screening tool for OVARIAN CANCER.

As a diagnostic procedure, laparoscopy is useful in taking BIOPSY of specimens as well as LYMPH NODE growths in the reproductive system. It can be used to determine the cause of pelvic pain or gynecological symptoms that cannot be confirmed by a physical exam or ultrasound.

Laparoscopic surgery is also used on a limited basis to remove cancerous tumors, surrounding tissues, and lymph nodes. Compared to open abdominal surgery, laparoscopy usually entails less pain, less risk, less scarring, and faster recovery. Because laparoscopy is much less invasive than traditional abdominal surgery, patients can leave the hospital sooner.

Procedure

Laparoscopy is a surgical procedure that is done in a hospital with anesthesia. Local anesthesia is sometimes used for biopsy and diagnosis; in operative procedures, general anesthesia is required. After the patient is anesthetized, a hollow needle is inserted into the abdomen in or near the navel, and carbon dioxide gas is pumped through the needle to expand the abdomen and give the surgeon a better view of the internal organs. The laparoscope is then inserted through this incision. The image from the camera attached to the end of the laparoscope is seen on a video monitor. Sometimes, additional small incisions are made to insert other instruments that are used to lift the tubes and ovaries for examination or to perform surgical procedures. If there are no complications, the patient may leave the hospital within four to eight hours. (Traditional abdominal surgery requires a hospital stay of several days.)

There may be some slight pain or throbbing at the incision sites in the first day or so after the procedure, and the gas that is used to expand the abdomen may cause discomfort under the ribs or in the shoulder for a few days. Depending on the reason for the laparoscopy in gynecological procedures, some women may experience vaginal bleeding. Many patients can return to work within a week of surgery, and most are back to work within two weeks.

Risk Factors

Laparoscopy is a relatively safe procedure, especially if the physician is experienced in the technique. The procedure carries a slight risk of puncturing a blood vessel or organ; and puncture could cause blood to seep into the abdominal cavity. Puncturing the intestines could allow intestinal contents to seep into the cavity. These are serious complications, and major surgery may be required to correct such problems. The rate of serious complications is only 0.2 percent. In some cases, laparoscopy may not be sufficient and standard surgery may be required.

Laparoscopy is generally not used for patients who have certain heart or lung conditions or for those who have some intestinal disorders, such as bowel obstruction.

laparotomy Surgery in which the abdomen is opened. The size, shape, and location of the actual incision vary with the type of surgery and the doctor's preference. Laparotomy is always performed with general anesthesia and is considered major surgery. It is used to diagnose and/or treat a variety of gynecologic cancers.

Laparotomy is often employed when the surgeon needs a more extensive view of the operating field. It is a far more extensive surgery than LAPAROSCOPY, a newer, alternate technique that involves smaller incisions and a shorter recovery time. (However, laparoscopy is not always appropriate.)

Sometimes either laparotomy or laparoscopy can be used to correct a condition. The choice of surgical technique may depend on the physician's training or preference and the particular needs of the patient.

lasers and cancer A treatment method that uses high-intensity light to destroy premalignant or malignant cells. The term *laser* stands for *light amplification by stimulated emission of radiation.* Whereas ordinary light occurs in many wavelengths and spreads in all directions, laser light is focused in a narrow high-energy beam. So powerful that it can cut through steel, a laser also can be used for precise surgical work. Lasers can treat cancer by shrinking or destroying a tumor with heat or by activating a photosensitizing agent that destroys cancer cells. It is a standard treatment for certain stages of precancerous conditions or cervical, vaginal, and VULVAR CANCERS. It is also used to ease the symptoms of cancer, such as bleeding or obstruction, especially when the cancer cannot be cured by other treatments.

These high-powered light beams have several advantages over standard surgical tools. Because they are more precise than scalpels, lasers can make an incision while avoiding tissue around the wound. And because the heat they produce sterilizes the surgery site, lasers can reduce the risk of infection. The laser is so precise that only a small incision is needed, so the operation is faster, and recovery is quicker because less bleeding, swelling, or scarring results.

The light from some lasers can be transmitted through a flexible endoscope fitted with fiber optics so that doctors can see to work in parts of the body that could not otherwise be reached except by surgery. Lasers also may be used with low-power microscopes, to provide a clear view of the site being treated. Used with other instruments, laser systems can produce a cutting area as small as 200 micrometers in diameter—less than the width of a very fine thread.

Although there are several different kinds of lasers, only three kinds have gained wide use in medicine: carbon dioxide (CO_2) lasers, argon lasers, and neodymium:yttrium-aluminum-garnet (Nd:YAG) lasers. CO_2 and Nd:YAG lasers are used to shrink or destroy tumors.

Carbon Dioxide (CO_2) Laser

The CO_2 laser can remove thin layers from the skin's surface without penetrating the deeper layers, a capacity that is especially useful for treating precancerous conditions and tumors that have not spread deeply into the skin. As an alternative to traditional scalpel surgery, the CO_2 laser is also able to make incisions in the skin.

Argon Laser

This laser can pass through only superficial layers of tissue. It is also used with light-sensitive dyes to treat tumors in a procedure known as photodynamic therapy, which is based on the property that certain chemicals can kill one-celled organisms in the presence of light. Some photosensitizing agents have a tendency to collect in cancer cells; when treated cancer cells are exposed to red light from a laser, the light is absorbed by the photosensitizing agent, which causes a chemical reaction that destroys the tumor. Photodynamic therapy is mainly used to treat tumors on or just below the skin or on the lining of internal organs.

Neodymium:Yttrium-Aluminum-Garnet (Nd:YAG) Laser

Light from the Nd:YAG laser can penetrate deeper into tissue than other lasers and can cause blood to clot quickly. It also can be carried through optical fibers to reach less accessible parts of the body.

Laser-Induced Interstitial Thermotherapy

Laser-induced interstitial thermotherapy is one of the newest techniques; it uses the same principle as the cancer treatment hyperthermia—use of heat to shrink tumors by damaging cells or depriving them of substances they need to live.

leiomyoma   See FIBROID TUMOR.

leiomyosarcoma (LMS)   A rare type of cancer that usually originates in the uterine muscle. This rare type of soft-tissue SARCOMA begins in smooth muscle cells. It occurs less often in the abdomen behind the intestines (retroperitoneal LMS) and in the skin (cutaneous LMS).

Smooth muscle cells make up the involuntary muscles, which are found in most parts of the body—in the uterus, stomach, intestines, blood vessel walls, and skin. A person cannot make an involuntary muscle move.

Treatment

LMS is a resistant cancer that is not very responsive to CHEMOTHERAPY, although surgery, chemotherapy, and RADIATION THERAPY are all typical treatments. The prognosis is best when the cancer is surgically removed with wide margins, while it is small and contained.

Surgery   Surgery is the most common treatment of adult soft tissue sarcoma. Currently, if the tumor can be removed completely, surgery is the treatment of choice. A doctor may remove the cancer and some of the healthy tissue around the cancer, but sometimes all or part of an affected limb may have to be amputated in order to ensure removal of all of the cancer. If cancer has spread to the LYMPH NODES, they are removed as well. If the cancer cannot be completely removed, other methods may also be used, depending on the number of tumors and their location.

Radiation   In situations in which a tumor is inoperable, radiation therapy can be used to shrink the growth so it can be surgically removed. Either internal or external radiation therapy is used to kill cancer cells and shrink tumors.

Prognosis

The prognosis for LMS depends on the patient's age and the size, grade, and stage of the tumor. Patients older than age 60 and patients who have tumors that are high grade or larger than five centimeters have a poorer prognosis.

leukapharesis   A method of removing GRANULOCYTES (white blood cells) from whole blood for transfusion into patients who are having CHEMOTHERAPY (which may lower the white blood cell count).

leukopenia   A condition in which there are too few white cells in a patient's blood supply, as the result of leukemia or lymphoma or as a side effect of chemotherapy treatment.

lifestyle and reproductive cancers   Scientists have identified many factors that contribute to the development of gynecologic cancers, including a number of avoidable lifestyle factors. Avoiding these risk factors whenever possible could lower a woman's chance of having cancer. The main risk factors fall in the following categories.

Infections

Several reproductive cancers have been linked to infectious agents, such as the HUMAN PAPILLO-MAVIRUS. Some cancers—including cervical, uterine, vaginal, and VULVAR CANCERS—may be prevented by practicing safe sex with a latex condom.

Diet

Researchers believe that what we eat makes a difference in the probability of developing a variety of cancers. The content of each meal, as well as the way it is prepared, influences cancer risk. For example, meat grilled on a barbecue may be more risky than meat prepared by baking or boiling. Cured meats that contain compounds such as nitrosamines have been linked to higher risk of cancers. Other evidence suggests that people who have a diet high in saturated fats have a higher cancer risk than those who have a lower-fat diet.

In some cases, insufficient consumption of certain foods can increase the risk of cancer. Eating a diet rich in fruits, vegetables, whole grains and other plant-based foods is associated with a reduced probability of cancer development.

Sedentary Lifestyle

Exercise has clearly been shown to lower cancer risk. In the 1990s, Harvard researchers found that women who played team sports reduced their lifetime risk of cervical, uterine and other reproductive cancers by 61 percent.

Obesity

Obesity does appear to be linked to some types of cancers including cancers of the endometrium, cervix, and ovary. In particular, there is a strong relationship between ENDOMETRIAL CANCER and obesity.

Although there are many theories about how obesity increases cancer risk, the exact mechanisms are not known. Many epidemiological studies have examined the impact of various aspects of diet on a woman's hormone levels. Studies in vegetarians who consumed low-fat diets have demon-strated increased urinary excretion of ESTROGENS and decreased plasma estrogen levels.

However, because obesity develops through a complex interaction of heredity and lifestyle factors determining whether obesity or another factor led to the development of cancer is not easy. Drawing conclusions from studies of obesity is made more difficult by the fact that definitions and measurements of *overweight* and *obese* vary from study to study; such variations have affected earlier study results and made comparing data across studies difficult.

According to a U.S. government panel and consistently with the recommendations of many other countries and the World Health Organization, *overweight* is defined as a body mass index (BMI) of 25 to 30, and *obese* as a BMI of 30 or more. Health risks increase gradually with increasing BMI. BMI is useful in tracking trends in the population because it provides a more accurate measure of who is overweight and obese than weight alone. By itself, however, this measurement cannot give direct or specific information about a person's health.

More studies are needed to evaluate the combined effects of diet, body weight, and physical activity on cancer, because it is not clear whether the increased cancer risk is due to extra weight, inadequate consumption of fruits and vegetables, or a high-fat, high-calorie diet.

Smoking

Quitting smoking can lower a woman's risk of CERVICAL CANCER or VAGINAL CANCER, because women who smoke are more likely to have these two types of cancer. The reason for this relationship is not known; some experts suspect that smoking causes some abnormal changes in cells, which then have a higher likelihood of becoming cancerous. A few studies have found a chemical by-product of nicotine (the addictive drug in cigarettes) in the secretions of the cervix. The poisons in cigarette smoke may also enter the cervix and vagina through the bloodstream.

Moreover, current and past smoking may increase the risk of cervical cancer among women who have been infected by human papillomavirus (HPV), according to a 2002 NATIONAL CANCER INSTITUTE study.

The only way to prevent these cancers caused by cigarettes is not to smoke. A smoker's risk of cancer development decreases dramatically after quitting and continues to decrease every year thereafter.

Hormones

Some types of malignant tumors need hormones to grow; therefore, an increase in the level of hormones in the body could increase the risk of certain cancers.

Birth control pills   Studies have consistently shown that using the Pill reduces the risk of OVARIAN CANCER, but there is some evidence that long-term use of these pills may increase the risk of cervical cancer.

Hormone replacement therapy   The estrogen and PROGESTIN component of the Women's Health Initiative concluded definitively in 2002 that postmenopausal women who use combined estrogen and progestin therapy have an increase in the risk of invasive breast cancer. Studies have also suggested an increased risk of ovarian cancer among longtime users of hormone replacement therapy.

After an average of five years of follow-up for each of more than 16,000 women in the study, the study found a 26 percent increase in breast cancer risk as compared to that in women taking a placebo. Research released in 2004 also found that women who took estrogen alone after menopause had a significantly increased risk of stroke and possibly a higher risk of dementia too, according to the National Institutes of Health. The NIH decided to stop the estrogen-only study a year before its planned completion because enough data had been collected to assess overall risks and benefits.

The government noted that estrogen alone is not as bad as combining it with the hormone progestin, but officials advise that estrogen still is too risky for long-term use.

However, estrogen alone did not increase the risk of breast cancer, a surprise to researchers because the estrogen-progestin combination had increased that risk by 26 percent.

For a long time, doctors had thought that using estrogen (alone or together with progestin) would keep women healthier after menopause by reducing heart attacks and keeping the brain sharp.

In stopping the estrogen-alone study, the government revealed that estrogen alone increased the risk of a stroke as much as combination estrogen-progestin does. For every 10,000 women, those taking hormones suffer eight more strokes per year than nonhormone users. At the same time, estrogen alone had no effect on heart disease. (In contrast, the estrogen-progestin combination increases heart attack risk by 29 percent.)

Neither type of hormone therapy seems good for women's brains. Preliminary data from a related study of women 65 and older suggest those taking estrogen alone were more likely to suffer some degree of dementia than those taking a placebo. Likewise, scientists announced in 2003 that the estrogen-progestin combination doubled the risk of Alzheimer's and other forms of dementia. Estrogen (and estrogen-progestin) decrease the risk of a hip fracture from bone-thinning osteoporosis, although only women who cannot take one of the nation's many other osteoporosis treatments should consider estrogen for that use, according to the government.

Fertility drugs   Some studies have found that certain FERTILITY DRUGS increase a woman's risk for ovarian cancer; others have shown no increased risk with use of fertility drugs. These studies and other recent research raise questions about whether infertile women who take fertility drugs and do not become pregnant and women who take certain fertility drugs for extended periods may be at increased risk of ovarian cancer. However, these links have not been proved, and more research is needed.

liver damage   Because the liver is the organ that breaks down most of the drugs used in CHEMOTHERAPY, it can be damaged by certain drugs, including methotrexate, high-dose CISPLATIN, high-dose cyclophosphamide (CYTOXAN), vincristine, and doxorubicin (ADRIAMYCIN). This damage is more likely in patients who are elderly or who have had hepatitis, which weakens the liver. However, symptoms of liver damage caused by chemotherapy usually end once the drug is stopped.

Symptoms of liver damage include yellowed skin and eyes (jaundice), fatigue, and pain below the right ribs or right upper abdomen. Blood tests are necessary to monitor the health of the liver.

Look Good . . . Feel Better (LGFB) program A free, nonmedical, national public service program founded in 1989 to help women deal with appearance-related changes caused by cancer treatment. The Look Good . . . Feel Better program was developed by the Cosmetic, Toiletry, and Fragrance Association, the AMERICAN CANCER SOCIETY, and the National Cosmetology Association. Today, LGFB group programs are held in every state and Puerto Rico, with products donated by 40 CTFA member companies. Teen and Spanish-language programs, self-help mailer kits, online programs, and a 24-hour hotline are also offered—and numerous independent international LGFB programs are available.

Luzca Bien . . . Siéntase Mejor, for example, offers bilingual group programs (English and Spanish) for Hispanic women in 14 locations: Albuquerque, Brownsville (Texas), Chicago, Dallas, Denver, Houston, Los Angeles, Miami, New York City, Phoenix, San Antonio, San Diego, San Francisco, and Washington, D.C. Spanish-language materials are available nationwide upon request.

Look Good . . . Feel Better for Teens offers programs for teen girls and boys in 13 cities—Boston, Columbus (Ohio), Denver, Durham (North Carolina), Houston, Memphis, New Haven, New York City, Palo Alto, Philadelphia, Rochester (Minnesota), Tampa, and Washington, D.C.—plus the 2bMe Web site with online demos.

Each two-hour, hands-on workshop includes a 12-step skin care/makeup application lesson, demonstration of options for dealing with HAIR LOSS, and discussion of nail-care techniques. Held at comprehensive care clinics, hospitals, ACS offices, and community centers, local group programs are organized by the American Cancer Society, facilitated by LGFB-certified cosmetologists, and aided by general volunteers. Patients in various stages of treatment receive makeover tips and personal attention from professionals trained to meet their needs. They also use and take home complimentary cosmetic kits in their appropriate skin tones (light, medium, dark, extra dark) with helpful instruction booklets. Professional advice is provided on wigs, scarves, and accessories. (Teen sessions also include social and health tips.) More than 40,000 individuals participate each year in small groups of five to 10, offering each patient a supportive circle, as well.

"Just for You" self-help kits in English or Spanish with 30-minute video and makeover tips booklet are offered free to patients who cannot locally access LGFB. For contact information, see Appendix I.

loop electrosurgical excision procedure (LEEP) A simple surgical procedure used to treat abnormal changes of the cells lining the cervix (a condition known as DYSPLASIA). The procedure is also used occasionally to treat carefully selected cases of CERVICAL CANCER.

In this technique, radio frequency current is used to remove abnormal tissues of the cervix. A chemical is applied afterward to prevent bleeding. LEEP has the advantage over other more destructive techniques (such as CO_2 laser or cryocautery) that an intact tissue sample for analysis can be obtained. LEEP is also popular because it is inexpensive and simple.

Complications occur in about 1 to 2 percent of women who have LEEP; they include bleeding and narrowing of the cervical opening.

lycopene One of more than 600 phytochemicals called CAROTENOIDS, which have very powerful disease-fighting capabilities. Lycopene is associated with the red color in tomatoes; tomato-based products such as sauce, soup, and juice have the most concentrated source of lycopene.

Cooked tomato sauces are associated with greater health benefits than uncooked foods, because the heating process makes lycopene more easily absorbed by the body. Also, lycopene is fat soluble, meaning that in order for the body to absorb it, it has to be eaten with at least a small amount of fat. Lycopene consumption has been associated with a reduced risk of many cancers.

lymphadenectomy Removal and biopsy of LYMPH NODES to check for the extent of the spread of cancer. When cancer is being staged to determine whether it has spread, the surgeon performs a BIOPSY of the lymph nodes to check for spread of malignant cells. Presence of cancer cells in the lymph nodes suggests that the cancer has spread from the primary site and is likely to spread to other parts of the body.

lymphatic system   A network of capillaries, vessels, ducts, nodes, and organs that produce, filter, and carry lymph, a colorless liquid that bathes the body's tissues and contains cells to help fight infection. As lymph is slowly moved through larger and larger lymphatic vessels, it passes through LYMPH NODES that filter out substances harmful to the body; these nodes also contain lymphocytes and other cells that activate the immune system to fight disease. Eventually, lymph flows into one of two large ducts in the neck. The right lymphatic duct collects lymph from the right arm and the right side of the head and chest and empties into the large vein below the right collarbone. The left lymphatic duct collects lymph from both legs, the left arm, and the left side of the head and chest and empties into the large vein below the left collarbone.

The lymphatic system collects excess fluid and proteins from the tissues and carries them back to the bloodstream. Swelling (LYMPHEDEMA) may occur if there is an increase in the amount of fluid, proteins, and other substances in the body tissues caused by problems in the blood capillaries and veins or by blockage in the lymphatic system.

lymphatic vessels   Thin, tubular structures that make up the lymph system, which removes cellular waste from the body by filtering it through the LYMPH NODES.

See also LYMPH NODE STATUS.

lymphedema   A fluid buildup that may collect in the arms or legs when lymph vessels or LYMPH NODES are blocked or removed. Although lymphedema is most often associated with breast cancer, it can also develop after treatment for other types of cancer as well. Left untreated, this stagnant fluid interferes with wound healing and provides a culture medium for bacteria that can result in infection in the lymph nodes (lymphangitis).

If lymph nodes are removed, there is always a risk of development of lymphedema, either immediately after surgery or weeks, months, even years later. Lymphedema can also develop if CHEMOTHERAPY is administered to the side of the body on which surgery was performed (such administration should be prevented) or after repeated aspirations of fluid in the underarms or in the groin area. Air travel has also been linked to the onset of lymphedema after cancer surgery, probably as a result of decreased cabin pressure. This is why cancer patients should always wear a compression garment (a special sleeve or stocking) when flying.

Risk Factors

There are a number of risk factors for the development of lymphedema:

- Surgical removal of lymph nodes in the underarm, groin, or pelvic regions
- Radiation therapy to the groin or pelvic regions
- Scar tissue in the lymphatic ducts or veins caused by surgery or radiation therapy
- Cancer spread to the lymph nodes in the pelvis or abdomen
- Tumors in the pelvis or abdomen that block lymph drainage
- Excessive thinness or heaviness, conditions that may delay recovery and increase the risk for lymphedema

Symptoms

Lymphedema can develop in any part of the body, causing symptoms such as a feeling of fullness in the limb, tightened skin, decreased flexibility in the ankle, or problems with fitting of clothing. A patient in the early stages of lymphedema has swelling that indents with pressure but remains soft. The swelling may be improved by supporting the leg in a raised position, gently exercising, and wearing elastic support garments.

However, continued problems with the lymphatic system cause the LYMPHATIC VESSELS to expand; as lymph flows back into the body tissues, the condition worsens. Pain, heat, redness, and swelling result as the body tries to get rid of the extra fluid. The skin becomes hard and stiff, and the symptom no longer improves with raised support of the leg, gentle exercise, or elastic support garments.

Stages

Lymphedema develops in a number of stages, from mild to severe (referred to as stages I, II, and III).

Stage I (spontaneously reversible): In the initial stage of lymphedema, tissue appears pitted when pressed by fingertips. Typically, on waking in the morning the affected area looks normal.

Stage II (spontaneously irreversible): In this intermediate stage, the tissue now has a spongy consistency and bounces back when pressed by fingertips, with no pitting. The area begins to harden and enlarge.

Stage III (lymphostatic elephantiasis): In this advanced stage, the swelling is irreversible and the affected area has usually grown quite large. The tissue is hard and unresponsive. Some patients consider reconstructive surgery ("debulking") at this stage.

Acute Lymphedema

There are four types of acute lymphedema, which may be treated with different aspects of decongestive therapy such as manual lymphatic drainage, bandaging, proper skin care and diet, compression garments (sleeves or stockings), or remedial exercises.

The first type of acute lymphedema is mild and lasts only a short time, appearing immediately after surgery to remove the lymph nodes. The affected limb may be warm and slightly red but is usually not painful. The limb generally improves within a week if it is supported in a raised position and if the patient periodically contracts the muscles in the affected arm or leg.

The second type of acute lymphedema occurs six to eight weeks after surgery or during RADIATION THERAPY. This type may be caused by inflammation of either lymphatic vessels or veins, producing a limb that is tender, warm, and red. It is treated by keeping the limb supported in a raised position and using anti-inflammatory drugs.

The third type of acute lymphedema occurs after an insect bite, minor injury, or burn that causes an infection of the skin and the lymphatic vessels near the skin surface in a leg that is chronically swollen. The affected area is red, very tender, and hot and is treated by supporting the affected arm or leg in a raised position and using antibiotics. Using a compression pump or wrapping the affected area with elastic bandages should not be done during the early stages of infection. Mild redness may continue after the infection.

The fourth and most common type of acute lymphedema develops very slowly and may become noticeable only two years or more after surgery—or many years after cancer treatment. The patient may experience discomfort of the skin or aching in the spine and hips caused by stretching of the soft tissues; overuse of muscles; or posture changes due to increased weight of the arm or leg.

Temporary versus Chronic Lymphedema

Temporary lymphedema lasts less than six months and does not involve hardening of the skin. A patient may be more likely to have lymphedema if there is

- A surgical drain that leaks protein into the surgical site
- Inflammation
- Inability to move the limb
- Temporary loss of lymphatic function
- Blockage of a vein by a blood clot or inflammation of a vein

Chronic (long-term) lymphedema is the most difficult of all types of swelling to treat; it occurs when the damaged lymphatic system of the affected area is not able to handle the increased need for fluid drainage from the body tissues. This may happen

- After a tumor recurs or spreads to the lymph nodes
- After an infection of the lymphatic vessels
- After periods of inability to move the limbs
- After radiation therapy or surgery
- When early signs of lymphedema have not been controlled
- When a vein is blocked by a blood clot

Patients who have chronic lymphedema are at increased risk of infection. No effective treatment is yet available for advanced chronic lymphedema.

Once the body tissues have been repeatedly stretched, lymphedema may recur more readily.

Prevention

Poor drainage of the lymphatic system due to radiation therapy or to surgery to remove the lymph nodes may make the affected leg more susceptible to serious infection. Even a small infection may lead to serious lymphedema.

It is important that patients take precautions to prevent injury and infection in the affected leg, since lymphedema can occur 30 years or more after surgery.

Because lymphatic drainage is improved during exercise, exercise can help prevent lymphedema. Women who have surgery that affects pelvic lymph node drainage should do leg and foot exercises.

lymph node   A small oval structure, ranging in size from a pinhead to a bean, that filters germs and foreign substances from lymph (the clear fluid that bathes many of the body's organs). When a lymph node traps germs, it swells; that is why a swollen lymph gland is often a sign of infection or disease. A valuable part of the immune system, lymph nodes are linked via LYMPHATIC VESSELS throughout the body. Lymph nodes can be found under the arms, behind the knee and ears, in the groin, and in the abdominal cavity.

See also LYMPHEDEMA; LYMPH NODE DISSECTION.

lymph node dissection   The removal of the LYMPH NODES from a specific area to check for malignant cells.

lymph node status   The determination of whether a LYMPH NODE contains malignant cells (positive result) or does not (negative result). Negative lymph node findings are associated with less aggressive types of cancer, and a better ultimate prognosis. During surgery, a number of lymph nodes are removed so the lab can check for malignant cells. More recently, sentinel node biopsy allows a surgeon to determine which node is the likely first one that cancer cells would reach; if this node is clear, it is likely that the rest are clear also.

Lynne Cohen Foundation for Ovarian Cancer Research   Nonprofit foundation created by the daughters of Lynne Cohen to support ground-breaking research to improve the survival rates of women who have OVARIAN CANCER. For contact information, see Appendix I.

macrobiotic diet   A mostly vegetarian diet whose advocates believe in preventing disease by adjusting food, lifestyle, relationships, and environment. Macrobiotic diet proponents believe that everything in the world (including cancer) has two opposite forces: yin and yang, an imbalance of yin and yang may cause cancer. The diet is planned to correct any imbalances of yin and yang that could lead to ill health or cancer.

The modern macrobiotic diet includes 50 percent whole grains and cereal, 20 percent to 30 percent vegetables, 5 percent to 10 percent soups, and 5 percent to 10 percent beans and sea vegetables. Foods that may occasionally be eaten include fish, seafood, seasonal fruits, nuts, seeds, and other natural snacks. Sugar and meat are not allowed in a macrobiotic diet.

The American Medical Association, the U.S. Food and Drug Administration, and nutrition experts believe a macrobiotic diet can be harmful. The NATIONAL CANCER INSTITUTE (NCI) and the AMERICAN CANCER SOCIETY believe adhering to a strict macrobiotic diet is not effective in treating or preventing cancer and that it poses certain risks.

Diet critics warn that the modern macrobiotic diet may not provide enough of certain nutrients, including protein, vitamins D and B_{12}, and the minerals zinc, calcium, and iron. An earlier version of the macrobiotic diet that included only grains has been associated with severe malnutrition and even death. There have been no randomized clinical studies to show the macrobiotic diet can be used to prevent or cure cancer. However, cancer experts believe that diets consisting primarily of plant products that are low in fat and high in fiber may reduce the risk of cardiovascular disease and some forms of cancer. One review concluded that dietary macro and micronutrients play an important role in estrogen metabolism, which may have an impact on hormone-related reproductive cancers.

The National Institutes of Health Office of Alternative Medicine has funded a pilot study to determine if a macrobiotic diet may prevent cancer.

magnetic resonance imaging (MRI)   A diagnostic technique that uses a magnetic field rather than radiation (as used in X-rays and radionuclide scans) to produce pictures of structures inside the body. It is used to diagnose and evaluate the extent of cancer and can produce images of blood vessels, cerebrospinal fluid, cartilage, BONE MARROW, muscles, ligaments, and the spinal cord.

An MRI is more expensive than a computed tomography (CT) scan, but it produces pictures that have greater clarity and definition. Because there are no dyes or radiation used, MRI is considered to be safer than X-rays and CT scans. However, patients who have any metal in their body (such as pacemakers, joint pins, surgical clips, artificial heart valves, an intrauterine device [IUD], or shrapnel) should not have MRI scans.

marijuana (*Cannabis sativa* L.)   A member of the cannabis plant family that can, when ingested, relax the mind and body, ease nausea, and heighten perception. One component of marijuana, delta-9-thiocarbanidin, is now available in synthetic form as the drug dronabinol (MARINOL) to treat nausea and vomiting in CHEMOTHERAPY patients. Although marijuana use is illegal in the United States, the U.S. Food and Drug Administration in 1985 approved Marinol for the treatment of nausea and vomiting associated with cancer chemotherapy in patients who did not respond to conventional antinausea treatments.

Although research has shown that THC is more quickly absorbed from marijuana smoke than from an oral preparation, any antinausea effects of smoking marijuana may not be consistent because of varying potency, depending on the source of the marijuana contained in the cigarette.

Eight states (Alaska, California, Colorado, Hawaii, Maine, Nevada, Oregon, and Washington) already allow gravely ill patients to use medical marijuana, usually through a doctor's recommendation and an independent board's certification. A similar bill that would have allowed medical marijuana in New Mexico was defeated in March of 2003.

The Marinol patient-assistance program is designed to help find potential insurance coverage for Marinol; for eligible patients with financial need, Marinol may be supplied free of charge. Information about the program is available by calling at (800) 256-8918.

Marinol (dronabinol)   A synthetic version of delta-9-thiocarbanidin, a component of MARIJUANA. It is used to treat nausea and vomiting of CHEMOTHERAPY patients who do not respond to any other antinausea medication.

Medicare   A federally subsidized insurance program for citizens older than age 65 that was established by Congress in 1965. Medicare has two parts: Part A, which is free, pays for 80 percent of inpatient hospital care and a variety of follow-up services. Part B, for which patients pay a monthly premium, pays for 80 percent of doctors' services, outpatient hospital care, and other medical expenses. Some people also decide to buy "Medigap" insurance to cover the unpaid 20 percent of medical costs.

Those who are older than age 65, who have permanent kidney failure, or are receiving Social Security Disability Income for 24 months are also eligible to enroll.

Cancer patients whose disease has spread are usually considered permanently disabled and are therefore also eligible for Medicare, regardless of their age. Generally, if cancer has spread to a major organ, such as the lung, liver, or brain, patients are accepted in the program.

menopause   The end of menstruation. Although the term specifically refers to a woman's final period, it is not an abrupt event, but a gradual process. It usually occurs naturally as a woman reaches her late 40s or early 50s, but it can also be surgically triggered by the removal of both ovaries (OOPHORECTOMY) or by CHEMOTHERAPY, which often destroys ovarian function.

Menopause is not a disease that needs to be cured, but a natural life-stage transition. However, some women need to make important decisions about treating symptoms that accompany menopause, including whether to use HORMONE REPLACEMENT THERAPY (HRT).

Many women have irregular periods and other problems for years before the end of their menstrual periods. Although it is not easy to predict when menopause begins, doctors agree that it is complete when a woman has not had a period for one year. Eight of every 100 women stop menstruating before age 40. At the other end of the spectrum, five of every 100 continue to have periods until they are almost 60. The average age at menopause is 51. There is no mathematical formula to determine when the function of the ovaries will begin to slow, although a woman can have a general idea of her body's timetable based on her family history, body type, and lifestyle. Women who began menstruating early do not necessarily stop having periods early as well, but it is true that a woman will likely enter menopause at about the same age as her mother. Menopause may occur later than average among smokers.

Once a woman enters puberty, each month her body releases one of the more than 400,000 eggs that are stored in her ovaries, and the lining of her uterus thickens in anticipation of receiving a fertilized egg. If the egg is not fertilized, progesterone levels drop and the uterine lining sheds and bleeds. By the time a woman reaches her late 30s or 40s, her ovaries begin to shut down, producing less estrogen and progesterone and releasing eggs less often. The gradual decline of ESTROGEN level causes a wide variety of changes in tissues that respond to estrogen, including the vagina, vulva, uterus, bladder, urethra, breasts, bones, heart, blood vessels, brain, skin, hair, and mucous membranes. Eventually, the lack of estrogen can make a woman more vulnerable to osteoporosis (which can begin in her 40s) and heart disease.

As the hormone levels fluctuate, a woman's menstrual cycle begins to change. Some women may have longer periods with heavy flow followed by shorter cycles and little bleeding. Others begin to miss periods completely. During this time, a woman finds it is more difficult to become pregnant.

Symptoms

The most obvious and common symptom of menopause is a change in the menstrual cycle, but there are a variety of other symptoms as well:

- Hot flashes
- Night sweats
- Insomnia
- Mood swings and irritability
- Memory or concentration problems
- Vaginal dryness
- Heavy bleeding
- Fatigue
- Depression
- Hair changes
- Headaches
- Heart palpitations
- Sexual disinterest
- Urinary changes
- Weight gain

Diagnosis

The clearest indication that menopause has occurred is the absence of a menstrual period for one year. However, it is also possible to diagnose menopause by testing a woman's HORMONE levels. One important test measures the levels of follicle-stimulating hormone (FSH), which decrease steadily as a woman ages. However, as a woman enters menopause, her hormone levels often fluctuate wildly from day to day. For example, if a woman's estrogen levels are high and progesterone levels are low, she may have mood swings, irritability, and other symptoms similar to those of premenstrual syndrome. As hormone levels shift and estrogen level falls, hot flashes occur. Because

of these fluctuations, a normal hormone level one day may not necessarily mean the level was normal the day before or that it will be the day after.

If it has been at least three months since a woman's last period, an FSH test may be more helpful in determining whether menopause has occurred. However, most doctors believe that the FSH test alone cannot be used as proof that a woman has entered early menopause. A better measure of menopause is a test that checks the levels of estrogen, progesterone, testosterone, and other hormones, in addition to FSH, at midcycle.

Treatment

Hormone replacement therapy When a woman enters menopause, her levels of estrogen drop and symptoms (such as hot flashes and vaginal dryness) begin. In the past, hormone replacement therapy was widely used to treat these symptoms by boosting the estrogen levels enough to suppress symptoms.

When hormone replacement therapy was first developed, doctors simply administered estrogen alone (ESTROGEN REPLACEMENT THERAPY, or ERT). ERT helped relieve the symptoms of menopause and appeared to protect against heart disease and bone fractures, problems that often occur in older women. But doctors discovered that it also increased the risk of cancer of the uterine lining. Adding progesterone to estrogen—and now calling it hormone replacement therapy—produced a combination that seemed to protect against endometrial cancer among women who had an intact uterus. Whether this conferred the other benefits seen with ERT, however, had not been known.

However, the largest randomized study ever to look at combined HRT in healthy postmenopausal women was stopped early, in July 2002, when researchers found an increased risk of breast cancer among participants. The study was stopped because of ethical concerns due to the clear risk for study subjects. At the time of the study, 38 percent of postmenopausal American women were using HRT.

Study participants receiving the estrogen/progesterone combination of HRT were also found to be at higher risk for coronary heart disease and blood clots, although HRT did seem to lower the risk of colorectal cancer and bone fractures. Overall, however, the risks outweighed the benefits, according to researchers. The Women's Health Initiative (WHI) study report, along with an editorial recommending against the long-term use of HRT in healthy postmenopausal women, was published in the July 17 *Journal of the American Medical Association.*

The 2002 study also did not look at short-term use of HRT to prevent menopausal symptoms, such as hot flashes, so it is difficult to draw conclusions about this.

The researchers looked at more than 16,000 healthy postmenopausal women who were part of the Women's Health Initiative (WHI), a trial funded by the National Institutes of Health. All of the women were between the ages of 50 and 79 and had an intact uterus. The women began taking either a combination estrogen–progestin pill or a placebo each day, starting in the mid-1990s. The women were supposed to be followed for an average of eight and a half years, and the researchers to study the results twice each year. The last scheduled review (May 2002) showed that the results were significant enough that the trial was stopped after just over five years.

The rate of breast cancers was 26 percent higher among those receiving HRT as opposed to those getting placebo. The rate for heart disease was 29 percent higher, stroke rate was 41 percent higher, and blood clot rate was more than twice as high in those having HRT.

HRT did have some benefits: rate of colorectal cancer was 37 percent lower in the HRT group, and the rate of bone fractures was 24 percent lower. Endometrial cancer rates were about the same in both groups.

By weighing each of these factors, researchers derived an overall *global index,* which showed that the risks outweighed the possible benefits for these serious conditions.

Given these results, researchers recommend that clinicians stop prescribing HRT for long-term use. Nonetheless, although the increased risk of breast cancer and other conditions may make HRT unsuitable for prevention in healthy people, the overall risk for each woman is still rather small. For example, the 36 percent increased risk of breast cancer is based on the fact that during one year, among 10,000 women receiving combination HRT there are 38 cases of breast cancer. Among 10,000 women taking a placebo, there are 30 cases. The same holds true for heart disease (37 cases per 10,000 women per year with HRT, versus 30 cases per 10,000 women per year with placebo) and blood clots (34 cases per 10,000 women per year with HRT, versus 16 cases per 10,000 women per year with placebo). Nevertheless, there is a risk, and it would probably increase as the time taking combination HRT increased.

The decision to pursue HRT should be made by a woman and her doctor after taking into consideration her medical history and situation. Women who choose to use hormones despite the risks should have an annual mammogram, breast exam, and pelvic exam and should report any unusual vaginal bleeding or spotting (a sign of possible uterine cancer).

Estrogen-only therapy   Women who have estrogen replacement therapy alone once (common therapy for women who have had a hysterectomy and have one or two ovaries) also have a higher risk of ovarian cancer, according to a 2002 study. This study included more than 44,000 postmenopausal women whose health histories were tracked for about 20 years. Compared to similar women not on hormone replacement therapy, those taking estrogen for 10 or more years had a 60 percent greater risk of development of ovarian cancer.

As early as the 1940s women began to use estrogen in high dosages to counteract some of the short-term discomforts of menopause; but after it became clear in the 1970s that estrogen use is associated with a high risk of uterine cancer, doctors began prescribing progestin, along with much lower dosages of estrogen. Estrogen-only therapy continued to be widely prescribed for women who had had a hysterectomy.

Hormone replacement therapy of both types was once used by an estimated 13.5 million women in the United States alone, nearly eight million estrogen-only and up to six million in combination with progestin. However, research released in 2003 and 2004 found that women who took either estrogen alone or the estrogen-progestin combination after menopause had a significantly increased risk of stroke, and possibly a higher risk of dementia too, according to the National Institutes of Health. In addition, the estrogen-progestin combination increased the risk of breast cancer by 26 percent. The NIH decided to stop studies of both types of hormone replacement therapy before the studies' planned completion because enough data had been collected to reveal serious risks. The government noted that estrogen alone isn't as risky for women as the estrogen-progestin combination, but officials advise that estrogen still is too risky for long-term use.

For a long time, doctors had thought that using estrogen (alone or together with progestin) would keep women healthier after menopause by reducing heart attacks and keeping the brain sharp.

Antiestrogens   A new type of hormone therapy offers some of the same protection against heart disease and bone loss as estrogen, but without the increased risk of breast cancer. This new class of drugs, known as antiestrogens, include the drug raloxifene. These drugs are called antiestrogens because for a long time they had been used to counter the effects of estrogen that cause breast cancer. However, in other parts of the body these drugs mimic estrogen, protecting against heart disease and osteoporosis without putting a woman at risk for breast cancer.

As estrogen does, raloxifene works by attaching to an estrogen receptor, much as a key fits into a lock. When raloxifene clicks into the estrogen receptors in the breast and uterus, it blocks estrogen at these sites. This is the secret of its cancer-fighting property. Many tumors in the breast are fueled by estrogen; if the estrogen cannot enter the cell, then the cancer stops growing.

Testosterone replacement   The ovaries also produce a small amount of male hormones, which decreases slightly as a woman enters menopause. The vast majority of women never need testosterone replacement, but it can be important if a woman has declining interest in sex. Testosterone can improve the libido as well as decrease anxiety and depression; adding testosterone especially helps women who have had hysterectomy. Testos-

terone also eases breast tenderness and helps prevent bone loss. However, testosterone does have side effects. Some women experience mild acne and some facial hair growth, but because only small amounts of testosterone are prescribed, most women do not appear to have extreme masculine characteristics.

Birth control pills   Women who are still having periods but who have annoying menopausal symptoms may take low-dosage birth control pills to ease the problems; this treatment has been approved by the U.S. Food and Drug Administration for perimenopausal symptoms of women younger than age 55.

Alternative treatments   Some women also report success in using natural remedies to treat the unpleasant symptoms of menopause. Herbs such as black cohosh have been used to relieve menopausal symptoms for centuries. In general, most herbs are considered safe, and there is no substantial evidence that herbal products are a major source of toxic reactions. But because herbal products are not regulated in the United States, contamination and accidental overdosage are possible. Herbs should be bought from a recognized company or through a qualified herbal practitioner. Women who choose to use herbs for menopausal symptoms should learn as much as possible about herbs and work with a qualified practitioner (an herbalist, a traditional Chinese doctor, or a naturopathic physician). Pregnant women should avoid herbs because of their unknown effects on a developing fetus.

Proponents of plant estrogens (including soy products) believe that plant estrogens are better than synthetic estrogen, but no one yet has proved that soy can provide all the benefits of synthetic estrogen without the negative effects. Nonetheless, the results of small preliminary trials suggest that the estrogen compounds in soy products can indeed relieve the severity of hot flashes and lower cholesterol level. It is also true that people in other countries who eat foods high in plant estrogens (especially SOY PRODUCTS) have lower rates of breast cancer and report fewer symptoms of menopause. In addition, whereas up to 80 percent of menopausal women in the United States experienced hot flashes, night sweats, and vaginal dryness, only 15 percent of Japanese women have similar problems. When all other factors are equal, it appears a soy-based diet may make a difference (and soy level is very high in plant estrogens).

However, "natural" or "plant-based" is not the same as "harmless." In large dosages, phytoestrogens can promote the abnormal growth of cells in the uterine lining. Estrogen alone of any type can lead to endometrial cancer; therefore, women on conventional ERT usually take progesterone (progestin) along with estrogen.

Exercise helps ease hot flashes by lowering the levels of circulating FSH and luteinizing hormone (LH) and by raising endorphin levels that drop during a hot flash. Even exercising 20 minutes three times a week can significantly reduce hot flashes.

Acupuncture is an ancient Asian art that involves placing very thin needles into different parts of the body to stimulate the system and unblock energy. It is usually painless and has been used for many menopausal symptoms, including insomnia, hot flashes, and irregular periods. Practitioners believe that acupuncture can facilitate the opening of blocked energy channels, allowing the life force energy (*chi*) to flow freely.

Therapeutic massage that includes acupressure can produce relief from a wide range of menopause symptoms by placing finger pressure at the same meridian points on the body used in acupuncture. There are more than 80 different types of massage, including foot reflexology, Shiatsu massage, and Swedish massage; they are all based on the principle that boosting the circulation of blood and lymph benefits health.

menopause, artificial The abrupt onset of MENOPAUSE as the result of removal of the ovaries (OOPHORECTOMY), CHEMOTHERAPY, RADIATION THERAPY of the pelvis, or any process that impairs ovarian blood supply. This type of menopause usually occurs immediately and has more severe symptoms than normally occur.

metastasis The spread of cancer cells to other areas of the body via the LYMPHATIC SYSTEM or the bloodstream.

mistletoe A semiparasitic plant that has been used for centuries to treat numerous human ailments; more recently, mistletoe extracts have been shown to kill cancer cells in the lab. It is used primarily as an injected prescription drug in Europe, but mistletoe extracts are not available in the United States. Although mistletoe plants and berries are considered poisonous, few serious side effects have been associated with mistletoe extract use.

The use of mistletoe as a treatment for cancer has been investigated in more than 30 clinical studies, but nearly all of the studies had major weaknesses that raise doubts about the reliability of the findings, according to federal researchers. At present, the U.S. government does not recommend the use of mistletoe by the general public.

Meanwhile, experts are investigating two components of mistletoe (viscotoxins and lectins) that they think may be responsible for certain anticancer effects. Viscotoxins are small proteins that can kill cells and possibly stimulate the immune system. Lectins are complex molecules of protein and carbohydrates that can trigger biochemical changes.

Because of mistletoe's ability to stimulate the immune system, it has been classified as a type of BIOLOGICAL RESPONSE MODIFIER (a diverse group of biological molecules that have been used to treat cancer or to lessen the side effects of anticancer drugs).

Commercially available extracts of mistletoe are marketed in Europe under a variety of brand names, including Iscador, Eurixor, Helixor, Isorel, Iscucin, Plenosol, and ABNOBAviscum. Some extracts are marketed under more than one name. For example, Iscador, Isorel, and Plenosol are also sold as Iscar, Vysorel, and Lektinol, respectively. All of these products are prepared from *Viscum album Loranthacea* (European mistletoe).

Mistletoe grows on several types of trees, and the chemical composition of extracts derived from it depends on the species of the host tree (such as apple, elm, oak, pine, poplar, and spruce), the time of year harvested, the way the extracts are prepared, and the commercial producer.

At least two researchers have received approval to study mistletoe as a cancer treatment.

Side Effects

Reported side effects of mistletoe extract have generally been mild, including soreness and inflammation at injection sites, headache, fever, and chills. A few cases of severe allergic reactions, including anaphylactic shock, have been reported.

However, mistletoe plants and berries are poisonous; and ingestion may cause seizures, vomiting, and death. The severity of the toxic effects associated with mistletoe ingestion may depend on the amount consumed and the type of plant.

mixed germ cell tumor   A tumor that contains more than one type of GERM CELL cancer (for example, TERATOMA and seminoma).

mixed tumors   Some tumors are made up of more than one type. For example, mixed müllerian tumors of the uterus are also called carcinosarcomas to indicate that they are derived both from epithelial and from connective tissues.

monoclonal antibodies (MOABs)   Synthetic antibodies produced by a single type of cell that are specific for a particular antigen. Researchers are examining ways to create MOABs specific to the antigens found on the surface of cancer cells.

MOABs are made by injecting human cancer cells into mice to cause the mouse immune system to produce antibodies against these cancer cells. The mouse cells producing the antibodies are then removed and fused with lab-grown cells to create "hybrid" cells (hybridomas) that can produce large quantities of pure antibodies. They may be used in cancer treatment in a number of ways:

- Reacting with specific types of cancer may enhance a patient's immune response to the cancer.
- They can be programmed to act against cell growth factors, interfering with the growth of cancer cells.
- They may be linked to anticancer drugs, radioisotopes (radioactive substances), or other toxins. When the antibodies latch onto cancer cells, they deliver these poisons directly to the tumor, helping to destroy it.

- They may help destroy cancer cells in BONE MARROW that has been removed from a patient in preparation for a BONE MARROW TRANSPLANT.
- MOABs carrying radioisotopes may also prove useful in diagnosis of certain cancers, such as ovarian cancer.

mouth sores   See STOMATITIS.

MUGA scan   Common term for "multiple-gated acquisition" scan, a noninvasive test using a radioactive technetium isotope designed to evaluate the functioning of the heart's ventricles. MUGA scans are given to some women to assess the health of their heart before starting treatment with certain kinds of chemotherapy, such as doxorubicin (ADRIAMYCIN), that may potentially damage the heart.

The scan takes about an hour. In this test, a small amount of radioactive material is injected into a vein, where it temporarily attaches to red blood cells. A camera that can detect the radioactive material takes pictures of the blood flow through the beating heart.

myelosuppression   A common side effect of CHEMOTHERAPY, in which the ability of the BONE MARROW to produce blood cells is damaged. The bone marrow produces three main types of mature blood cells: platelets, red blood cells, and white blood cells. A complete blood count measures the levels of the three basic blood cells. During the period of myelosuppression, patients may have an increased risk of infection, bleeding, or anemia symptoms.

A low white blood cell count is called NEUTROPENIA; this condition lowers a patient's resistance to bacterial infection and may prevent a patient from receiving cancer chemotherapy at the prescribed times and dosages. A low red blood cell count, called ANEMIA, may cause fatigue, heart palpitations, shortness of breath, and a pale complexion. A low platelet count is called THROMBOCYTOPENIA. Platelets prevent bleeding by causing blood clots to form at the site of an injury; thrombocytopenia may cause bruising, nosebleeds, or excessive bleeding from minor wounds or mucous membranes.

Myelosuppression is the most common side effect that causes chemotherapy treatment delays or dosage reductions. Several drugs can be used to prevent or decrease the severity of myelosuppression caused by chemotherapy.

myomectomy The removal of FIBROID TUMORS (noncancerous tumors) from the wall of the uterus. Myomectomy is the preferred treatment for fibroids in women who want to keep their uterus. Larger fibroids must be removed with an abdominal incision, but small fibroids can be taken out by using LAPAROSCOPY or hysteroscopy. A myomectomy is an alternative to HYSTERECTOMY that can relieve fibroid-induced menstrual symptoms that have not responded to medication.

Usually, fibroids are buried in the outer wall of the uterus, and abdominal surgery is required. If they are on the inner wall of the uterus, uterine fibroids can be removed by hysteroscopy. Fibroids on a stalk (pedunculated) on the outer surface of the uterus can be removed with laparoscopy. Removal of fibroids through abdominal surgery is a more difficult and slightly more risky operation than hysterectomy because the uterus bleeds from the sites where the fibroids were, and stopping the bleeding may be difficult or impossible. This surgery is usually performed with general anesthesia, although some patients may be given spinal or epidural anesthesia. The incision may be horizontal (the "bikini" incision) or a vertical incision from the navel downward.

After separating the muscle layers below the skin, the surgeon makes an opening in the abdominal wall. Next, the surgeon makes an incision over each fibroid, grasping and pulling out each growth. Each opening in the uterine wall is then stitched with sutures. The uterus must be meticulously repaired in order to eliminate potential sites of bleeding or infection. Then the surgeon sutures the abdominal wall and muscle layers above it with absorbable stitches and closes the skin with clips or nonabsorbable stitches.

When appropriate, a laparoscopic myomectomy may be performed; in it the surgeon removes fibroids with the help of a laparoscope inserted into the pelvic cavity through an incision in the navel. The fibroids are removed through a tiny incision below the navel that is much smaller than the four- or five-inch opening required for a standard myomectomy.

If the fibroids are small and located on the inner surface of the uterus, they can be removed with a thin telescopelike device called a hysteroscope, which is inserted into the vagina through the cervix and into the uterus. This procedure does not require abdominal incision, so hospitalization is shorter.

Surgeons often recommend hormone treatment with a drug called leuprolide (Lupron) two to six months before surgery in order to shrink the fibroids so they are easier to remove. In addition, Lupron stops menstruation, so women who are anemic have an opportunity to build up their blood count. Although the drug treatment may reduce the risk of excess blood loss during surgery, there is a small risk that temporarily smaller fibroids may be missed during myomectomy, only to enlarge later after the surgery is completed.

Patients may need four to six weeks of recovery after a standard myomectomy before they can return to normal activities, but women who have had laparoscopic or hysteroscopic myomectomies can leave the hospital the same day.

There is a risk that removal of the fibroids may lead to such severe bleeding that the uterus itself has to be removed. Because of the risk of blood loss during a myomectomy, patients may want to consider banking their own blood before surgery.

National Alliance for Caregiving A nonprofit organization dedicated to providing support to family caregivers and the professionals who help them and to increasing public awareness of issues facing family caregiving. They offer reports or informational products for in-depth analysis of current caregiving research, reviews of books and videos that deal with today's caregiving issues, researched links to organizations that focus on different aspects of caregiving, and "Tips for Family Caregivers," to help caregivers help themselves.

Created in 1996, the group was founded by a partnership that includes the American Society on Aging, the Department of Veterans Affairs, and the National Association of Area Agencies on Aging. The founding sponsor is Glaxo Wellcome. Current membership includes more than 30 national organizations. For contact information, see Appendix I.

National Asian Women's Health Organization (NAWHO) A nonprofit organization founded in 1993 to achieve health equity for Asian Americans. NAWHO's goals are to raise awareness about the health needs of Asian Americans through research and education and to support Asian Americans as decision makers via leadership development and advocacy. Through its innovative programs, NAWHO is increasing knowledge of breast cancer and CERVICAL CANCER, training violence-prevention advocates, expanding access to immunizations, changing attitudes about reproductive health care, and erasing stigma related to depression. For contact information, see Appendix I.

National Bone Marrow Transplant Link A national clearinghouse that provides information about a variety of BONE MARROW TRANSPLANT issues.

Services include patient advocacy, research funding, referrals, and a resource guide. For contact information, see Appendix I.

National Breast and Cervical Cancer Early Detection Program (NBCCEDP) A U.S. government program that helps women gain access to lifesaving early detection screening programs for breast cancer and CERVICAL CANCER. The program offers free or low-cost screenings to uninsured, low-income, elderly, minority, and Native American women nationwide.

Many deaths that result from these cancers— which occur disproportionately among women who are uninsured or underinsured—could be prevented by increasing cancer screening rates among all women at risk. PAP TESTS are underused by women who have less than a high school education, are older, live below the poverty level, or are members of certain racial and ethnic minority groups.

To help improve access to early detection screening for cervical cancers for underserved women, Congress passed the Breast and Cervical Cancer Mortality Prevention Act of 1990, which created the Centers for Disease Control and Prevention's National Breast and Cervical Cancer Early Detection Program. This program, currently funded at $192.6 million, provides both screening and diagnostic services, including the following:

- Clinical breast exams
- Mammograms
- Pap tests
- Surgical consultation
- Diagnostic testing for women whose screening outcome is abnormal

Under the program, almost 1.5 million women have been screened and more than 48,170 precancerous cervical lesions and 831 cervical cancers have been diagnosed. The NBCCEDP is improving health care for underserved women through outreach, public and professional education, improved access to services, diagnostic evaluation, case management, treatment services, and quality assurance measures.

National Cancer Institute (NCI)   A component of the National Institutes of Health, the NCI was established under the National Cancer Act of 1937 as the federal government's principal agency for cancer research and training. The National Cancer Act of 1971 broadened the scope and responsibilities of the NCI and created the National Cancer Program, which conducts and supports research, training, and health information dissemination, as well as other programs related to the cause, diagnosis, prevention, and treatment of cancer; rehabilitation from cancer; and the continuing care of cancer patients and their families. The NCI is responsible for coordinating the National Cancer Program.

Services include the NCI's comprehensive database, which contains peer-reviewed summaries and the most current information on cancer treatment, screening, prevention, genetics, and supportive care. The NCI also maintains a registry of cancer clinical trials being conducted worldwide; directories of physicians and professionals who provide genetic counseling services; and organizations that provide care to people with cancer. For contact information, see Appendix I.

National Cancer Institute Cancer Centers Program   A program that comprises more than 50 National Cancer Institute (NCI)–designated CANCER CENTERS engaged in multidisciplinary research to reduce cancer incidence, morbidity, and mortality rates. Through Cancer Center Support grants, this program supports three types of centers:

- COMPREHENSIVE CANCER CENTERS conduct programs in basic research, clinical research, and prevention and control research, as well as programs in community outreach and education.

- CLINICAL CANCER CENTERS conduct programs in clinical research and some programs in other research areas.

- CANCER CENTERS focus on basic research or cancer control research but do not have clinical oncology programs.

Several cancer centers existed in the late 1960s. The National Cancer Act of 1971 strengthened the program by authorizing the establishment of 15 new cancer centers and continued support for existing centers. The passage of the act also dramatically transformed the centers' structure and broadened the scope of their mission to include all aspects of basic, clinical, and cancer control research. Today, more than 40 cancer centers meet the NCI criteria for comprehensive status. Each type of cancer center has specific characteristics and capabilities for organizing new programs of research that can exploit important new findings and address timely research questions. All NCI-designated cancer centers are reevaluated each time their cancer center support grant is up for renewal (generally every three to five years).

Since the passage of the National Cancer Act, the Cancer Centers Program has continued to expand. Today, NCI-designated cancer centers continue to work toward creating new and innovative approaches to cancer research. Through interdisciplinary efforts, cancer centers can effectively move this research from the laboratory into clinical trials and into clinical practice. Patients who seek clinical oncology services (screening, diagnosis, or treatment) can obtain those services at Clinical Cancer Centers or Comprehensive Cancer Centers. They can also participate in clinical trials (research studies that have human subjects) at these types of cancer centers. Information about referral procedures, treatment costs, and services available to patients can be obtained from the individual cancer centers; for contact information, see Appendix II.

Comprehensive Cancer Center

To attain recognition from NCI as a Comprehensive Cancer Center, an institution must pass rigorous peer review. Under guidelines revised in 1997, a Comprehensive Cancer Center must perform research in three major areas: basic research; clinical research; and cancer prevention, control, and population-based research. It must also have a strong body of interactive research that bridges these research areas. In addition, a Comprehensive Cancer Center must conduct activities in outreach, education, and information provision, which are directed toward and accessible to both health care professionals and the lay community.

Clinical Cancer Centers

These centers must have active programs in clinical research, and may also have programs in another area (such as basic research; or prevention, control, and population-based research). Clinical Cancer Centers focus on both laboratory research and clinical research within the same institutional framework. This interaction of research and clinical activities is a distinguishing characteristic of many Clinical Cancer Centers.

Cancer Center

The general term *cancer center* refers to an organization with scientific disciplines outside the specific qualifications for a comprehensive or clinical center. Such centers may, for example, concentrate on basic research, epidemiology and cancer control research, or other areas of research.

National Cervical Cancer Coalition (NCCC) A coalition of women and family members concerned with CERVICAL CANCER issues. Members include women's groups, cytotechnologists, pathologists, laboratories, technology companies, cancer researchers, hospitals, and organizations that provide cervical cancer screening programs. Members hope to educate the public about cervical cancer prevention and outreach, new screening and treatment options, cervical cancer screening and follow-up programs, the human papillomavirus, and PAP TEST.

The NCCC has special, personal focus on providing outreach support to women battling cancer and family members. The NCCC has developed outreach, prevention, awareness, and education efforts, such as the nation's first cervical cancer hotline, the cervical cancer quilts project, and the free "Pap Smear Day" held the second Friday of January for women who have not had a Pap smear for three years. For contact information, see Appendix I.

National Coalition for Cancer Survivorship (NCCS) The only patient-led advocacy organization working on behalf of U.S. survivors of all types of cancer and those who care for them to ensure high-quality cancer care for all Americans. Founded in 1986, NCCS continues to lead the cancer survivorship movement. By educating all those affected by cancer and speaking out on issues related to quality of cancer care, NCCS hopes to empower every survivor. NCCS serves a key role in policy-making in Washington, D.C., as well as providing a source of support for thousands of survivors and their families. Services include referrals, information, education, and advocacy. For contact information, see Appendix I.

National Comprehensive Cancer Network (NCCN) A nonprofit alliance of the world's leading CANCER CENTERS, established in 1995 to support member institutions in the evolving managed-care environment. NCCN goals are to strengthen the mission of member institutions by providing state-of-the-art cancer care, advance cancer prevention, screening, diagnosis, and treatment through excellence in basic and clinical research and to enhance the effectiveness and efficiency of cancer-care delivery.

The NCCN develops programs and products that, in partnerships with managed-care companies, employers, and unions, offer people greater access to leading doctors, superior treatment, programs that continuously improve the effectiveness of treatment, and management that enhances the efficiency of cancer-care delivery. For contact information, see Appendix I.

National Family Caregivers Association A nonprofit association that provides educational and emotional support for family caregivers of cancer patients. Services include advocacy and individual, family, group, peer, and bereavement counseling. For contact information, see Appendix I.

National Hospice and Palliative Care Organization   The largest nonprofit membership organization that represents HOSPICE and palliative care programs and professionals in the United States. The organization is committed to improving end-of-life care and expanding access to hospice care with the goal of profoundly enhancing quality of life for those who are dying and their loved ones.

Considered to be the model for high-quality, compassionate care at the end of life, hospice care involves a team-oriented program of expert medical care, pain management, and emotional and spiritual support expressly tailored to patients' wishes. Emotional and spiritual support are also extended to the family and loved ones. Health-care professionals who specialize in hospice and palliative care work closely with staff and volunteers to address all of the symptoms of illness, with the aim of promoting comfort and dignity. Generally, this care is provided in the patient's home or in a homelike setting operated by a hospice program. Medicare, private health insurance, and Medicaid, in most states, cover hospice care for patients who meet certain criteria. In recent years, many hospice-care programs added *palliative care* to their names to reflect that they also provide care and services to people earlier in their illness than traditional hospice programs.

Those offering "palliative care" seek to address not only physical pain, but also emotional, social, and spiritual pain to achieve the best possible quality of life for patients and their families. Palliative care extends the principles of hospice care to a broader population that could benefit from receiving this type of care earlier in their illness or disease process.

To better serve individuals who have advanced illness or are terminally ill and their families, many hospice programs encourage access to care earlier in the illness or disease process.

The National Hospice and Palliative Care Organization was founded in 1978 as the National Hospice Organization and changed its name in 2000. With headquarters in Alexandria, Virginia, the organization advocates for the terminally ill and their families. It also develops public and professional educational programs and materials to enhance understanding and availability of hospice and palliative care, convenes frequent meetings and symposia on emerging issues, provides technical informational resources to its membership, conducts research, monitors congressional and regulatory activities, and works closely with other organizations that share an interest in end-of-life care. For contact information, see Appendix I.

National Lymphedema Network (NLN)   A nonprofit organization that provides support, education, and information on LYMPHEDEMA. This internationally recognized organization, founded in 1988, is a driving force behind the movement in the United States to standardize quality of treatment for lymphedema patients nationwide. In addition, the NLN supports research into the causes of and possible alternative treatments for this often incapacitating condition. The NLN has a toll-free recorded information line; offers referrals to lymphedema treatment centers, health-care professionals, training programs, and support groups; publishes a quarterly newsletter with information about medical and scientific developments, support groups, and pen pals/net pals; offers educational courses; conducts a biennial national conference on lymphedema; and maintains an extensive computer database. For contact information, see Appendix I.

National Marrow Donor Program   A national group that maintains a registry of BONE MARROW donors, provides information on the way to become a donor, and organizes donor recruitment drives. For contact information, see Appendix I.

National Ovarian Cancer Association   A Canadian organization dedicated to overcoming OVARIAN CANCER, supporting women who are living with the disease, building awareness among the general public, encouraging research into early detection and improved treatment, and ultimately, finding a cure. Education and support include two Web sites with resource information and a package of general information and a video about ovarian cancer. The association also funds a chair in ovarian cancer research at the University of Ottawa and sponsors a national forum on the disease. For contact information, see Appendix I.

National Ovarian Cancer Coalition (NOCC)
The leading OVARIAN CANCER public information and education organization in the United States. NOCC initiated the first toll-free ovarian cancer information line (1-888-OVARIAN) and maintains a comprehensive Web site for ovarian cancer support (www.ovarian.org). The NOCC's missions are to raise awareness of ovarian cancer and to promote education about this disease. By dispelling myths and misunderstandings, the coalition is committed to improving the overall survival rate and quality of life of those affected by ovarian cancer. For contact information, see Appendix I.

National Patient Advocate Foundation A
national network for health-care reform that supports legislation to enable cancer survivors to obtain insurance funding for medical care and participation in clinical trials. The foundation provides referrals, information, advocacy, and health insurance assistance. For contact information, see Appendix I.

National Patient Air Transport Hotline A clearinghouse used to arrange air transportation for cancer patients who cannot afford travel for medical care. For contact information, see Appendix I.

Native American/Alaska-Native women Native
American/Alaska-Native women are members of more than 550 tribes that range in size from 20 to 250,000 people. Descending from the original inhabitants of the United States, they face new health risks associated with cultural dislocation, poverty, and the historical neglect of Native American/Alaska-Native rights and treaties.

The lack of comprehensive health insurance limits Native American and Alaska-Native women's access to regular health services for disease prevention, screening, diagnosis, treatment, and management of chronic and acute conditions. For example, an estimated 40 percent of Native American/Alaska-Native women who have INDIAN HEALTH SERVICE (IHS)–provided health care had not been screened

for CERVICAL CANCER within the last year. Recent estimates suggest that 73 percent of Native American/Alaska-Native women do not have annual blood pressure screenings. Overall, uninsured women are more likely than insured women to go without needed preventive health-care services.

The IHS is a program of the U.S. Department of Health and Human Services that provides hospital and ambulatory medical care as well as preventive and rehabilitative health-care services for Native Americans and Alaska Natives who are members of a federally recognized tribe.

Cervical Cancer
Native American women have the lowest cervical cancer incidence rate among U.S. population groups, according to 2000 statistics (7.7 per 100,000, compared to 17.5 for Hispanics, 13.3 for African Americans, and 9.6 for Caucasians). On the other hand, because so few of these women are screened for cervical cancer, the death rate for this type of cancer is higher (3.3) than that for Asians and Pacific Islanders (3.1) and Caucasians (2.8). Only African Americans and Hispanics have a higher death rate. Socioeconomic factors, including lack of education about PAP TESTS and poor access to transportation systems, contribute to this problem.

Endometrial Cancer
Native American and Alaska-Native women have some of the lowest rates of ENDOMETRIAL CANCER of all Americans.

Ovarian Cancer
Rates of OVARIAN CANCER are high among Native American and Alaska-Native women.

natural killer cells (NK cells) White blood cells
that can kill tumor cells and infected body cells. NK cells kill on contact by binding to the target cell and releasing a burst of toxic chemicals. Normal cells are not affected by NK cells, which play a major role in cancer prevention by destroying abnormal cells, preventing them from causing damage.

nausea and cancer treatment Feelings of nausea
may start within one to four hours of receiving

CHEMOTHERAPY for cancer; the worst nausea occurs during the first 12 to 24 hours. After that, occasional or unexpected episodes of mild nausea or vomiting may occur. Fortunately, since the mid-1990s several very strong antinausea medicines that reduce or eliminate this side effect have become available.

A few chemotherapy drugs—vincristine, carboplatin, bleomycin, FLUOROURACIL (5-FU), methotrexate, and VP 16—do not usually cause nausea. If a woman's particular drug regimen is likely to cause significant nausea, intravenous (IV) drugs are given with chemotherapy to prevent this side effect.

Preventing Nausea

Patients should eat lightly before and for one to two days after chemotherapy, avoiding fried food, fruit juice, spicy foods, and foods such as hamburger, steak, or hot dogs.

Patients who are prescribed chemotherapy that is likely to cause nausea are given medicine to prevent nausea before the drugs are administered and given prescriptions for medicines to prevent nausea at home. Typically antinausea medications include prochlorperazine (COMPAZINE), lorazapam (Ativan), dexamethasone (DECADRON), aprepitant (Emenol) ondansatron (Zofran), granisetron (Kytril), and dolasetron (Anzemet). All of these medications work well for nausea, but certain drugs may work better for one person than another.

Easing Nausea

Eating certain foods, such as crackers, toast, oatmeal, soft bland vegetables and fruits, clear liquids, and skinned baked chicken, can help ease nausea. Foods to be avoided include fatty, greasy, or fried foods; sweets; and hot or spicy foods. Patients should not force themselves to eat during periods of nausea because doing so may trigger aversions to favorite foods. Patients who experience nausea should sip cool liquids between meals, not during meals. It may also help to eat in a room other than the kitchen if cooking smells make nausea worse.

needle biopsy See BIOPSY.

neoadjuvant therapy Administration of chemotherapy treatment before surgery with the goal of decreasing the size of a cancerous tumor so that it is easier to remove. With the development of new chemotherapy drugs and radiation therapy, clinical trials of neoadjuvant therapy are currently ongoing.

neoplasm Any abnormal growth. Neoplasms may be benign or malignant, but the term is usually used to describe a cancer.

neutropenia A blood condition characterized by low blood levels of white blood cells called neutrophils that are important in fighting infection. About 60 percent of all white blood cells are neutrophils. Because they are very important to fighting infection, when these vital white blood cells diminish in number, a person is much more likely to contract infections.

Neutropenia can be caused by CHEMOTHERAPY or RADIATION THERAPY or by cancer cells that directly infiltrate the BONE MARROW, interfering with the production of blood cells. Neutropenia may also be caused by BONE MARROW TRANSPLANT.

People who have neutropenia contract infections readily and often, usually in the lungs, mouth and throat, sinuses, and skin. Painful mouth ulcers, gum infections, ear infections, and periodontal disease are common. Severe, life-threatening infections may occur.

In general, the blood of healthy adults contains about 1,500 to 7,000 neutrophils per cubic millimeter (mm^3) (children younger than age six may have a lower neutrophil count). The severity of neutropenia generally depends on the absolute neutrophil count (ANC), as follows:

- *Mild neutropenia:* an ANC between $1,500/mm^3$ and $1,000/mm^3$
- *Moderate neutropenia:* an ANC between $500/mm^3$ and $1,000/mm^3$
- *Severe neutropenia:* an ANC below $500/mm^3$

Treatment

Often a person who has neutropenia must be hospitalized and receive intravenous antibiotics. Neutropenia caused by chemotherapy is treated by stopping the drugs until the white blood cell count increases (usually within a week).

nicotine See SMOKING.

Nurses' Health Study (NHS) One of the largest prospective investigations into the risk factors for major chronic diseases in women, sponsored by Brigham and Women's Hospital in Boston. The study includes the dietary and health records of nearly 89,000 female nurses across the United States and has provided important information about the development of reproductive cancers.

The Nurses' Health Study was established in 1976 and a second study of younger nurses (the Nurses' Health Study II) was established in 1989. The studies have grown to include a team of clinicians, epidemiologists, and statisticians at the Channing Laboratory, along with collaborating investigators and consultants in the surrounding medical community of the Harvard Medical School, Harvard School of Public Health, Brigham and Women's Hospital, Dana-Farber Cancer Institute, Boston Children's Hospital, and Beth Israel Hospital.

The primary motivation in starting the first NHS was to investigate the potential long-term consequences of the use of birth control pills, a potent drug that was being prescribed to hundreds of millions of normal women. Registered nurses were selected because experts believed their nursing education would allow them to respond accurately to brief, technically worded questionnaires. The first study included 122,000 nurses, who are contacted every two years to answer a follow-up questionnaire regarding diseases and health-related topics such as smoking, hormone use, and menopausal status.

Because researchers recognized that diet and nutrition would play important roles in the development of chronic diseases, in 1980 the first food-frequency questionnaire was collected. Subsequent diet questionnaires were collected in 1984, 1986, and every four years since. Questions related to quality of life were added in 1992 and repeated every four years. Because certain aspects of diet cannot be measured by questionnaire (especially minerals that become incorporated in food from the soil in which it is grown), the nurses submitted 68,000 sets of toenail samples between the 1982 and 1984 questionnaires.

To identify dietary mineral levels, and potential biomarkers such as hormone levels and genetic markers, the nurses have at times also submitted toenail and blood samples.

Nurses' Health Study II

The primary motivation for developing the NHS II was to study oral contraceptives, diet, and lifestyle risk factors in a population younger than that of the original study. This younger generation included women who started using oral contraceptives during adolescence and who were therefore exposed to these hormones during their early reproductive life. Several studies, suggesting such exposures might be associated with substantial increases in risk of breast cancer, provided a strong justification for investment in this large cohort. In addition, researchers planned to collect detailed information on the type of oral contraceptive used, which was not obtained in the original Nurses' Health Study.

The initial target population included women between the ages of 25 and 42 years in 1989; the upper age was to correspond with the lowest age group in the NHS. A total of 116,686 women remain in the second NHS.

Every two years, nurses receive a follow-up questionnaire with questions about diseases and health-related topics including smoking, hormone use, pregnancy history, and menopausal status. In 1991, the first food-frequency questionnaire was collected, and subsequent food-frequency questionnaires are administered at four-year intervals. A two-page quality-of-life supplement was included in the first mailing of the 1993 and 1997 questionnaires. Blood and urine samples from approximately 30,000 nurses were collected in the late 1990s.

nutrition and cancer treatment Although good nutrition may not cure cancer, dietary factors do play an important role in cancer treatment. A patient battling a severe disease such as cancer needs adequate nutrition to maintain strength and overall well-being, keep the IMMUNE SYSTEM functioning, prevent the breakdown of body tissue, and help the body heal. A well-nourished person is better able to tolerate treatment side effects and may be able to handle more aggressive treatments.

Good nutrition may also increase a patient's odds of survival. In general, a cancer patient should eat the best possible mix of nutrients without too much fat.

However, nutrition can be a problem for women who have cancer for several reasons. If the cancer has spread, it may interfere with eating and digestion as a result of problems in chewing and swallowing, gastrointestinal tract blockages, or interference with digestive enzymes and hormones. In addition, cancer treatment such as RADIATION THERAPY and CHEMOTHERAPY can cause nausea, vomiting, swallowing problems, painful mouth sores and sore throat, and dry mouth. Treatment may alter a patient's ability to taste or smell. Depression and lack of energy may make a person unwilling to eat, and appetite and metabolism may change.

Loss of appetite can be caused by the cancer itself, cancer treatment, or depression. CACHEXIA is the medical term for the wasting and dramatic weight loss seen in many cancer patients. Patients who have cachexia have body organs that starve and waste along with muscle and fat. Nearly all who have cancer that has spread experience weight loss due to appetite loss or cachexia. Although this loss may not be preventable, attention to eating and good nutrition allows a better quality of life, helps the body tolerate treatment, and can contribute to improvement in resistance to infection.

Improving Nutrition

There are a number of lifestyle changes that reproductive cancer patients can make to try to improve their nutrition:

- *Relaxation.* Patients should choose a quiet place to eat, listen to soothing music, and lessen distractions.
- *Presentation.* Patients can try to make eating a more pleasurable experience by preparing and presenting food in appetizing, attractive ways.

- *Spontaneous mealtimes.* Patients should eat when they are hungry and should not wait for mealtime. Because nausea or lack of appetite may come and go, patients should eat whenever they feel they can.
- *Small meals.* Patients often prefer to eat many small meals throughout the day instead of loading the stomach with three big meals.
- *Snacks.* Patients should keep snacks accessible and eat between meals.
- *Favorite foods.* Breast cancer patients should concentrate on having favorite foods available; availability can sometimes improve appetite.
- *Change of diet.* Sometimes eating a different type of food can stimulate the appetite.
- *Watch temperature.* Patients should pay attention to the temperature of the food they eat and notice what works better. Some patients find that warm or room-temperature food is better tolerated; others find that cold foods are more soothing. In general, hot and spicy foods are not well tolerated by most patients.
- *Avoidance of strong smells.* Patients should avoid cooking foods that have unpleasant smells. It may be better to eat food that has little or no odor, such as cottage cheese or crackers.
- *Loading of calories.* Patients can get extra calories by adding dry milk, honey, jam, or brown sugar to food whenever possible.

Nausea Tips

Patients who feel nauseated should call their doctor for antinausea medication. Taken as directed, it is often quite effective. Patients who are vomiting should not try to eat or drink until vomiting has stopped. Good diet choices for nausea include crackers, toast, oatmeal, soft bland vegetables and fruits, clear liquids, and skinned baked chicken. Foods to be avoided are fatty, greasy, and fried foods; sweets; and hot or spicy foods. Patients should not force themselves to eat during periods of nausea because doing so may trigger aversions to favorite foods.

Patients who experience nausea should drink liquids between meals, not during meals. It is sometimes helpful to eat in a room other than the kitchen if cooking odors worsen nausea.

Physical Eating Problems

Some patients may have trouble with eating due to physical problems related to the spread of their cancer or to the effects of chemotherapy. If this is the case, they should

- Avoid foods that may irritate the mouth, such as spicy, acidic, citrus, or salty foods

- Take very small bites of food
- Cook foods until they are very tender
- Puree foods in a blender or food processor
- Mix foods with broth, sauces, or thin gravies to make them easier to swallow
- Drink through a straw

obesity and cancer A number of factors have been linked to a woman's risk of developing cancer of the reproductive organs, including obesity—an abnormally high, unhealthy proportion of body fat more severe than simply being overweight. Obesity appears to increase the risk of cancers of the uterine lining, cervix, and ovary; in fact, there is a strong relationship between ENDOMETRIAL CANCER and obesity.

This is of particular concern because by the early 2000s, more than 60 percent of American adults were considered to be overweight to some extent, and almost 25 percent were obese. This was a dramatic increase from the early 1980s, when only about 15 to 20 percent of Americans were overweight. Each year since the late 1970s, Americans have been getting heavier; from 1991 to 1998, the obesity rate increased in every state in the United States across all races, age levels, and educational levels.

Although there are many theories about how obesity increases cancer risk, the exact mechanisms are not known. In addition, because obesity develops through a complex interaction of heredity and lifestyle factors, determining whether obesity or another factor led to the development of cancer is not easy. Making conclusions from studies of obesity more difficult is that definitions and measurements of *overweight* and *obese* vary from study to study; that variability has affected earlier study results and made comparison of data across studies difficult.

Most researchers who study obesity as a risk factor for cancer currently use a formula based on weight and height, known as body mass index (BMI). According to a U.S. government panel and consistently with the recommendations of many other countries and the World Health Organiza-tion, *overweight* is defined as a BMI of 25 to 30, and *obese* as a BMI of 30 or more. Health risks increase gradually with increasing BMI. BMI is useful in tracking trends in the population because it provides a more accurate measure of who is overweight and obese than measurement of weight alone. By itself, however, this measurement cannot give direct or specific information about a person's health.

More studies are needed to evaluate the combined effects of diet, body weight, and physical activity on cancer because the increase in cancer risk may be due to extra weight, inadequate consumption of fruits and vegetables, or a high-fat, high-calorie diet.

In the future, researchers may measure physical fitness rather than level of physical activity as a way to predict health risks. The complex relationship between physical activity and obesity necessitates that researchers include both factors in future epidemiological investigations.

A panel of experts who met at the International Agency for Research on Cancer (IARC) in Lyon, France, concluded that being overweight and having a sedentary lifestyle are associated with several diseases. The panel recommended preventing obesity early in life by establishing healthy eating habits and regular physical activity. The panel advised women who are overweight or obese to avoid gaining weight and to lose weight through diet changes and exercise. The IARC, which is part of the World Health Organization, coordinates and conducts research on the causes of cancer and develops scientific strategies for cancer control.

oncogenes Genes that may trigger or allow cancer to grow. Some genes contain instructions that control when a person's cells grow and divide; those that promote cell division are called oncogenes. Normally these genes are responsible for helping cells to grow and spread, but when damaged in some way, they can cause cells to become malignant. Cancers can be caused by DNA mutations that activate oncogenes.

Genes known to have an effect on reproductive cancers include HER2-NEU, RAS family genes, and AICT2 genes.

See also TUMOR SUPPRESSOR GENES.

oncogenic virus   A virus that can help stimulate cancer growth. More than 100 of these viruses are known to exist; many are "slow viruses" that live in the body for years and that are believed to be linked to human cancer. The HUMAN PAPILLOMAVIRUS is one type of oncogenic virus; it is linked to almost all cases of CERVICAL CANCER.

oncologist   A physician whose primary interest is cancer. In most cases, when a woman is diagnosed with cancer of the reproductive organs, a clinical oncologist takes charge of her overall care through all phases of the disease. Within the field of clinical oncology there are three primary disciplines—medical oncology, surgical oncology, and radiation oncology.

- *Medical oncologists* are physicians who specialize in treating cancer with medications and CHEMOTHERAPY.
- *Surgical oncologists* are physicians who specialize in surgical aspects of cancer including BIOPSY, STAGING, and surgical removal of tumors.
- *Radiation oncologists* are physicians who specialize in treating cancer with therapeutic radiation.

Some doctors also specialize in GYNECOLOGIC ONCOLOGY. A gynecologic oncologist is an obstetrician or gynecologist who specializes in the diagnosis and treatment of women with gynecologic cancers. After completion of medical school, they must have two to four years of structured training in all of the effective forms of treatment of gynecologic cancer (surgery, radiation therapy, chemotherapy, and experimental treatments) as well as the biological and pathological characteristics of

gynecologic cancer. This training takes place in a limited number of medical centers. The unique aspect of this training is that it allows patients to receive treatment (surgery, chemotherapy, or radiation therapy) or combinations of therapy most likely to be successful without fragmenting their care among many physicians. Gynecologic oncologists practice in teaching hospitals, cancer centers, and regional and local hospitals.

Education and Training

Clinical oncologists complete four to seven years of postgraduate medical education depending on their primary discipline. In the United States, medical, radiation, and pediatric oncology are recognized as medical specialties by the American Board of Medical Specialties.

In order to become practicing cancer specialists, medical oncologists usually take board exams administered by the American Board of Internal Medicine, and radiation oncologists usually take board exams administered by the American Board of Radiology. Surgical oncologists do not have an equivalent specialty board, but general surgeons are certified by the American Board of Surgery; those surgeons who choose to specialize further in oncology receive a *certificate of special competence* after they complete the oncology training program.

Regardless of their particular discipline, medical, radiation, and surgical oncologists are broadly trained in all three areas of oncology and are knowledgeable about the appropriate use of each treatment approach. Within the three disciplines, oncologists usually choose to specialize further in specific types of cancer, such as reproductive cancers.

oncologist, gynecologic   See GYNECOLOGIC ONCOLOGIST; ONCOLOGIST.

oncologist, medical   See ONCOLOGIST.

oncologist, radiation   See ONCOLOGIST.

oncologist, surgical   See ONCOLOGIST.

oncology   The branch of medicine related to the study of cancerous tumors.

oncology clinical nurse specialist (CNS) An advanced practice nurse who has a master's degree and extensive education in the needs of cancer patients. A CNS specializing in oncology works primarily in hospitals to provide and supervise care for cancer patients who are either chronically or critically ill. Oncology CNSs monitor their patients' physical condition, prescribe medication, and manage symptoms. They are trained to apply nursing theory and research to clinical practice and may function as researchers, administrators, consultants, and educators in this field.

The CNS can help women who are trying to deal with their diagnosis and/or treatment regimen. Managing symptoms, maintaining health and wellness during treatment, and coping with information about reproductive cancer and its treatment are all areas of expertise that the clinical nurse specialist can share with patients and families. The oncology CNS works closely with the entire health-care team to ensure that a plan of care is comprehensive, identifies the patient's needs, and is clear to and manageable by the patient and family. The CNS can help the patient and family understand and cope with a cancer diagnosis.

Oncology Nursing Society (ONS) The largest professional membership oncology association in the world. ONS initiates and actively supports educational, legislative, and public-awareness efforts to improve the care of people with cancer. This professional organization of more than 30,000 registered nurses and other health-care providers is dedicated to excellence in patient care, education, research, and administration in oncology nursing. ONS, which was established in 1975, has grown to include more than 218 chapters and 32 special interest groups. It provides information and education to nurses around the world. In addition, the society plays an active role in advocacy activities at the local, state, national, and international levels. For contact information, see Appendix 1.

oophorectomy The surgical removal of one or both ovaries (also called ovariectomy). An oophorectomy is performed to remove cancerous ovaries or remove the source of ESTROGEN that stimulates some cancers, among other reasons. If one ovary is removed, a woman may still menstruate and have children, but if both ovaries are removed, menstruation stops and a woman can no longer have children naturally.

An oophorectomy may include the complete removal of one or two ovaries, or just a portion. However, when the procedure is done to treat OVARIAN CANCER or other spreading cancers, both ovaries are always removed. This procedure is a bilateral oophorectomy.

Oophorectomies are sometimes performed on premenopausal women who have been diagnosed with estrogen-sensitive breast cancer in an effort to remove the main source of estrogen from the body. However, this procedure is now performed less commonly than it was in the 1990s.

Today, chemotherapy drugs that alter the production of estrogen are available; TAMOXIFEN, for example, blocks any of the effects any remaining estrogen may have on cancer cells.

Until the 1980s, women older than age 40 who had a HYSTERECTOMY (the surgical removal of the uterus) also routinely had both healthy ovaries and fallopian tubes removed at the same time, in an operation called a bilateral SALPINGO-OOPHORECTOMY. Many physicians reasoned that a woman older than 40 was approaching menopause and soon her ovaries would stop secreting estrogen and releasing eggs. Removing the ovaries would therefore eliminate the risk of ovarian cancer and accelerate menopause by only a few years.

However, by the 1990s doctors began to have second thoughts about routine oophorectomies. Reasoning that the risk of ovarian cancer in women with no family history of the disease is less than 1 percent, doctors also realized that removing the ovaries increases the risk of cardiovascular disease and speeds osteoporosis unless a woman takes replacement hormones.

Of course, under certain circumstances an oophorectomy may still be the treatment of choice to prevent breast and ovarian cancer in certain high-risk women. A study done at the University of Pennsylvania and released in 2000 showed that among healthy women who carried the *BRCA1* or *BRCA2* genetic mutations that predisposed them to breast cancer the risk of breast cancer dropped from 80 percent to 19 percent when the ovaries were removed before age 40. Women between the ages of 40 and 50 had less of a risk reduction with the surgery, and there was no significant reduction of breast cancer risk in women who had the surgery after age 50.

Overall, ovarian cancer still ranks low on a normal woman's list of health concerns: it accounts for only 4 percent of all cancers in women. But the lifetime risk for development of ovarian cancer in women who have mutations in *BRCA1* is significantly higher than that of the general population: a 30 percent risk of ovarian cancer by age 60. For women at increased risk, oophorectomy may be considered after the age of 35 if childbearing is complete.

Although the value of ovary removal in preventing both breast and ovarian cancer is clear, scientists do not agree about when and at what age this treatment should be offered. In addition, preventative oophorectomy, also called prophylactic bilateral oophorectomy (PBO), is not always covered by insurance. One study conducted in 2000 at the University of California at San Francisco found that only 20 percent of insurers paid for PBO; another 25 percent had a policy against paying for the operation; and the remaining 55 percent said that they would decide about payment on an individual basis.

There are situations in which oophorectomy is a medically wise choice for women who have a family history of breast or ovarian cancer, but women with healthy ovaries who are having a hysterectomy for reasons other than cancer should discuss with their doctors the benefits and disadvantages of having the ovaries removed at the time of the hysterectomy.

The Procedure

Oophorectomy is performed with general anesthesia through the same type of incision (either vertical or horizontal) used for abdominal hysterectomy. Horizontal incisions leave a less noticeable scar; vertical incisions give the surgeon a better view of the abdominal cavity. After the incision is made, the abdominal muscles are pulled apart so that the surgeon can see the ovaries. Then the ovaries (and often the fallopian tubes) are removed.

An oophorectomy can be done laparoscopically. In this procedure, a tube containing a tiny lens and light source is inserted through a small incision in the navel. A camera can be attached to allow the surgeon to see the abdominal cavity on a video monitor. When the ovaries are detached, they are removed though a small incision at the top of the vagina. The ovaries can also be cut into smaller sections and removed.

The benefit of an abdominal incision is that the ovaries can be removed even if a woman has many adhesions from previous surgery, and the surgeon can check the surrounding tissue for disease. If cancer is suspected, a vertical abdominal incision must be used. The disadvantages of abdominal surgery are that bleeding is more likely to be a complication of this type of operation, it is more painful, and the recovery period is longer. A woman can expect to be in the hospital two to five days and to need three to six weeks to return to normal activities.

There is some discomfort after surgery, but the degree of discomfort varies and is generally greater with abdominal incisions, because the abdominal muscles must be stretched out of the way so that the surgeon can reach the ovaries. If even part of one ovary remains, it produces enough estrogen that a woman continues to menstruate, unless her uterus has been removed in a hysterectomy.

CHEMOTHERAPY or RADIATION THERAPY is often administered in addition to surgery for cancer. Some women find that losing their ovaries is emotionally upsetting; they can benefit from counseling and support groups.

Although an oophorectomy is a relatively safe operation, as all major surgery does, it entails some risks. The patient may have an unanticipated reaction to anesthesia, internal bleeding, blood clots, accidental damage to other organs, and postsurgical infection. Complications after an oophorectomy if both ovaries are removed include changes in sex drive, hot flashes, and other symptoms of menopause.

oophorectomy, prophylactic Surgical removal of both healthy ovaries as a way of preventing OVARIAN CANCER. It generally is recommended only for certain very high-risk patients older than age 40, such as women who carry the *BRCA1* or *BRCA2* gene. Recent studies suggest that removal of both ovaries can also lower the risk of development of breast cancer of women who have *BRCA* gene mutations.

Although this operation significantly lowers ovarian cancer risk, it does not entirely eliminate it. In some women at a very high risk of ovarian cancer (due to a strong family history) who have had both ovaries removed, cancers can still form from the lining cells of the pelvic cavity where the ovaries were previously located. This type of cancer, known as primary PERITONEAL CARCINOMA, occurs more often in women who have *BRCA* gene mutations.

osteopontin   A protein that appears to occur in high levels in women who have early OVARIAN CANCER, according to a 2002 Boston study. Detecting this protein could provide a way to diagnose ovarian cancer in its earliest stages—a potentially lifesaving event. What is particularly important is that the high readings occur whether the tumor is at an early or later stage of development.

Researchers hope they will be able to develop a screening test to search for osteopontin and other markers of ovarian cancer, helping to identify tumors before they spread. That would be a major turning point in efforts to combat ovarian tumors, which are among the deadliest cancers in the United States. Each year, 25,000 women are diagnosed with ovarian cancer and 15,000 die.

However, although scientists at Brigham and Women's Hospital and at Dana-Farber Cancer Institute are optimistic about their findings, more tests are needed and it will be years before an ovarian screening test is in widespread use.

As a marker for the disease, osteopontin is not reliable enough that doctors can use it to make decisions about surgery, but used in combination with other markers, including a protein called prostasin, a screening test could be almost 100 percent accurate. The need for such a test is urgent, because most ovarian cancer patients are diagnosed at a late stage, when the prognosis is poor. By the time symptoms appear, the disease has often spread. If ovarian cancer is not detected until it has progressed to its third or fourth stage, less than one in three patients survives five years or longer.

ovarian ablation   Inactivation of the ovaries as a method of treating or preventing cancer. Ovarian ablation can be achieved by surgery, radiation treatment, or HORMONE manipulation.

Surgery

The ovaries can be removed during a surgical procedure called OOPHORECTOMY, usually performed during LAPAROSCOPY, which produces only one or two small scars near the navel. This operation is usually done with general anesthesia and necessitates a one- or two-day hospitalization.

In some cases it may not be possible for the ovaries to be removed in this way (for example, if a woman has had previous abdominal surgery). In this situation, the ovaries are removed through a short incision directly below the navel; this surgery may require a longer hospital stay. The operation produces an immediate and permanent ovarian ablation.

Radiation Treatment

RADIATION TREATMENT aims high-energy X-rays at the ovaries, stopping their functioning. After an ultrasound precisely locates the ovaries, the outpatient radiation treatment can begin; it continues over a period of a few days. In some cases radiation may be administered on alternate days to reduce the likelihood of side effects such as nausea and tiredness.

Irradiating the ovaries produces a much slower ovarian ablation than oophorectomy; a woman's periods gradually stop during the first few months after treatment.

Possible side effects of radiation treatments include diarrhea, nausea, and abdominal discomfort. These symptoms are usually temporary; sometimes they may continue for a week or more.

There is a small possibility that radiation treatment will not be effective. It may be necessary to use a higher dosage of radiation to ensure that the ovaries are completely ablated.

Another potential but rare risk of an ovarian ablation by irradiation is the possibility of radiation damage that appears months or years after the treatment in organs and tissues near the ovaries. This risk can be minimized by careful planning and low radiation dosages.

Hormone Manipulation

Hormone manipulation stops the ovaries' production of ESTROGEN by interfering with other hormones from the brain that control ovarian function. The drug most commonly used to do this is goserelin (Zoladex), which is injected into the abdomen once a month.

Estrogen production usually drops to levels similar to those after surgery within three weeks of drug treatment. This effect continues as long as the treatment does. Zoladex is commonly given for two to five years.

The advantage of using drug treatment to stop estrogen production is that the effects are potentially reversible. Once therapy is stopped, most women's ovaries begin to function again within five to six months.

One side effect of ovarian ablation is early MENOPAUSE, which may cause symptoms such as hot flushes, sweats, vaginal dryness, and loss of sex drive. In contrast to those of natural menopause, these symptoms tend to begin abruptly and more intensely.

ovarian cancer Cancer that starts in the cells of the ovaries. There are many types of tumors that can originate in the ovaries, many of which are harmless. For example, OVARIAN CYSTS are not usually malignant and usually fade away without treatment. However, a doctor may recommend they be removed, especially if they are growing, to make sure they do not become malignant.

Ovarian cancer is a serious and underrecognized threat to women's health—the deadliest of the gynecologic cancers and the fifth leading cause of cancer death among U.S. women. Overall, it is the sixth most common type of cancer to affect women, excluding nonmelanoma skin cancer. Ovarian cancer occurs in every one of 57 women; about 25,500 American women are diagnosed each year, and about 16,090 die each year.

The good news is that the ovarian cancer incidence rate has been slowly decreasing since 1991. (The incidence rate is a precise way for scientists to describe how common or rare a disease is.) The *ovarian cancer incidence rate* is defined as the number of new cases diagnosed each year per 100,000 women.

The five-year survival rate for ovarian cancer at all stages is 37 percent. If a woman is still alive five years after the date of her diagnosis, she is considered to have the greatest chance of cure. Current data suggest that the risk of recurrence after five years, and of subsequent death of this type of cancer, is no greater than a woman's risk of dying naturally.

Although ovarian cancer is very treatable when it is detected early, the vast majority of cases are not diagnosed until cancer has spread beyond the ovaries. When ovarian cancer is detected before it has spread beyond the ovaries, more than 90 percent of women survive longer than five years. Only 25 percent of ovarian cancer cases in the United States are diagnosed in the early stages. When ovarian cancer is diagnosed in advanced stages, the chance of five-year survival is only about 25 percent.

Risk Factors
All women are at risk for ovarian cancer; some factors may put some women at higher risk for the disease.

History of cancer Having a family or personal history of ovarian, breast, or colon cancer is the most significant risk factor for ovarian cancer. Approximately 5 to 10 percent of ovarian cancer cases are associated with hereditary risk. Women can inherit risk from either parent, particularly if a first-degree relative has or has had breast, ovarian, colon, or UTERINE CANCER. Some researchers believe that a family history of prostate cancer may also be linked to increased risk for ovarian cancer. Women who have a personal or family history of these types of cancer are more likely to have ovarian cancer before the age of 50.

BRCA1/BRCA2 genes About one in every 10 ovarian cancer cases is hereditary, usually attributed to mutations in one of two genes: *BRCA1* and *BRCA2*. Women who inherit a mutation in either of these genes have a higher risk of development of epithelial ovarian cancer (as well as breast cancer). Although having these mutations increases risk for the disease, it does not guarantee that a woman who has the gene will have ovarian cancer.

Women who have a family history of breast and ovarian cancer or a personal history of either, particularly if diagnosed before age 50, should be aware of increased risk for the other. Women who have had breast cancer before the age of 50 are twice as likely to have ovarian cancer as women who have not. Ovarian cancer has also been linked to colon cancer (via different genes, however).

Hereditary nonpolyposis colon cancer (HNPCC or Lynch syndrome II) This genetic cancer syndrome that has been linked to a 12 percent risk of ovarian cancer and a 40 to 60 percent risk of endometrial cancer. (See HEREDITARY NONPOLYPOSIS COLON CANCER for more information.)

Age Up to 56 percent of women diagnosed with ovarian cancer are older than age 65. Although ovarian cancer can strike women at any age, the incidence increases dramatically after the age of 50, peaking between the ages of 55 and 65. Nearly two-thirds of the women diagnosed with ovarian cancer after age 50 are detected in late stage, when the five-year survival rate is only about 25 percent. As a result, it is important that women continue to have regular gynecologic exams after childbearing is complete.

No children Because ovarian cancer risk drops with each subsequent pregnancy, women who do not bear children appear to be at higher risk for ovarian cancer. Women who have had problems with conception are also at an increased risk of the disease.

Endometriosis Women who have endometriosis have a 50 percent higher risk of ovarian cancer than women without the condition. Endometriosis is a chronic, progressive disease that develops when tissue lining the inner surface of the uterus starts to grow outside the uterus. These implants occur most frequently in the pelvic area and on the reproductive organs, although they can appear in other areas as well. Between 20 and 40 percent of women diagnosed with this chronic disease are infertile, and researchers suspect that the most likely link between endometriosis and ovarian cancer is the association between endometriosis and infertility. It is well established that ovarian cancer risk is reduced with each pregnancy. Consequently, women who do not bear children, whether by choice or as a result of infertility, are believed to be at greater risk for ovarian cancer.

Possible Causes

Hormone replacement therapy (HRT) Experts are not sure whether HORMONE REPLACEMENT THERAPY (HRT) has been linked to ovarian cancer, but a 2002 study of hormone therapy that replaced only ESTROGEN did find a link between the treatment and ovarian cancer. About 40 percent of postmenopausal American women had used HRT to relieve the symptoms of menopause until a study released in May 2002 showing that women who had estrogen plus PROGESTIN HRT had a higher risk of heart disease, stroke, and invasive breast cancer. Although therapy that replaces estrogen alone has been proved to increase ovarian cancer risk in some studies, more research is needed to determine whether there is a link between combination HRT and the disease.

Talc products Some research has shown a potential link between talc exposure in the genital area and a slightly increased risk of ovarian cancer. Talcum powder is produced from talc, which in its natural form may contain asbestos (a known carcinogen). Because of this association with asbestos, all talc products marketed for use in the home, including baby powders, body powders, and facial powders, have been required to be asbestos free since 1973.

Studies suggest that talcum powder (including "asbestos-free" talc) may affect the outer layer of the ovaries when applied to the genital area, sanitary napkins, diaphragms, or condoms. Although several studies have examined the relationship between talcum powder and ovarian cancer, findings are mixed. Some experts recommend that women consider avoiding talc products until more conclusive research is available.

Fertility drugs Since the 1980s, more and more American women have taken fertility drugs in the hope of becoming pregnant. There are conflicting results of studies checking a possible link between fertility drugs and a higher risk of ovarian cancer. Whereas several studies in the early 1990s identified certain fertility drugs as increasing a woman's risk for ovarian cancer, a study published in February 2002 reported that ovarian cancer risk was not increased by use of fertility drugs but rather by infertility itself. In this study, researchers compared 5,207 women who had ovarian cancer and 7,705 women who did not have the disease and found that women who had endometriosis or unexplained fertility problems were 73 percent and 19 percent respectively. Although more likely to have the disease, this study was significantly larger than previous studies, more research is needed to rule out a connection between ovarian cancer and fertility drugs definitively.

Acquired genetic changes Most DNA mutations of ONCOGENES or TUMOR SUPPRESSOR GENES related to ovarian cancer occur during a woman's life, they are caused by radiation or cancer-causing chemicals. So far, studies have not been able to identify any single chemical in the environment or in a woman's diet that causes mutations. The cause of most acquired mutations remains unknown.

Most ovarian cancers have several acquired gene mutations. Research has suggested that tests to identify acquired changes of certain genes in ovarian cancers, such as the *p53* tumor suppressor gene or the *HER-2* oncogene, may aid prognosis. The role of these tests is still not certain, and some cancer specialists feel that more research is needed.

Recently, a MONOCLONAL ANTIBODY therapy called trastuzumab (Herceptin) that specifically interrupts the growth-promoting action of the *HER-2* oncogene has been developed. This new treatment has been approved as a treatment for breast cancer and is currently being tested in clinical trials to determine whether it will be effective in treating ovarian cancer.

Types of Ovarian Cancer

There are three different types of ovarian cancer, which are classified according to the type of cell from which they start: EPITHELIAL OVARIAN CARCINOMA, GERM CELL TUMOR, and ovarian STROMAL CARCINOMA.

Epithelial ovarian carcinoma The most common type of ovarian cancer, epithelial ovarian carcinoma begins in cells on the surface of the ovaries (epithelial cells). This type accounts for between 65 and 90 percent of all ovarian cancers. Epithelial ovarian carcinomas are further divided into types, including serous (40 percent), endometrioid (20 percent), undifferentiated (15 percent), borderline (15 percent), clear cell (6 percent), and mucinous (1 percent).

Epithelial carcinomas are further divided into grades according to the aggressiveness of the cells, ranging from grade 0 (tumors of low malignant potential) to grade III (poorly differentiated). The lower the grade number, the better the prognosis.

Clear cell, grade III carcinomas have a poorer prognosis than the other cell types.

Germ cell carcinoma Germ cell carcinoma is an ovarian cancer that begins in the cells that form the eggs and makes up about 5 percent of ovarian cancer cases. Germ cell carcinoma can occur in women of any age; however, it tends to be found most often in women in their earlier 20s. There are six main types of germ cell carcinomas, of which the three most common types are TERATOMAS, DYSGERMINOMAS, and endodermal sinus tumors. There are also many benign tumors that begin in the germ cells.

Stromal carcinoma Ovarian stromal carcinoma develops in the connective tissue cells that hold the ovary together and those that produce the female hormones estrogen and progesterone; it accounts for the remaining three percent of ovarian cancer cases. The two most common types are granulosa cell tumors and Sertoli's and Leydig's cell tumors. Unlike the more common epithelial ovarian carcinoma, 70 percent of the cases of stromal carcinoma are diagnosed early (by stage I).

Symptoms

Although many women assume there are no symptoms of ovarian cancer, in fact there are several indications of problems. The type of symptoms a woman has are often associated with the location of the tumor and its impact on the surrounding organs. They tend to be general and can mimic nongynecologic conditions such as irritable bowel syndrome. Symptoms include the following:

- Abdominal pressure, bloating, or discomfort
- Abnormal bleeding
- Constipation or diarrhea
- Fatigue
- Nausea, indigestion, or gas
- Shortness of breath
- Unexplained weight gain or loss
- Urinary frequency

Diagnosis

There are no completely foolproof screening tools to identify ovarian cancer, and it is hard to diagnose because symptoms are easily confused with those of other diseases.

CA 125 An elevated CA 125 blood level, though an indicator of ovarian cancer, is not a foolproof. In premenopausal women, for example, it is not uncommon for a CA 125 count to be higher than normal as a result of benign conditions unrelated to ovarian cancer, such as uterine fibroids, liver disease, or inflamed fallopian tubes. Other types of cancer can also elevate a woman's CA 125 level. The CA 125 test is more accurate in postmenopausal women. In about 20 percent of cases of advanced stage disease, and half of all early stage disease, the CA 125 level is not elevated. As a result, CA 125 level is usually only one of several tools used to diagnose ovarian cancer. (Among the most important uses of the CA 125 test are evaluation of tumor response of patients who are undergoing treatment and monitoring of the levels of women who are in remission for evidence of disease recurrence.)

LPA blood test Lysophosphatidic acid (LPA) stimulates the growth of ovarian tumors, and one small study found that levels of LPA in blood plasma are elevated in about 90 percent of women who have early ovarian cancer. Clinical trials are ongoing to determine the effectiveness of LPA in detecting ovarian cancer; it is still too early to know whether this test will be a good screening tool. This test is not yet available to the public.

DNA blood test A successful blood test for abnormal DNA shed by ovarian tumors has been developed by Johns Hopkins scientists. The test is based on a digital analysis of single nucleotide polymorphisms, or "SNPs"; called digital SNP which separates the two strands of code found in every gene to search for imbalances that are a hallmark of cancer cell DNA.

In a 2002 study, the Hopkins team looked at 54 blood samples from late- and early-stage ovarian cancer patients. Using digital SNP analysis, they found imbalances in 87 percent (13 of 15) of early-stage ovarian cancers and 95 percent (37 of 39) of late-stage disease. No imbalances were detected in 31 blood samples from healthy individuals. The researchers also compared the type of genetic imbalance found in 17 of the samples with the corresponding tumor tissue and found that 15 of these had matching imbalance patterns. Digital SNP appears to detect ovarian cancers very well and is far more precise than other available tests, but the

testing is too expensive and labor-intensive to serve as a general screening test. Although there still is no useful way to screen all women for ovarian cancer, this test may be appropriate for women at high risk.

The Hopkins group also is investigating ways of achieving the same accurate detection rate with a less costly, more efficient test that could be used on a broader scale for ovarian and a variety of other cancers.

In normal cells, DNA has two versions (alleles)—one from the mother's copy of the gene and the other from the father's copy. Tumor cells, however, have an unequal ratio of maternal and paternal alleles. Digital SNP analysis counts the alleles present in each blood sample. In looking at the ovarian cancer samples, the team found high total amounts of DNA in 47 percent of women with early-stage ovarian cancers and in 56 of those with late-stage disease.

Laparotomy An exploratory surgical procedure, LAPAROTOMY is usually required to confirm an ovarian cancer diagnosis. During this procedure, cysts or other suspicious areas must be removed and biopsied. After the incision is made, the surgeon assesses the fluid and cells in the abdominal cavity. If the lesion is cancerous, the surgeon continues with a process called surgical staging to figure out how far the cancer has spread.

Staging

The initial surgery and staging of ovarian cancer are critical to determining the best course of treatment and prognosis. Ovarian cancer is staged at surgery on the basis of classifications devised by the International Federation of Gynecology and Obstetrics.

Stage I: Cancer is limited to one or both ovaries.

Stage IA: Cancer is limited to the inside of just one ovary, with no cancer on the outer surface of the ovary. There are no ascites containing malignant cells, and the tumor has not ruptured.

Stage IB: Cancer is limited to both ovaries without any malignant cells on the outer surfaces. There are no ascites containing malignant cells, and the tumor has not ruptured.

Stage IC: The tumor is classified as either stage 1A or stage 1B, and malignant cells have appeared on the outer surface of one or both ovaries, or at least one of the tumors has ruptured, or there are ascites.

Stage II: The tumor involves one or both ovaries, and it has spread to other pelvic structures.

Stage IIA: The cancer has spread to the uterus, the fallopian tubes, or both.

Stage IIB: The cancer has spread to the bladder or rectum.

Stage IIC: The tumor is classified as either stage IIA or stage IIB and either it is also on the outer surface of one or both ovaries, or at least one of the tumors has ruptured, or there are ascites containing malignant cells.

Stage III: The tumor involves one or both ovaries and has spread beyond the pelvis to the lining of the abdomen and/or the lymph nodes. The tumor is limited to the true pelvis but has also spread to the small bowel or omentum.

Stage IIIA: During the staging operation, the surgeon can see cancer involving one or both of the ovaries, but no cancer is grossly visible in the abdomen, and it has not spread to the lymph nodes. However, when biopsy samples are checked under a microscope, very small deposits of cancer are found in the abdominal surfaces.

Stage IIIB: The tumor is in one or both ovaries, and cancer in the abdomen is large enough for the surgeon to see, but not larger than two centimeters in diameter. The cancer has not spread to the lymph nodes.

Stage IIIC: The tumor involves one or both ovaries, it has spread to the lymph nodes, and/or the deposits of cancer are larger than two centimeters in diameter and are found in the abdomen.

Stage IV: Growth of the cancer involves one or both ovaries and has spread to the liver or lungs. Presence of ovarian cancer cells in the excess fluid accumulated around the lungs (pleural fluid) is also evidence of stage IV disease.

Prevention

Although there is currently no way to prevent ovarian cancer, there are several ways a woman may reduce the risk of development of the disease.

Birth control pills Oral contraceptives can cut the risk of ovarian cancer in half if taken for at least five years, probably because of the protective effect of higher PROGESTIN levels, breaks in the ovulation cycle, or a combination of both. In addition, several clinical studies have reported that the effects last for years after Pill use has ceased.

However, some studies have indicated that oral contraceptives may increase breast cancer risk in women who have a strong family history of breast cancer. Other studies, on the other hand, have not found any increase in breast cancer risk among women with *BRCA* mutations who take oral contraceptives. Recent studies of the risk reduction value of birth control pills in women who carry the *BRCA1* or *BRCA2* gene mutation—and are therefore at high risk for breast and ovarian cancer—have reached conflicting conclusions. Whereas a 1998 study reported that birth control pills reduce risk for women who have *BRCA1* or *BRCA2* genetic mutations, a study published in July 2001 found that the pills do little to reduce risk in these women. Further research is required to determine the effect of oral contraceptives on women who have *BRCA1* or *BRCA2* mutations.

Pregnancy and breast-feeding Pregnancy and prolonged breast-feeding significantly lower the risk of ovarian cancer, although it is unclear whether the protective effect of pregnancy relates to hormonal factors or to the suppression of ovulation. Studies show a 40 percent reduction in risk for women who bear at least one child, an additional 10 to 15 percent risk reduction with each successive term pregnancy. However, the risk reduction does not appear to extend beyond the fourth pregnancy.

Tubal ligation/hysterectomy Tubal ligation and hysterectomy may help prevent ovarian cancer in women who carry the *BRCA1* or *BRCA2* gene mutations, although scientists are not sure why. Some studies suggest that tubal ligation moderately disrupts blood flow to the ovary, in turn diminishing the number of menstrual cycles. Other studies propose that both operations, either by tying the tubes or by removing the uterus, block the passage of cancer-causing materials from the vagina to the ovaries. However, the impact of these operations on ovarian cancer risk is relatively small, and they cannot prevent all or even most cases. Experts believe therefore that these operations should be performed only when there is a valid medical reason, and not exclusively for their possible effects in preventing ovarian cancer.

Prophylactic ovary removal   Removing healthy ovaries (OOPHORECTOMY) reduces the incidence of ovarian cancer by about 99 percent. This procedure is usually suggested only for women at very high risk—those who have two or more first-degree relatives who have ovarian cancer (or ovarian and breast cancer) or those who have a *BRCA1* or *BRCA2* gene mutation who are past their childbearing years. However, even after oophorectomy, women (including those who have *BRCA1* and *BRCA2* gene mutations) still have about a 1.8 percent risk of primary PERITONEAL CARCINOMA—cancer of the abdominal lining, a close relative to ovarian cancer. Although this type of cancer is rare, it can develop even in a woman who does not have ovaries. It appears to be the same as epithelial ovarian cancer under a microscope, has the same symptoms, spreads in a similar pattern, and is treated the same way as ovarian cancer.

Diet   Some studies suggest that a high-fat diet may increase ovarian cancer risk, but other studies disagree. The AMERICAN CANCER SOCIETY recommends choosing fruits, vegetables, and whole grain products to make up most of the diet and limiting intake of high-fat foods, especially those from animal sources. Even though the impact of these dietary recommendations on ovarian cancer risk remains uncertain, following these recommendations can help prevent several other diseases, including some types of cancer.

See also OVARIAN CANCER–BREAST CANCER LINK.

ovarian cancer–breast cancer link   Most known genetic mutations that increase breast cancer risk also appear to increase risk of OVARIAN CANCER. In 1994, two breast cancer susceptibility genes were identified: *BRCA1* on chromosome 17 and *BRCA2* on chromosome 13. When a woman carries a mutation in either *BRCA1* or *BRCA2,* she is at an increased risk of breast cancer (and, to a lesser extent, of ovarian cancer) at some point in her life. Experts estimate that for women in the general population the lifetime risk for ovarian cancer is 1.7 percent, whereas for women with altered *BRCA1* or *BRCA2* genes, the risk is 16 to 60 percent.

BRCA1 and *BRCA2* normally help to suppress cell growth which is why a person who inherits either gene in an altered form has a higher risk of getting breast or ovarian cancers. In fact, experts believe that inherited alterations in the *BRCA1* and *BRCA2* genes are responsible for nearly all cases of familial ovarian cancer and about half of all cases of familial breast cancer.

The likelihood that breast and/or ovarian cancer is associated with *BRCA1* or *BRCA2* is highest in families who have

- A history of multiple cases of breast cancer
- Cases of both breast and ovarian cancer
- One or more family members who have two primary cancers (original tumors at different sites)
- An Ashkenazi (Eastern European) Jewish background

However, not every woman in such families has an alteration in *BRCA1* or *BRCA2,* and not every cancer in such families is linked to alterations in these genes.

Genes are small pieces of DNA, the material that acts as a master blueprint for all the cells in the body. A person's genes determine such characteristics as hair and eye color, height, and skin color. Any mistakes in a gene that interfere with its function can lead to disease.

Both men and women carry two copies of each *BRCA* gene in their cells. One copy of the *BRCA1* gene is present on each of a person's two chromosome 17s, and one copy of the *BRCA2* gene is present on each of a person's two chromosome 13s. People inherit one copy of each of their genes from their mother and another copy of each gene from their father. If one parent has a defective *BRCA1* or *BRCA2* gene, there is a 50 percent chance the child may inherit this defective copy and a 50 percent chance the child may inherit the normal copy. If a person inherits a defective *BRCA1* or *BRCA2* gene, then each of that person's children likewise has a 50 percent chance of inheriting it.

The *BRCA1* and *BRCA2* genes produce a chemical substance that helps the body prevent cancer. Most women have two normal copies of both the *BRCA1* and *BRCA2* genes, both of which produce this cancer-preventing substance. However, some women have a genetic defect in one copy of their two *BRCA1* and *BRCA2* genes; as a result, their body does not produce a normal amount of this cancer-fighting substance. These women are at very high risk of breast or ovarian cancer.

Women who have an inherited alteration in one of these genes have an increased risk of having ovarian or breast cancer at a young age (before menopause) and often have multiple close family members who have the disease.

Some evidence suggests that there are slight differences in patterns of cancer between people with *BRCA1* alterations and people with *BRCA2* alterations, and even between people with different alterations in the same gene. For example, one study found that alterations in a certain part of the *BRCA2* gene were associated with a higher risk for ovarian cancer than alterations in other areas of *BRCA2*.

Most research related to *BRCA1* and *BRCA2* has been done on large families with many affected individuals. Estimates of breast and ovarian cancer risk associated with *BRCA1* and *BRCA2* alterations have been calculated from studies of these families. Because family members share a proportion of their genes and, often, their environment, it is possible that the large number of cancer cases seen in these families may be partly due to other genetic or environmental factors. Therefore, risk estimates that are based on families who have many affected members may not accurately reflect the levels of risk in the general population.

Genetic Testing

It is possible to diagnose an altered *BRCA1* gene with a blood test, although the cost for genetic testing can range from several hundred to several thousand dollars, and not all insurance policies cover the test. Some people may choose to pay for the test, even when their insurer would be willing to cover the cost, to protect their privacy. From the date that blood is drawn, it can take several weeks or months for test results to become available. It may be possible to have the genetic test performed for free as part of a clinical study at a comprehensive cancer center.

If the Test Is Positive

If a patient tests positive for altered *BRCA1* or *BRCA2* genes, there are several possible approaches to take. Careful monitoring for symptoms of cancer may result in a diagnosis of disease at an early stage, when treatment is more effective. Surveillance methods for breast cancer may include mammography and a clinical breast exam. For ovarian cancer, surveillance methods may include transvaginal ultrasound, CA125 blood testing, and clinical exams.

Patients may also choose prophylactic surgery, in which the doctor removes as much of the at-risk tissue as possible in order to reduce the chance of cancer. However, preventive mastectomy (removal of healthy breasts) and preventive salpingo-oophorectomy (removal of healthy fallopian tubes and ovaries) are not guarantees against development of cancers in these areas. Because not all at-risk tissue can be removed by these procedures, some women have had breast cancer, ovarian cancer, or a type of cancer similar to ovarian cancer even after prophylactic surgery.

Ovarian Cancer Canada/Cancer de l'Ovaire Canada A nonprofit organization dedicated to improving the quality and length of life of women diagnosed with OVARIAN CANCER, to educating healthy women and the medical community about this disease, and to raising funds for research. For contact information, see Appendix I.

Ovarian Cancer National Alliance A national organization dedicated to placing ovarian cancer education, policy, and research issues prominently on the agendas of national policy makers and women's health-care leaders. The group was formed in September 1997, when leaders of seven ovarian cancer groups joined forces. The alliance founders were the newsletter *Conversations!;* the National Ovarian Cancer Coalition; Ovar'coming Together; the Ovarian Cancer Coalition of Greater Washington, D.C., the Ovarian Cancer Survivors Quilt Project; Ovarian Plus International; and SHARE: Self-Help for Women with Breast or Ovarian Cancer.

Since its founding, the Ovarian Cancer National Alliance has continued to raise awareness of ovarian cancer, the deadliest of the gynecologic cancers. The group supports research, advocacy, information, and patient support. For contact information, see Appendix I.

Ovarian Cancer Research Fund   A nonprofit organization dedicated to creating early diagnostic treatment programs and research directed to finding a cure for OVARIAN CANCER. This group works to raise public awareness of ovarian cancer while helping patients and their loved ones understand this disease and its treatment. They also provide educational information, including resource materials and a free video about ovarian cancer. For contact information, see Appendix I.

ovarian cysts   Small fluid-filled sacs on the surface of an ovary that are quite common in women during their childbearing years but that are not usually malignant. Most CYSTS result from the changes in HORMONE levels that occur during the menstrual cycle and the production and release of eggs from the ovaries. Most are harmless and recede spontaneously; however, some cysts produce severe symptoms that can be life-threatening.

The normal ovary produces a normal cyst with each menstrual cycle during a woman's reproductive years. The normal cyst (follicle) contains the egg and usually is less than three centimeters. After ovulation, this cyst remains behind but is rarely bigger than five centimeters and disappears with each menstrual cycle. Cysts are considered to be abnormal if they persist throughout multiple cycles, are six centimeters or larger, or are formed during childhood or after menopause. Nevertheless, the vast majority of these abnormal cysts are benign.

Although cyst formation is a normal part of ovulation in premenopausal women, cysts that do not disappear or that occur after menopause need to be evaluated. Doctors do not know whether these benign ovarian cysts can develop into OVARIAN CANCER; to be sure, experts usually recommend that they be removed.

Types of Ovarian Cysts

There are two types of functional cysts—follicular cysts and corpus luteum cysts. The follicle releases an egg when the pituitary gland sends a burst of hormone called luteinizing hormone (LH). A follicular cyst begins when LH does not surge, and the chain reaction does not start. The result is a follicle that does not rupture or release its egg; instead it grows until it becomes a cyst. Follicular cysts are usually harmless, rarely cause pain, and often disappear within two or three menstrual cycles.

If the LH does surge and an egg is released, the follicle responds to LH by producing large quantities of estrogen and progesterone in preparation for conception. This change in the follicle is called the corpus luteum. However, sometimes after the egg's release, its escape hole seals off and tissues accumulate inside, causing the corpus luteum to expand into a cyst. Although this cyst usually disappears in a few weeks, it can grow to almost four inches in diameter and has the potential to bleed into itself or twist the ovary, causing pelvic or abdominal pain. If it fills with blood, the cyst may rupture, causing internal bleeding and sudden, sharp pain.

Benign cysts do not invade neighboring tissue as malignant tumors do, but if a benign ovarian cyst is large, it can cause abdominal discomfort and may interfere with the production of ovarian hormones, causing irregular vaginal bleeding or an increase in body hair. If a large tumor or cyst presses on the bladder, a woman may need to urinate more frequently.

Some women have less common types of cysts that in rare cases can become cancerous. Women who have such cysts between the ages of 50 and 70 are at higher risk of ovarian cancer. Women who have or who are at increased risk of breast cancer also are at higher risk of OVARIAN CANCER. The following types of cysts are less common. These may form on the ovaries and increase the risk of ovarian cancer:

Dermoid cysts are actually benign tumors called teratomas that may contain hair, skin, or teeth, because they form from cells that produce human eggs. Although they are rarely malignant, they can become large and cause painful twisting of the ovary and fallopian tube.

Endometriomas form in women who have endometriosis, a condition in which uterine cells grow outside the uterus. Occasionally, some endometrial tissue may attach to the ovary and form a cyst.

Cystadenomas develop from ovarian tissue and may be filled with a watery liquid or mucus. They can grow up to 12 inches or more, twisting the ovary and fallopian tube.

Symptoms

An ovarian cyst may not cause any symptoms at all, or it may trigger the following symptoms:

• Menstrual irregularities

• Pelvic pain—constant or intermittent dull ache that may radiate to the back and thighs

• Pelvic pain shortly before a menstrual period begins or ends

• Pelvic pain during sex

• Nausea, vomiting, or breast tenderness similar to the discomfort experienced during pregnancy

• Abdominal fullness or heaviness

• Rectal or bladder pressure

• Difficulty in emptying the bladder completely

A woman who experiences severe or spasmodic pain in the lower abdomen, accompanied by fever and vomiting, should see a doctor. These symptoms and symptoms of shock (cold, clammy skin; rapid breathing; lightheadedness or weakness) require immediate emergency medical attention.

Diagnosis

A cyst on the ovary may be found during a PELVIC EXAM, during which the doctor feels the ovaries. If a cyst is suspected, doctors often advise further testing to determine which type it is and whether treatment is necessary. To identify the type, a doctor may perform a pelvic ultrasound. In this painless procedure, a transducer is inserted into the vagina to create a video screen image of the uterus and ovaries. This image can then be photographed and analyzed by the doctor to confirm the presence of a cyst, help identify its location, and determine whether it is solid or fluid-filled. Fluid-filled cysts tend to be benign; solid material in cysts may indicate the need for further evaluation.

Alternatively, a doctor may insert a laparoscope into the abdomen through a small incision to view the ovaries, drain fluid from a cyst, or take a sample for biopsy.

The following factors may indicate that a cyst may be cancerous:

• *Size.* About 5 percent of growths smaller than about two inches are cancerous, but the likelihood of cancer increases from 10 percent to 20 percent when the growth is between two and four inches, and risk increases again from 40 percent to 65 percent when the tumor is bigger than four inches.

• *Age.* The chance a cyst is malignant is about 25 percent at age 50 but gradually increases, so that by age 80, the chance that a cyst is malignant is about 60 percent.

• *Postmenopause.* Only about 10 percent of postmenopausal ovarian cysts are functional cysts; the other 90 percent are tumors with cysts that can be either benign or malignant. Doctors do not know why ovarian cysts form after menopause, but they do know that the number of years a woman has been postmenopausal and her use of hormone replacement therapy have no relation to the development of ovarian cysts.

Treatment

Treatment depends on a woman's age, the type and size of the cyst, and symptoms. Functional ovarian cysts typically disappear within 60 days without any treatment. Oral contraceptive pills may be prescribed to help establish normal cycles and decrease the development of functional ovarian cysts. Ovarian cysts that do not seem normal may require surgical removal by laparoscopy or exploratory laparotomy. Surgical removal is often necessary if a cyst is larger than six centimeters or lasts longer than six weeks. Treatment may include:

Watchful waiting A woman can wait and be reexamined in four to six weeks if she is not yet menopausal, ovulates and has no symptoms, and an ultrasound reveals a simple, fluid-filled cyst. Follow-up pelvic ultrasounds at periodic intervals are usually recommended to determine whether the cyst has changed in size. Watchful waiting, including regular monitoring with ultrasound, also is a common treatment option recommended for postmenopausal women if a cyst is fluid-filled and less than two inches in diameter.

Birth control pills If a woman has a benign cyst that is large and causes symptoms, birth control pills may help shrink it. Use of birth control pills may also reduce the chance of cyst growth.

Women who have used birth control pills for more than three years also may have half the risk of development of ovarian cancer.

Surgery   A doctor may recommend removing a cyst that is bigger than two inches in diameter or is solid, filled with debris, growing, or persisting through two or three menstrual cycles. Cysts also may be removed if they are irregularly shaped, cause pain or other symptoms, and can be found on both ovaries. If a cyst is not cancerous, it can be removed and the ovaries left intact in a procedure known as a cystectomy. It is also possible to remove the one affected ovary and leave the other intact in a procedure known as OOPHORECTOMY.

Leaving at least one ovary intact also enables the body to keep producing estrogen. However, if a cyst is cancerous, the doctor may advise a hysterectomy to remove both ovaries and uterus. Because the risk of ovarian cancer increases after menopause, doctors more often recommend surgery when a cystic mass develops on the ovaries at that time.

Prevention

There is no way to prevent the growth of ovarian cysts, but regular pelvic examinations can ensure that ovarian changes are diagnosed as early as possible. In addition, women should note any changes in their monthly cycle, including atypical symptoms that may accompany menstruation or that persist over more than a few cycles.

ovarian germ cell tumor   A type of rare OVARIAN CANCER that affects specific cells from which the ovaries develop before birth. The most common germ cell tumors (found primarily in teenage girls and young women) are DYSGERMINOMA, endoder-mal sinus tumor, EMBRYONAL CARCINOMA, malignant TERATOMA, and CHORIOCARCINOMA.

Symptoms

There are very few symptoms at the beginning of this condition; later on, symptoms may include abdominal swelling without weight gain in other places or vaginal bleeding after menopause.

Diagnosis

Ovarian germ cell tumor can be diagnosed with a PELVIC EXAM, blood tests and urinalysis, ultrasound, and computed tomography CT scans.

Treatment

Treatment depends on the stage of the disease; typically it involves surgery, RADIATION THERAPY, and CHEMOTHERAPY.

ovarian stromal carcinoma   See STROMAL CARCINOMA, OVARIAN.

ovaries   A pair of almond-sized organs in the female reproductive system located on each side of the uterus that produce eggs and female hormones. Each month during a woman's menstrual cycle, an egg is released from one ovary in a process called ovulation. The egg travels from the ovary through the fallopian tube to the uterus, where it implants if it has been fertilized by sperm.

The ovaries are also the main source of the female hormones ESTROGEN and progesterone, which influence the development of a woman's breasts, body shape, and body hair. They also regulate the menstrual cycle and pregnancy.

ovaries, removal of   See OOPHORECTOMY.

pain control   Controlling REPRODUCTIVE CANCER pain is a key component of any overall treatment plan; the most successful methods combine multiple therapies to prevent pain. When pain does break through, the proper dose of pain reliever should be taken immediately. Many patients have a tendency to wait until the pain is excruciating before seeking relief, but waiting too long often necessitates use of more pills and less effective pain control.

Estimates of persistent pain among cancer patients range from about 14 percent to almost 100 percent. The most common estimates found that pain was poorly controlled in 26 to 41 percent of all cancer patients.

One obstacle to measuring the scope of the problem is that patients themselves often give their doctors poor insight into their pain; some believe that pain is just part of the cancer experience and must be tolerated. Others have an unrealistic fear of opiates and often choose to suffer instead of asking for the drugs.

The best pain treatment depends on the level of pain and its cause. Mild pain often can be treated with acetaminophen, aspirin, or a nonsteroidal anti-inflammatory drug (NSAID). Ibuprofen and naproxen are two NSAIDs frequently suggested for mild cancer pain. Moderate to severe pain usually requires an opioid, usually beginning with codeine and progressing to other options, such as oxycodone, morphine, and hydromorphone.

Long-acting narcotics, such as methadone and sustained-release morphine sulfate, are used when breakthrough pain is a problem. For patients who have problems in swallowing pills, options include liquid morphine and a fentanyl skin patch.

Although pain is not always a prominent feature of cancer, it is one of the most feared symptoms. Today, however, there is no reason most who have cancer pain cannot be made comfortable.

The first step in managing cancer pain is proper evaluation. There are various types of pain in cancer, whether caused by injury of tissues around the tumor (nociceptive pain), tumor's stimulation of nerves (neuropathic pain), or individual mental responses to sensation from the tumor (psychogenic pain).

Not surprisingly, self-reporting by the patient is the most important way to assess the pain. A full history, physical exam, and appropriate lab and imaging studies (X-ray, computed tomography [CT], MAGNETIC RESONANCE IMAGING [MRI]) should reveal how the disease process is producing pain. But the pain's intensity, and features and the factors affect it are all important in helping decide the best strategy for treatment.

Acute Pain

Certain procedures involved in cancer diagnosis or treatment can sometimes produce acute pain, including BONE MARROW BIOPSY, needle aspiration, CHEMOTHERAPY (especially by injection), immunotherapy (pain in the joints or muscles), and RADIATION THERAPY. Such attacks can usually be managed with adequate doses of nonmorphine painkillers.

Chronic Pain

The most common chronic cancer pain occurs when the cancer spreads to the bone. Experts do not known why some bone metastases are painless and others are terribly painful. If the spine is involved, there may be damage to the spinal cord or nerve roots.

Other types of chronic pain conditions are due to nerve pain after surgery, node biopsy, or radiation. Chemotherapy can sometimes cause persistent nerve pain, which stops when the drug is discontinued.

Opioid Drugs

The most typical way to ease pain of women who have cancer is to use the derivatives of morphine, called opioid derivatives. The choice of drug depends on the woman's age, whether she also has liver or kidney disease, and potential for interactions with other medications. Although taking drugs orally is usually preferred, other methods (such as the transdermal skin patch) can be used if there is difficulty in swallowing or any severe gastrointestinal upset.

For continuous or frequently recurring pain, it is usually better to have a fixed dosage schedule (such as every four hours) than to administer the drug "as needed." Starting at a low dosage, the dosage is increased until pain stops or side effects prevent an increase. If pain "breaks through" the schedule, a rescue dose can be added immediately; rescue dose levels are typically 5 to 15 percent of the total daily dosage of the drug.

Oral doses can be given more often, if necessary, with as little as two hours between doses; the minimal interval between intravenous administrations can be as short as 10 to 15 minutes. It is important to know that there is no "correct" or "maximal" dosage for cancer patients—the correct dosage is whatever prevents pain.

In many cases, the development of side effects does not prevent further increase in dosage; the treating physician can prescribe medications or other therapies to counteract the most common problems seen with opioids, such as nausea, vomiting, and constipation.

Nonopioid Analgesics

Acetaminophen and NSAIDs are good painkillers, but they have a maximal dose level above which no more benefit can be expected. These medications are most useful for people who have bone pain or inflammatory pain in which the affected area is warm, red, and swollen. A newer type of NSAID, cyclooxy-genase-2 (COX-2) inhibitors, may be superior to other NSAIDs in preventing stomach or kidney toxicity.

In addition, certain types of cancer may do well with a particular drug directed at the tissue involved, such as treating bone pain with BISPHOS-PHONATES (Fosamax) or calcitonin.

Adjuvant Drugs

Adjuvant medications are drugs that help analgesics work more effectively. Some drugs that are not primarily painkillers may have pain-relieving activity as well as their main effect. For instance, steroids, antidepressants, some anesthetics, anti-epilepsy drugs, and major tranquilizers may each be helpful in various cases of nerve pain. They are usually given after opioid therapy has been stabilized. Adjuvant drugs include the following:

- *Tricyclic antidepressants* such as amitriptyline and doxepin, which can improve the action of opioids
- *Benzodiazepines* such as lorazepam and diazepam, which control anxiety to help reduce dosage of pain pills
- *Selective serotonin reuptake inhibitors* and other antidepressants, which improve mood
- *Nerve-pain modulators* such as gabapentin, which control pain but do not affect opioid brain receptors

Radiation Therapy and Chemotherapy

In addition to its main use as a way of destroying cancer cells, radiation therapy is often used to control pain, chiefly in managing the spread of cancer from the original site to the bone. Chemotherapy can provide pain relief in pancreatic cancer by shrinking a tumor, but there is often a problem of balancing this sort of improvement against the toxic effects that chemotherapy can produce.

Nondrug Therapy

There are many alternative treatments for cancer patients whose pain is not adequately controlled by medication, provided primarily by specialists in hospital settings. A cancer treatment center or pain clinic is the best place to get information and advice about these therapeutic approaches, if the patient's cancer-management team does not offer them. The following are the most common:

- Acupuncture
- Exercise
- Heat or cold treatment
- Massage

- Breathing exercises
- Relaxation techniques
- Hypnosis
- Individual, group, or family psychological therapy

Papanicolaou's stain   See PAP TEST.

Pap test (Papanicolaou's stain)   A simple, painless screening test used to detect CERVICAL CANCER, which strikes 10,520 American women a year and kills 3,900 of them. Because this type of cancer usually grows slowly, regular Pap tests can identify it early, when cells are just beginning to become malignant. This testing can help doctors cure or even prevent cervical cancer. However, although a Pap test result is useful for early detection of cervical cancer, it cannot detect most OVARIAN CANCER.

No cancer screening test in history is as effective as the Pap test for the early detection of cancer. In fact, since the Pap exam began to be used after World War II, deaths of cervical cancer have dropped 70 percent in the United States. And 80 percent of women who die of cervical cancer have not had a Pap test in the previous five years.

During the Pap test, the doctor or other healthcare professional obtains some cells from the cervix for lab analysis.

Pap Test Drawbacks

Pap tests are not perfect. The test can result in many false-negative rates (finding no cancer where malignancy is actually present).

Because any single Pap test can miss up to 40 percent of abnormalities, the more Pap tests a woman has, the better chance she has of maintaining her health. In addition, since precancerous and cancerous changes of the cervix develop slowly, the annual Pap test is the best way to prevent cervical cancer, by catching abnormal cells before they become malignant.

If the Test Result Is Abnormal

Results of more than two million Pap tests a year are considered to be inconclusive—that is, some cells appear abnormal, but it is unclear whether this abnormality is caused by a harmless benign condition or a precancerous condition. Adoption of new Pap test guidelines issued by a panel of U.S. experts from 29 professional groups, including the AMERICAN CANCER SOCIETY and the American College of Obstetricians and Gynecologists, could lead to a decrease in the number of return visits to the doctor and a reduction of anxiety for the millions of women whose cervical cancer results are "inconclusive."

In the past, many American women who had abnormal but inconclusive results had at least two follow-up Pap tests within a year, a colposcopy test to examine and biopsy the cervix, or a test for the HUMAN PAPILLOMAVIRUS (HPV), the chief cause of cervical cancer.

HPV is a sexually transmitted virus. It is believed that at any one time, some 40 million Americans are infected. For most people the body quickly eliminate the infection, and most HPV strains are harmless and cause no symptoms. But a few types of HPV can cause cervical cancer if infection lingers.

The new Pap test guidelines recommend that when test results are inconclusive, HPV testing alone be the preferred next step for many women. In many cases, the HPV test can use the same Pap test sample. If the HPV test is negative for the riskiest forms of the virus—as it is for about half of these women—the patient can be assured she does not have cancer or precancerous cells and does not need more follow-up testing.

The recommendations reflect a better understanding in recent years that only a few high-risk strains of HPV are the primary cause of cervical cancer. Until now, there had been no consensus among doctors on which follow-up test was the best response to abnormal findings. The new guidelines note that all three follow-up methods are safe and effective; however, HPV testing is preferred if Pap tests are done with liquid-based screening, which is becoming increasingly popular at labs around the United States. In this liquid technique, cells scraped from the cervix are collected in liquid instead of being smeared between two slides. Liquid-based screening makes more cells available for HPV testing.

Preparing for a Pap Test

For the best sample, a woman should schedule a Pap test during the two weeks after the end of her menstrual period. She should neither have sex nor douche 48 hours before the test. Pap smears should be done by labs accredited by the College of American Pathologists or another accrediting group. If the doctor's lab is not accredited, the patient can ask that the sample be sent to an accredited institution.

In the spring of 2003, the U.S. Food & Drug Administration (FDA) approved a test for HPV to be included in every regular Pap smear for women older than age 30. However, the new addition to the Pap smear is not automatically used—women have to choose to add the HPV test, which costs about $50. Automatic HPV screening is not recommended for women younger than 30 because they are the most likely to have transient, harmless HPV infections.

The new test requires some patient education, because millions of women will learn they have HPV even though their Pap results are negative. However, most of those infections are harmless and the women affected will be infection free within the year. Women diagnosed with HPV should be monitored and having another Pap test within six to 12 months; retesting can identify the few who will have problems. Women whose Pap smear results shows no sign of cancer and who are free of HPV can safely wait three years to be rechecked, according to new physician guidelines distributed after the FDA ruling. Women who do not choose to have HPV testing or who have signs of infection need more frequent Pap tests.

Experts do not know how many cases of cervical cancer the new test will help detect or prevent, but it is expected to help detect the rare fast-growing cervical cancer that occurs between regular Pap tests.

Patient Advocate Foundation A national network advocating health-care reform. Its primary function is to support legislation that enables cancer survivors to obtain insurance funding for medical care and participation in clinical trials. The group also serves as an active liaison between patients and insurers, employers, and/or creditors. In doing so, they resolve insurance, job retention, and/or debt crisis matters related to patients' diagnosis. Other services include referrals, information, advocacy, and health insurance assistance. For contact information, see Appendix I.

pelvic examination Internal examination of the reproductive organs to check the pelvic area inside and out. This is usually combined with a PAP TEST. Pelvic exams, which take only about five minutes, should begin at age 18 or when a woman becomes sexually active (whichever occurs first). Routine pelvic examination is recommended because it can detect some reproductive system cancers at an early stage. A number of health-care specialists, who have specialized training in the health and diseases of a woman's reproductive organs, can conduct pelvic examinations. They include gynecologists, nurse midwives, and gynecological nurse practitioners.

During the exam, the health-care specialist first examines the external genitalia to make sure there are no sores or swelling. Next, the specialist inserts a speculum into the vagina to inspect for inflammation, discharge, and sores. At this point, he or she usually obtains a Pap smear by gently scraping cells from the outside of the cervix as well as from the cervical canal. The cells are sent to a lab for analysis to make sure there are no abnormalities.

Next, the specialist feels the woman's uterus and ovaries by inserting two fingers into the vagina; with the other hand, he or she presses on the outside of the lower abdomen. This process helps indicate whether the organs are the right size and at normal locations. Next is a rectal exam to check for polyps, hemorrhoids, or other rectal problems. A test for occult blood also can be done at this time.

Most health-care specialists also conduct a breast exam at the time of a pelvic examination.

peritoneal carcinoma Cancer of the abdominal lining, which is closely related to OVARIAN CANCER. It develops from cells that line the pelvis or abdomen, which are very similar to epithelial cells on the surface of the ovaries. Although this type of cancer is rare, it can develop even in a woman who does not have ovaries. It appears almost identical to the epithelial ovarian cancer under a microscope, it has the same symptoms, it spreads in a similar pattern, and it is treated in the same way as ovarian cancer. The lining of the peritoneal cavity and the surface of the ovary have the same embryonic origin; therefore, the two cancers appear almost identical and are treated in the same way.

Primary peritoneal carcinoma is also called extraovarian primary peritoneal carcinoma (EOPPC) or serous surface papillary carcinoma. Because it tends to spread along the surfaces of the pelvis and abdomen, determining exactly where the cancer started is often difficult.

Symptoms

Symptoms of EOPPC are similar to those of ovarian cancer, including abdominal pain or bloating, nausea, vomiting, indigestion, and a change in bowel habits. Also as ovarian cancer can, EOPPC may trigger a rise in blood level of the TUMOR MARKER CA 125.

Genetic Links

Scientists consider it possible that the *BRCA1* gene mutation, which is associated with both breast and ovarian cancers, may function similarly in primary peritoneal carcinoma. However, not all peritoneal cancers are genetic—most cases are not.

Treatment

Treatment for EOPPC usually includes surgery to remove as much of the cancer as possible, followed by the same type of CHEMOTHERAPY used to treat ovarian cancer.

Prognosis

Information on prognosis is limited for this newly recognized type of cancer; early studies suggest that prognosis is similar to that of ovarian cancer.

Phase I trial   A study in which researchers test a new drug or treatment in a small group of people (between 20 and 80 subjects) for the first time to evaluate its safety, determine a safe dosage range, and identify side effects.

See also CLINICAL TRIALS; PHASE II TRIAL; PHASE III TRIAL; PHASE IV TRIAL.

Phase II trial   A clinical study with a larger group of participants than in a PHASE I TRIAL (between 100 and 300 subjects) in which researchers test a drug or treatment to determine whether a drug or treatment is effective and to evaluate its safety further.

See also CLINICAL TRIALS; PHASE I TRIAL; PHASE III TRIAL; PHASE IV TRIAL.

Phase III trial   A clinical study with a larger group of participants than in a PHASE I TRIAL or a PHASE II TRIAL (between 1,000 and 3,000 subjects) in which researchers test a drug or treatment to confirm effectiveness, monitor side effects, compare the treatment to commonly used methods, and collect safety information.

See also CLINICAL TRIALS; PHASE I TRIAL; PHASE II TRIAL; PHASE IV TRIAL.

Phase IV trial   A postmarketing study that provides more information about a drug or treatment, including its risks, benefits, and optimal use, than a Phase I, II, or III trial.

See also CLINICAL TRIALS; PHASE I TRIAL; PHASE II TRIAL; PHASE III TRIAL.

phenolics   A category of more than 2,000 PHYTOCHEMICALS, or plant chemicals. The chemical structure of these phytochemicals gives them the ability to mop up many FREE RADICALS as they circulate through the bloodstream. For this reason, phenolics are considered to be among the most powerful antioxidants and are studied for their ability to interfere with tumors.

phenoxodiol   A synthetic experimental anticancer drug that in studies has killed 100 percent of OVARIAN CANCER cells, including those cells resistant to "gold standard" chemotherapy drugs such as paclitaxel and carboplatin. The tests were conducted on human cell lines at Yale University School of Medicine.

The drug induces ovarian cancer cell death by changing a signal pathway in cancerous cells that would otherwise not allow the unhealthy cells to die. All cells in the human body must eventually die and be replaced. But when cancer cells do not die, problems occur. A key objective in cancer therapy is to find a way to trigger natural cell death (called APOPTOSIS) in cancer cells.

Phenoxodiol could be successful in treating other cancer types as well, according to a study published in the May 1, 2003 issue of *Oncogene*. The researchers also tested phenoxodiol in mice and found a threefold reduction in the size of tumors compared to those of a control group. No side effects were noted.

A PHASE II TRIAL using phenoxodiol for women with chemoresistant ovarian cancer is under way at Yale University. Five Phase I human trials with phenoxodiol have been completed; they have shown few side effects. Preliminary results of a trial conducted at the Cleveland Clinic found that more than half of the 10 patients tested on the experimental drug had some response. These patients had different types of advanced cancer that did not respond to conventional chemotherapy.

Ovarian cancer is the most lethal gynecological malignancy and the fifth leading cause of all cancer deaths of women. Although the initial response to chemotherapy is better than 80 percent, most ovarian cancer recurs because of chemotherapy resistance.

Phenoxodiol will most likely become available once it has been thoroughly investigated in clinical trials, submitted in an INVESTIGATIONAL NEW DRUG application to the U.S. Food and Drug Administration (FDA), and approved by the FDA as a safe and effective drug.

Physician's Data Query (PDQ) A comprehensive cancer database maintained by the NATIONAL CANCER INSTITUTE (NCI) and distributed since 1984 to doctors and the public. It is now available in multiple forms including fax, e-mail, conventional mail, and the Internet, in both English and Spanish. The PDQ contains peer-reviewed summaries about cancer treatment, screening, prevention, genetics, and supportive care and directories of physicians, professionals who provide genetics services, and organizations that provide cancer care.

The PDQ also contains the world's most comprehensive cancer clinical trials database, with about 1,800 abstracts of trials that are open and accepting patients, including trials for cancer treatment, genetics, diagnosis, supportive care, screening, and prevention. In addition, there is access to about 12,000 abstracts of clinical trials that have been completed or are no longer accepting patients.

The PDQ cancer-information summaries are peer reviewed and updated monthly by six editorial boards composed of specialists in adult treatment, pediatric treatment, complementary and alternative medicine, supportive care, screening and prevention, and genetics. The boards review current literature from more than 70 biomedical journals, evaluate its relevance, and synthesize it into clear summaries.

phytochemicals Natural compounds found only in plants that protect them from the ravages of sunlight and other environmental threats. Phytochemicals are currently being studied for their roles in blocking the formation of some cancers. They may also protect against some forms of heart disease, arthritis, and other degenerative diseases.

All fruits, vegetables, grains, oils, nuts, and seeds contain varying amounts of phytochemicals; some of these foods have levels that are higher, which make them a better choice for a healthy diet. Among the thousands of different phytochemicals, each one potentially has some benefit to humans. Some of these phytochemicals are currently being studied for their potential to prevent reproductive cancers.

Many studies have already provided evidence that eating more fruits and vegetables decreases the risk of cancer. In fact, phytochemical research helped prompt the NATIONAL CANCER INSTITUTE to initiate its Five-a-Day program for healthy eating, in which consumers are urged to eat more foods such as garlic, broccoli, onions, and soy products.

Phytochemicals, which represent thousands of different components in plant foods, differ from vitamins and minerals in that they are not considered essential nutrients. Yet a diet that includes phytochemicals from a wide range of fruits and vegetables has been associated with the prevention and treatment of cancer. Since different phytochemicals are present in different foods, eating a varied diet is important to ensure maximal potential cancer protection.

The specific phytochemical content of different fruits and vegetables tends to vary by color, and each has particular functions. Some phytochemicals act as ANTIOXIDANTS, some protect and regenerate essential nutrients, and others work to deactivate cancer-causing substances. Phytochemicals include allium compounds, CAROTENOIDS, glucosinolates, polyphenols, and flavonoids.

Allium compounds   Allium compounds such as allyl sulfides may help detoxify and rid the body of some carcinogenic compounds. Food sources include onions, garlic, scallions, and chives.

Carotenoids   Carotenoids such as alpha-carotene, beta-carotene, cryptoxanthin, lycopene, and lutein work as antioxidants, helping to offset harm caused by environmental pollutants such as pesticides and cigarette smoke. Food sources include dark green, orange, or red fruits and vegetables, especially carrots, sweet potatoes, tomatoes, spinach, broccoli, cantaloupe, and apricots.

Glucosinolates   Glucosinolates such as glucobrassicin are metabolized to produce two other phytochemicals—isothiocyanates and INDOLES—which trigger production of enzymes that block cell damage due to carcinogens. Food sources include cruciferous vegetables such as broccoli, broccoli sprouts, cabbage, and brussels sprouts.

Polyphenols   Polyphenols such as ellagic acid and ferulic acid are thought to prevent conversion of substances into carcinogens and to inhibit mutations. Food sources include oats, soybeans, and fruits and nuts—especially strawberries, raspberries, blackberries, walnuts, and pecans.

Flavonoids   Flavonoids include more than 2,000 powerful antioxidants from sources such as coffee, tea, cola, berries, tomatoes, potatoes, broad beans, broccoli, Italian squash, onions, and citrus fruits.

In the Future

Some day, scientists may develop "super breeds" of certain foods that contain higher levels of beneficial phytochemicals. Seed catalogs already offer home gardeners the opportunity to buy seeds of several of these supervegetables. For example, sulforaphane has been identified as a potent inducer of detoxifying enzymes (broccoli is a good source, and three-day-old broccoli sprouts is even better—they contain between 20 and 50 times more sulforaphane than do mature broccoli). In one study, rats fed sulforaphane had fewer malignant tumors, and their tumors developed at a slower rate.

In addition to high-sulforaphane broccoli sprouts, consumers can now buy high-lycopene tomatoes and high-beta-carotene cauliflower. Soon, some package labels may even list the amounts of dominant protective substances, just as food labels today list the amounts of calories or carbohydrates.

See also PHYTOESTROGENS.

phytoestrogens   ESTROGEN-like compounds found in plants. Many different plants produce compounds that may mimic or interact with estrogen HORMONES in animals. At least 20 compounds have been identified in at least 300 plants of more than 16 different plant families. These compounds, which are weaker than estrogens that occur naturally in humans, can be found in more than 300 foods, including garlic, parsley, soybeans, wheat, vegetables, fruits, and coffee.

Some phytoestrogens consumed at the levels in the typical American-style diet are associated with a reduced risk of ENDOMETRIAL CANCER, a new study has found.

Phytoestrogens can be divided into three chemical classes: the isoflavonoids, the lignans, and the coumestans. *Isoflavonoid* phytoestrogens occur primarily in soybeans and SOY PRODUCTS. *Lignan* phytoestrogens are found in high-fiber foods such as cereal brans and beans; flaxseeds contain large amounts of lignans. The *coumestan* phytoestrogens are found in various beans such as split peas, pinto beans, and lima beans; alfalfa and clover sprouts are the foods with the highest levels of coumestans.

Because scientists have found phytoestrogens in human urine and blood samples, they know that these compounds can be absorbed into the human body. Phytoestrogens differ remarkably from synthetic ENVIRONMENTAL HORMONES in that they are readily broken down, are not stored in tissue, and are quickly excreted.

How Phytoestrogens Work

Phytoestrogens may have different effects, depending on the dose. At low doses phytoestrogens can act as estrogen does; at high doses they block estrogen.

Phytoestrogens that mimic estrogen may affect the production or the breakdown of estrogen by the body, as well as the level of estrogen carried in the bloodstream.

Phytoestrogens that act differently than estrogen does may affect communication pathways between cells, preventing the formation of blood vessels to tumors or altering the processing of DNA for cell multiplication. Which of these effects occurs is unknown. It is possible that more than one of them may be working, affecting various parts of the body.

Phytoestrogens and Health

Scientists do not agree about the role of phytoestrogens in human health. When consumed as part of an ordinary diet, phytoestrogens are probably safe and may even help protect against certain cancers, such as endometrial cancer.

However, eating too many phytoestrogens may cause some health problems. Laboratory animals, farm animals, and wildlife whose entire diet was made up of phytoestrogen-rich plants had reproductive problems. Although humans almost never have a diet made up exclusively of phytoestrogen-rich foods, those who eat uncooked soy or use phytoestrogen pills may be exposing themselves to some health risks. Many natural compounds, especially hormones, can be potent and can have both good and bad health effects, depending on their level in the body. These substances should always be used in moderation to prevent unintentional health consequences.

History of Phytoestrogens

Humans have used plants for medicinal and contraceptive purposes for thousands of years. Many plants historically used to prevent pregnancies or cause abortions contain phytoestrogens and other hormonally active substances. Modern scientists know that its seeds contain a chemical that blocks progesterone, a hormone that is necessary for establishing and maintaining pregnancy.

Cancer Prevention

Phytoestrogens have been investigated as possible cancer preventives. In one recent study, women who had a diet higher in certain phytoestrogens had endometrial cancer less often than women whose diet was lower in those substances. The development of endometrial cancer is related to prolonged exposure to estrogens without cyclic exposure to progesterone. Estrogen is primarily responsible for directing endometrial cells to multiply or proliferate. Proliferation is necessary during the "buildup" phase of the endometrium's cycle; however, the hormone's effects must be cyclically constrained by other hormones, such as progesterone. Estrogen stimulation that continues unchecked can lead to ENDOMETRIAL HYPERPLASIA, which is a known risk factor for the later development of endometrial cancer. There is evidence that phytoestrogens in the diet may help counteract the proliferative effects of estrogen.

Phytoestrogens compete with estrogen for cell-receptor binding sites, helping to control the level of estrogen circulating in the blood. Phytoestrogens' "antiestrogen effect" may block the development of endometrial cancer by reducing hormonal activities that cause endometrial cells to proliferate uncontrollably.

In the study, consumption of isoflavones and lignans—but not for coumestans—was associated with a lower risk of endometrial cancer, particularly among postmenopausal women. Obese postmenopausal women who consumed relatively low amounts of phytoestrogens had the highest risk of endometrial cancer; however, the interaction between obesity and phytoestrogen intake was not statistically significant.

The health effects of phytoestrogens may depend on the kind and amount of phytoestrogens eaten and the age, gender, and health of the diner. Women who ate the highest amount of foods rich in these compounds had a 54 percent reduction in cancer risk, compared with that of those who consumed the least.

Cancer Risks

Though some level of phytoestrogens may protect against cancer, higher exposure to any type of estrogen over a lifetime is linked with an increased breast cancer risk. It is currently unclear whether phytoestrogens in soy foods affect breast cancer risk. Results of studies looking directly at breast cancer risk and soy in the diet conflict: almost half of the studies have reported no effect of soy on breast cancer risk. In addition, animal and cellular studies of soy phytoestrogens have generated both enthusiasm and concern. Animal studies have shown that soy phytoestrogens can decrease breast cancer formation in rats, but other animal and human studies suggest that soy phytoestrogens can behave as estrogen does and potentially increase breast cancer risk.

Some scientists have suggested that women be cautious about eating large amounts of soy products or soy supplements because of the possible harmful effects of soy phytoestrogens.

Recommendations

Experts suggest that women be careful how they use phytoestrogen supplements that may contain phytoestrogens at levels far higher than those found in food. Since phytoestrogens can have estrogen-like effects in humans, use of these supplements for a long time could increase breast cancer risk. Moderate consumption of foods high in phytoestrogens is unlikely to have any adverse effects.

Birth Control Pills and Hormone Therapy

The effects of phytoestrogens on women who are taking birth control pills or being treated with postmenopausal hormonal therapy have not been examined. Both of these treatments use estrogen, and since phytoestrogens can act as the hormone estrogen acts, a diet very high in phytoestrogens may disrupt or amplify the estrogen's effect. However, such effects have not been reported in groups of women who consume a diet high in phytoestrogens.

Children and Teens

Experts in several nations, including Great Britain, Switzerland, Australia, and New Zealand, have suggested that soy infant formulas be used only for children who are not breastfed and who are definitely intolerant to cow's milk. Soy formulas contain much higher amounts of phytoestrogens than those found in human breast milk. In addition, infants fed soy formula have blood levels of phytoestrogens that are far greater than normal levels of estrogen in infants. No studies have examined the health effects of children's eating phytoestrogen-rich foods.

Pregnancy and Breast-feeding

Pregnant or breast-feeding women should not use phytoestrogen supplements or consume substantial amounts of flaxseeds on a regular basis. In animal studies, the phytoestrogens found in high amounts in flaxseeds have caused developmental problems; some studies of soy phytoestrogens have shown a possible increase in susceptibility to cancer in offspring. However, eating moderate amounts of soy or flax products should present no problem. Women in China and Japan regularly eat foods that contain soy phytoestrogens during pregnancy and breast-feeding, and to date no adverse health effects have been reported in these countries.

See also PHYTOCHEMICALS.

placental alkaline phosphatase   A tumor marker sometimes used to test for GERM CELL CANCER, particularly seminoma.

pleural effusion, malignant   A buildup of fluid in the space between the lungs and the interior walls of the chest (the pleural cavity) that can be caused by the spread of OVARIAN CANCER, among other malignancies.

Treatment

Malignant pleural effusion should be treated aggressively as soon as it is diagnosed because if a malignant pleural effusion is left untreated, the underlying lung will become encased by tumor and fibrous tissue. Once this has occurred, the underlying lung is trapped and will no longer re-expand. Multiple chemical agents have been used, but the most common treatment in the United States has been tetracycline.

port   Also called a life port or port-a-cath, this device is surgically implanted under the skin (usually on the chest) so that medication, CHEMOTHERAPY, and blood products can be given easily. A port is usually inserted if the veins in a woman's arm are difficult to use for treatment, or if certain types of chemotherapy drugs are to be administered.

An implantable port has a thin, soft plastic tube (a catheter) that is threaded into a vein, with its opening (port) just under the skin on the chest or arm. The catheter is long, thin, and hollow and is usually inserted under the skin of the chest. The tip of the catheter lies in a large vein just above the heart, and the other end connects with the port under the skin on the upper chest. The port will show as a small bump underneath the skin, but nothing is visible on the outside of the body.

Ports also can be used when it is necessary to take samples of blood for testing. This means it is possible for a patient to have treatment without having to have frequent injections. The patient can go home with the port in place, where it may be left in place for weeks or months. A port may be very useful if doctors or nurses find it difficult to inject needles into a patient's veins, or if the walls of the veins have been hardened by previous treatment.

The port will be implanted at the hospital by a surgeon or a radiologist, usually in an operating room while the patient is under a general anesthetic.

pregnancy Pregnancy and prolonged breast-feeding significantly lower the risk of several types of reproductive cancers, including OVARIAN CANCER, although it is unclear whether the protective effect of pregnancy relates to hormonal factors or to the suppression of ovulation. Studies show a 40 percent reduction in risk of ovarian cancer in women who bear at least one child, and an additional 10 to 15 percent risk reduction with each successive term pregnancy. However, the risk reduction does not appear to extend beyond the fourth pregnancy.

In addition, women who have never been pregnant have a higher probability of development of UTERINE CANCER, perhaps because high levels of PROGESTINS are produced during pregnancy. If a woman does not ovulate regularly during her reproductive years, lack of ovulation can upset the delicate balance between estrogenic hormones that encourage the development of cancer and the progestigenic hormones that protect against cancer.

primary site The original site where a cancer tumor appeared.

See also SECONDARY BONE CANCER; SECONDARY BRAIN TUMOR; SECONDARY LIVER CANCER; SECONDARY LUNG CANCER.

progestin The hormonal ingredient in oral contraceptive pills that provides the highest level of protection against OVARIAN CANCER.

Past studies have suggested that using oral contraceptives for three or more years may be associated with a 30 to 50 percent lower risk of developing ovarian cancer, but the exact relationship between HORMONE concentration and ovarian cancer risk had remained unclear.

In a new study, Duke University researchers analyzed oral contraceptive use among 390 women between the ages of 20 and 54 years who had been diagnosed with epithelial ovarian cancer. The researchers separated the women into four categories depending on the formulations of contraceptives they used: high progestin/high estrogen, high progestin/low estrogen, low progestin/high estrogen, and low progestin/low estrogen.

Compared with women who took high progestin/high estrogen contraceptives, women taking low progestin/high estrogen contraceptives were more than twice as likely to develop ovarian cancer; women taking low progestin/low estrogen contraceptives were 60 percent more likely to develop ovarian cancer; and women taking no contraceptives were nearly three times as likely to develop ovarian cancer. The scientists report that the reduction in ovarian cancer risk appeared to be related to the concentration of progestin; the concentration of estrogen in the formulations did not appear to be related to ovarian cancer risk.

The Duke researchers note that the oral contraceptives they studied existed more than 20 years ago and that newer formulations of oral contraceptives are less potent, and therefore, may be less likely to reduce the risk of ovarian cancer.

Prostate, Lung, Colorectal and Ovarian (PLCO) Cancer Screening Trial A large-scale study evaluating the usefulness of a blood test for the TUMOR MARKER known as CA 125 and a test called TRANSVAGINAL ULTRASOUND. Both CA 125 and transvaginal ultrasound are used in OVARIAN CANCER screening.

protocol The treatment plan for using an experimental drug or therapy that outlines the treatment hypothesis and goals. A drug protocol includes details on drug administration, dosage, and duration. *Protocol* also may refer to a standardized treatment program.

pyelogram, intravenous (IVP) A procedure used to diagnose any urologic complications and for staging CERVICAL CANCER. In this procedure, a dye is injected into a vein, which then passes into the urine through the kidneys. It accumulates in the center of the kidney, the bladder and ureters, outlining the kidneys, ureters, and bladder on X-ray.

When some cervical cancers spread beyond the cervix, they may press on the ureters and block the flow of urine, causing kidney damage. The IVP is important in detecting this rare but serious complication.

R. A. Bloch Cancer Foundation   A nonprofit foundation that offers a cancer hotline, home volunteers who have had diagnoses similar to those of clients, support groups, educational and special-interest presentations, and a list of medical multidisciplinary second-opinion boards. The foundation's toll-free hotline matches newly diagnosed patients with someone who has survived the same cancer. For contact information, see Appendix I.

race and reproductive cancer   A woman's race appears to affect her rates of diagnosis and survival directly. Members of minorities tend to receive substandard medical care because of racial discrimination in health-care settings, time pressures on health-care workers, and low-end health insurance plans, according to a landmark 2002 report by the Institute of Medicine (*Unequal Treatment: Confronting Racial and Ethnic Disparities in Health Care*). As a result, more members of minority groups die of cancer than do Caucasians. Lower-quality medical care was found even when minority patients' income, age, medical condition, and insurance coverage were similar to those of white patients.

Early detection could lower the high cancer death rates among minorities, since regular cancer-related checkups, blood testing, and other testing detect cancer early, when treatment is more successful. About half of all cancers can now be discovered early by such screening methods. Unfortunately, people in too many minority groups are not getting this preventive care.

See also AFRICAN-AMERICAN WOMEN; ASIAN WOMEN; HISPANIC/LATINA WOMEN; NATIVE AMERICAN/ALASKA-NATIVE WOMEN.

radiation oncologist   See ONCOLOGIST.

radiation therapy   Women who have had surgery for REPRODUCTIVE CANCER are almost always candidates for radiation therapy, after the surgery has healed, as a means of killing any remaining cancer cells. The radiation may be directed externally by a machine (external radiation) or may be administered by radioactive material in thin plastic tubes that are placed internally (implant radiation). Some women have both kinds of radiation therapy.

In external radiation therapy, the patient usually goes to the hospital five days a week for several weeks. For implant radiation, a woman stays in the hospital for several days while the implants remain in place; they are removed before the woman goes home. In some hospitals high dose rate brachytherapy is performed by placing an implant for three to five weeks.

Radiation therapy is sometimes used before surgery to kill cancer cells, or after surgery and CHEMOTHERAPY or HORMONAL THERAPY to destroy cancer cells and shrink tumors. This therapy is most often selected in cases in which the tumor is large or not easily removed by surgery.

During the course of radiation therapy women may be extremely tired, especially after several treatments. This fatigue may continue after treatment. Resting is important, but research has suggested that trying to stay reasonably active can help fend off fatigue.

It is also common for the skin in the treated area to become red, dry, tender, and itchy. Toward the end of treatment, the skin may become moist; exposing this area to air as much as possible helps the skin to heal. These effects of radiation therapy on the skin are temporary, and the area gradually heals once treatment ends. However, there may be a permanent change in the color of the skin that was irradiated.

radiologist A medical doctor who specializes in radiology and who diagnoses diseases of the human body by using X-rays, ultrasound, radio waves, and radioactive materials. To become a radiologist, a student must complete medical school and then spend four additional years as a resident in radiology.

radiotherapy See RADIATION THERAPY.

recurrence The return of cancer after treatment, which may occur either at the original site of the disease, or at another location (metastasis). In a local recurrence, cancerous tumor cells remain in the original site and regrow over time. A regional recurrence of cancer is more serious than a local recurrence, because it usually indicates that the cancer has spread past the original site and the nearby lymph nodes. A distant cancer recurrence (also known as a metastasis) is the most dangerous type of recurrence. In this case, the cancer cells have spread to distant regions of the body, such as the bone, lung, liver, or brain.

Treatment, which depends on the type and severity of the cancer recurrence, may include more surgery, chemotherapy, radiation therapy, or other drug therapies.

red blood cell A type of blood cell that carries oxygen from the lungs to other parts of the body. Red blood cells contain hemoglobin, an iron-rich protein that is responsible for absorbing oxygen in the lungs and later releasing it to the body's tissues. Chemotherapy drugs kill rapidly dividing cells, including red blood cells. This is why more than 60 percent of chemotherapy patients eventually have a deficiency of red blood cells called ANEMIA, which leads to fatigue, dizziness, headaches, and shortness of breath.

During chemotherapy treatment patients have regular blood tests to check the number of red cells in the blood; the next chemotherapy treatment may be postponed, and a blood transfusion given, if the count is very low. Other treatments for anemia include injections of ERYTHROPOIETIN (EPO), which can boost red blood cell count.

Erythropoietin is the major blood growth factor that encourages the BONE MARROW to produce more red blood cells. Although it is a naturally occurring substance, it can now be made in the laboratory in much larger quantities than the body normally produces. EPO is often administered near the end of chemotherapy treatment to patients who are anemic, very tired, or breathless. EPO can cause side effects, including flu symptoms, rashes, and high blood pressure.

relapse See RECURRENCE.

Relief Band Explorer A patented watchlike electronic medical device that provides drug-free, non-invasive relief from nausea and vomiting by gently stimulating nerves on the underside of the wrist. When activated, the device emits a low-level electrical current across two small electrodes on its underside. It is available by prescription for the treatment of nausea and vomiting caused by chemotherapy. The band is the only medical device to be approved by the U.S. Food and Drug Administration for use in hospitals and doctors' offices for the treatment of severe forms of nausea and vomiting caused by CHEMOTHERAPY.

remission The complete or partial disappearance of signs and symptoms of cancer in response to treatment; the period in which a disease is under control. Remission of a cancer does not necessarily indicate cure.

reproductive cancer The uncontrolled growth and spread of abnormal cells originating in the female reproductive organs, including the cervix, ovaries, uterus, fallopian tubes, vagina, and vulva. Of the approximately 3.9 million women alive today who have a history of any type of cancer, nearly 20 percent have been diagnosed with a cancer of the reproductive system.

ENDOMETRIAL CANCER is the most common cancer of the female reproductive organs: 40,320 new cases are diagnosed each year in the United States and about 7,090 women die annually. Although the survival rate is high, African-American women are nearly twice as likely to die of the disease as are Caucasian women.

OVARIAN CANCER is the sixth most common cancer among women; 25,580 new cases of ovarian cancer are diagnosed each year in the United States. Although ovarian cancer accounts for 4 percent of all new cancers in women, it causes more deaths than any other cancer of the female reproductive system—making it the fifth leading cause of cancer death among women. About 16,090 women die each year of ovarian cancer.

The death rate for CERVICAL CANCER has dropped sharply as the routine PAP TEST has become more common. Still, about 10,520 cases of invasive cervical cancer are diagnosed in the United States each year. Although increasingly less common in the United States because of prevalent early detection and treatment of precancerous lesions, it remains a major global health concern, particularly in the developing world. Some researchers estimate that noninvasive cervical cancer (CARCINOMA IN SITU) is nearly four times more common than invasive cervical cancer.

When VULVAR CANCER is detected early, it is highly curable; about 3,970 cases of vulvar cancer are diagnosed each year. VAGINAL CANCER is relatively rare, responsible for about 2 percent of cancers of the female reproductive system. It is estimated that approximately 2,160 cases of vaginal cancer are diagnosed in the United States each year.

Symptoms

Symptoms of one of the reproductive cancers may include any of the following:

- Unusual vaginal bleeding or discharge
- A sore that does not heal
- Pain or pressure in the pelvic area
- A persistent change in bowel or bladder habits
- Frequent indigestion or abdominal bloating
- A thickening or lump that either causes pain or can be seen or felt

See also FALLOPIAN TUBE CANCER; UTERINE CANCER.

rhabdomyosarcoma A childhood cancer, usually diagnosed before the age of three, that may appear in the vagina, vulva, or uterus. Tumors in the vagina or genital area, as opposed to those in other parts of the body, are associated with a more favorable outcome.

This fairly rare soft tissue cancer is the most common soft tissue SARCOMA in children; it accounts for up to 13 percent of the malignant tumors in childhood. Embryonal rhabdomyosarcoma, the most common type, usually occurs in children younger than age six. Alveolar rhabdomyosarcoma occurs in older children and accounts for about 20 percent of all cases. Although rhabdomyosarcoma is not common in adults, it can occur in people in their 40s and 50s. About 250 American children are diagnosed with rhabdomyosarcoma each year; usually they are between the ages of two and 20 years.

Symptoms

Symptoms vary, depending on the part of the body where the tumor appears; in the genital area, it may involve swelling, bleeding from the vagina, or a solid tumor.

Cause

The vast majority of cases of rhabdomyosarcoma occur sporadically with no recognized risk factor, although a small proportion are associated with genetic conditions. Some experts believe that some rhabdomyosarcoma tumors begin developing before birth, as immature rhabdomyoblasts begin to mature and develop into muscles. Much research has focused on the genetic structure of these rhabdomyoblasts and possible detection of a gene error that can produce the disease later in development.

Rhabdomyosarcomas usually have chromosome abnormality in the cells of the tumor. In children who have an embryonal rhabdomyosarcoma, there is usually an abnormality of chromosome 11. In alveolar rhabdomyosarcoma, there is usually a rearrangement in the chromosome material between chromosomes 2 and 13. This rearrangement changes the position and function of genes, causing a fusion called a fusion transcript. Patients have an abnormal fusion transcript involving two genes, known as *PAX3* and *FKHR*. This important discovery has led to improvements in diagnosis of rhabdomyosarcoma.

Rhabdomyosarcomas are also more common in children who have the genetic disorders neurofibromatoses and Li-Fraumeni syndrome. The neurofibromatoses (NF) are a set of genetic disorders that prompt tumors to grow along various types of nerves and that can affect the development of tissues such as bones and skin. NF causes tumors to grow anywhere on or in the body, which can lead to developmental abnormalities. Li-Fraumeni syndrome is a clustering of soft tissue cancers in a family, caused by mutations in a tumor suppressor gene called *p53,* which results in uncontrolled cell growth. There has been no association established between rhabdomyosarcoma and environmental exposures.

Diagnosis

After a complete medical history and physical examination, the doctor may consider taking a biopsy of the tumor, or performing blood and urine tests or multiple scans (computed tomography, magnetic resonance imaging, ultrasound, bone scans, BONE MARROW aspiration, lumbar puncture, or X-ray).

Staging

Staging is the process of finding out whether or how far the cancer has spread. There are various staging systems used for rhabdomyosarcoma:

- *Stage 1:* This early stage is characterized by cancer involving the head and neck, or nonbladder/nonprostate genitourinary region, or biliary tract. These are considered to be "favorable sites" with a better prognosis.
- *Stage 2:* Localized disease of any primary sites not included in the stage 1 category; these are considered to be "unfavorable sites." Primary tumors must be less than or equal to five cen-

timeters in diameter, and there must be no clinical regional lymph node involvement by tumor.

- *Stage 3:* Localized disease of any other primary site with tumors larger than five centimeters and/or regional node involvement.
- *Stage 4:* Metastatic disease at diagnosis.

Treatment

Specific treatment for rhabdomyosarcoma is determined by the physician on the basis of the child's age, overall health, and medical history; extent of disease; tolerance for specific medications, procedures, or therapies; course of the disease; and parents' preferences. Treatment may include combination therapy, including surgery followed by chemotherapy, followed by second-look surgery for some patients whose tumors could not be removed initially. Radiation treatment may be given, depending on the type of tumor, the extent of the disease, and the extent of the surgical site.

For patients who have tumors of the vagina, vulva, and uterus, the initial surgical procedure is usually transvaginal biopsy. The responsiveness of tumors of the vagina and vulva to chemotherapy generally precludes the need for radical surgery. Conservative surgical intervention for vaginal rhabdomyosarcoma, with primary chemotherapy and adjunctive radiation when necessary, appears to be very effective.

Because of the smaller number of people who have uterine rhabdomyosarcoma, experts are less sure about treatment; chemotherapy is considered to be as effective as radiation therapy.

S

salpingectomy   The removal of one or both of a woman's fallopian tubes. A bilateral salpingectomy (removal of both tubes) is usually done if the ovaries and uterus are also to be removed; if a fallopian tube and an ovary are both removed at the same time, this procedure is called a SALPINGO-OOPHORECTOMY. A salpingo-oophorectomy is necessary when treating OVARIAN CANCER and ENDOMETRIAL CANCER because the fallopian tubes and ovaries are the most common sites to which cancer may spread.

Regional or general anesthesia may be used. Often a laparoscope (a hollow tube with a light on one end) is used in this type of operation, because the incision can be much smaller and the recovery time much shorter. In this procedure, the surgeon makes a small incision just beneath the navel. The surgeon inserts a short hollow tube into the abdomen and, if necessary, pumps in carbon dioxide gas in order to move intestines out of the way and view the organs better. After a wider double tube is inserted on one side for the laparoscope, another small incision is made on the other side, through which other instruments can be inserted. After the operation is completed, the tubes and instruments are withdrawn. The tiny incisions are sutured and there is very little scarring. In the case of a pelvic infection, the surgeon makes a horizontal (bikini) incision four to six inches (10 to 15 cm) long in the abdomen directly above the pubic hairline. This allows the doctor to remove the scar tissue. (Alternatively, a surgeon may use a vertical incision from the pubic bone toward the navel; this incision is less common).

Most women are out of bed and walking around within three days. Within a month or two, a woman can slowly return to normal activities such as driving, exercising, and working.

salpingo-oophorectomy   The surgical removal of a fallopian tube and an ovary to treat ovarian or other gynecological cancers. If only one tube and ovary are removed, the woman may still be able to conceive and carry a pregnancy to term.

If the procedure is performed through a laparoscope, the surgeon need not make a large abdominal incision and can shorten recovery time. In this technique, the surgeon makes a small cut through the abdominal wall just below the navel. When the laparoscope is used, the patient can have either regional or general anesthesia; if there are no complications, the patient can leave the hospital in a day or two. In this procedure, the recovery time can be much shorter than that of standard surgery. There may be some discomfort around the incision for the first few days after surgery, but most women are walking by the third day. Patients can gradually resume normal activities such as driving, exercising, and working.

If a laparoscope is not used, the surgery involves an incision four to six inches (10 to 15 cm) long into the abdomen either extending vertically up from the pubic bone toward the navel or horizontally (the "bikini incision") across the pubic hairline. The scar from a bikini incision is less noticeable, but some surgeons prefer the vertical incision because it provides greater visibility while operating. This method is major surgery that requires three to six weeks for full recovery.

Immediately after the operation, patients should avoid sharply flexing the thighs or the knees. Persistent back pain or bloody or scanty urine indicates that a ureter may have been injured during surgery.

Surgical Menopause

If both ovaries of a premenopausal woman are removed as part of the operation, the sudden loss of

ESTROGEN triggers an abrupt premature menopause that may entail severe symptoms of hot flashes, vaginal dryness, painful intercourse, and loss of sex drive. In addition to these symptoms, women who lose both ovaries lose the protection these hormones provide against heart disease and osteoporosis many years earlier than if they had experienced natural menopause. Women who have had their ovaries removed are seven times more likely to have coronary heart disease and much more likely to have bone problems at an early age than are premenopausal women whose ovaries are intact.

Reaction to the removal of fallopian tubes and ovaries depends on a wide variety of factors, including the woman's age, the condition that required the surgery, her reproductive history, her social support, and any previous history of depression. Women who have had many gynecological surgeries or chronic pelvic pain seem to have a higher tendency to experience psychological problems after the surgery.

Risks

Major surgery always involves some risk, including infection, reactions to anesthesia, hemorrhage, and scars at the incision site. Almost all pelvic surgery causes some internal scars, which, in some cases, can cause discomfort years after surgery.

sarcomas Cancers that develop in bone, muscle, and connective tissue. About 5 percent of all UTERINE CANCER and between 2 to 3 percent of VAGINAL CANCER and VULVAR CANCER are sarcomas. Sarcoma generally has a less favorable prognosis than CARCINOMA.

See also UTERINE SARCOMA.

secondary bone cancer Cancer in the bone that has spread from a different primary site, such as an area of the reproductive system. A malignant tumor is made up of millions of cancer cells. Some of these can break away from the original site and spread to other parts of the body through the lymphatic and blood systems; this process is called metastasis or cancer recurrence. Areas of the bone most commonly affected are the spine, skull, pelvis, hipbones, and upper bones of the arms and legs.

Bone contains two types of living cells—*osteoclasts,* which destroy and remove small amounts of old bone, and *osteoblasts,* which help build up new bone. In secondary bone cancer, the cancer cells that have spread to the bone produce chemicals that interfere with this process, prompting the osteoclasts to become overactive and destroy more bone than can be replaced. This process can lead to some of the symptoms of secondary bone cancer.

Symptoms

Secondary bone cancer can cause a number of symptoms, including pain, presence of calcium in the blood, fractures, or anemia.

Pain Pain in the affected bone can range from mild to severe. Some bone pain may cause a dull ache over the affected area, or a burning or a stabbing pain that may be either persistent or worse at night. Certain movements may affect the pain, and there may be tenderness at the site.

Bone pain can almost always be relieved or controlled, and a number of effective pain relievers are available. A mild painkiller such as a nonsteroidal anti-inflammatory drug may be tried first. If this is not enough to relieve the pain, a stronger painkiller such as dihydrocodeine may be used. In cases in which the pain is severe, a morphine-based drug is often prescribed. Sometimes a combination of drugs may be needed. These medications should be taken at specified times rather than when pain is unbearable.

In some cases, these drugs may not control the pain fully. The patient may need to be admitted to a hospital or into a hospice for an assessment by a specialist palliative-care pain team.

Hypercalcemia Sometimes secondary bone cancer can alter the bone structure so that calcium is released into the bloodstream. If the calcium level is too high, it may cause nausea, vomiting, constipation, or drowsiness. In more severe cases, a woman may be very thirsty, weak, or confused. Symptoms can be relieved by drinking plenty of water or having intravenous fluids to flush the calcium out of the body. BISPHOSPHONATES may also help (see later discussion).

Fractures Secondary bone cancer may weaken the bone, potentially increasing the risk of fracture in some circumstances. Radiation treatment can help prevent a weak bone from fracturing. Alternatively, an orthopedic surgeon can try to prevent fractures by securing the bone with a metal screw or plate or by replacing a joint. The implants that are used are designed to last indefinitely.

If a bone has already fractured, the orthopedic surgeon attempts to repair the fracture by using a metal screw or pin or joint replacement. In rare cases, a whole section of bone can be replaced (endoprosthesis).

If an area of vertebrae fractures or collapses, pressure on the spinal cord that may require emergency surgery may result. If the symptoms appear gradually, radiation treatment may be recommended first. With either treatment, steroids are administered to help reduce inflammation. Sometimes a combination of all three treatments may be used.

Anemia In rare cases, the secondary cancer cells may invade the bone marrow, where blood cells are made. This process may trigger the release of immature blood cells into the bloodstream, causing anemia, with symptoms of tiredness or shortness of breath. Blood tests and a bone marrow biopsy may be needed to make a diagnosis. The anemia can be corrected by regular blood transfusions.

Diagnosis

Secondary bone cancer can be diagnosed with X-rays or a bone scan that can detect small areas of cancer cells that have migrated to the bones.

Bone X-ray A bone X-ray can reveal certain changes in the bone, although it may not identify small areas of secondary bone cancers.

Bone scan A bone scan is a more sensitive test than an X-ray, which can highlight any abnormal areas of bone more clearly. A bone scan reveals the entire skeleton; X-rays highlight only one particular area. A scan is not painful, but the patient must lie flat and still for about half an hour. A few hours before the scan, a small amount of a weak, harmless radioactive substance is injected into a patient's vein. Any areas of bone cancer appear as an increased uptake of the radioactive substance in the affected area. It is important to remember that people with other bone conditions, such as osteoporosis and arthritis, also may have positive bone scan findings without secondary bone cancer.

Magnetic resonance imaging (MRI) MRI scan uses magnetism instead of X-rays to provide a detailed picture of an area of bone. As with a bone scan, the MRI is not painful, but patients must lie flat and still.

Treatment

Secondary bone cancer can be treated and pain eased, but it cannot be cured. The aim is to relieve symptoms and improve quality of life by controlling the growth of the cancer. Treatments may include HORMONE THERAPY, CHEMOTHERAPY, RADIATION THERAPY, or surgery, either alone or in combination. The treatment offered depends on a number of factors, including symptoms, extent of cancer spread in the bones, whether or not a woman is postmenopausal, the type of tumor, and the woman's general health.

Hormone therapy Hormone therapy may be the first choice of treatment for secondary bone cancer. A number of hormone therapies are available, the drug most commonly used first is the antiestrogen drug tamoxifen. Women who are already taking tamoxifen when they have secondary bone cancer may be prescribed other hormone drugs known as aromatase inhibitors.

Chemotherapy If secondary bone cancer does not respond to hormone treatment or has stopped responding to it, chemotherapy drugs may be tried next. They may be given alone or in combination. Secondary bone cancer can be slow to respond to chemotherapy, however, and a woman may need several cycles at three- or four-week intervals before any benefit can be seen.

Radiation therapy The aim of radiation treatment is to improve quality of life by improving mobility, decreasing pain, and preventing fractures. Radiation therapy for secondary bone cancer can be given in a single dose, or in divided dosages over a few days to ensure that side effects will be mild.

Radiation therapy may also be given internally, by injecting a radioisotope into a vein. The radioisotope travels through the bloodstream and delivers radiotherapy to the bones affected by the cancer cells. It is sometimes useful when the secondary cancer is widespread.

Bisphosphonates Bisphosphonates are drugs that target the parts of the skeleton where there is high bone turnover; they do not treat the cancer directly but may help reduce the breakdown of the bone by restricting the action of the osteoclasts. Given in tablet form or through a drip into the vein, they work by reducing high blood levels of calcium and easing pain that has not responded well to painkillers or that is too widespread for local radiation therapy. Long-term use of bisphosphonates reduces the risk of bone fractures and may delay the spread of secondary bone cancer.

secondary brain tumor   Cancer in the brain that has spread from a different primary site, such as an area in the reproductive system (ovaries, cervix, uterus, fallopian tubes, vagina, or vulva). This also may be described as metastasis or recurrent reproductive cancer.

Symptoms

Symptoms that reproductive cancer has spread to the brain depend on the area of the brain affected. Women who have this condition may have some of these symptoms but are unlikely to experience all of them.

The most common symptom of secondary brain cancer is a headache different from other headaches. It is generally worse in the morning and gradually decreases during the day, or it may be continuous and worsen over time. The headache may occur with nausea, vomiting, or fatigue. Other possible symptoms include general weakness or weakness down one side of the body, unsteadiness, seizures, and double vision. Less common symptoms include behavior changes, confusion, and speech problems. Although these symptoms can begin suddenly, they more typically develop slowly.

Diagnosis

During a physical exam, the physician may check the eyes for swelling caused by pressure from the brain; examine the arms and legs for changes in sensation, strength, and reflexes; and evaluate the woman's balance and walking ability.

A computed tomography (CT) scan can take a three-dimensional picture of the brain to check for lesions. A MAGNETIC RESONANCE IMAGING scan, which uses magnetic waves instead of X-rays, is an effective method of brain tumor diagnosis. On rare occasions it may be necessary to take a BIOPSY specimen of the tumor to confirm the diagnosis.

Treatment

Cancer that has spread to the brain cannot be cured, so any treatment aims to control the symptoms to improve quality of life. Treatments may include radiation therapy, use of steroid drugs, or surgery.

Radiation therapy   RADIATION THERAPY is the most commonly used treatment for secondary brain cancer. It is given in daily dosages over about five days. Fatigue is a common side effect of radiation therapy, especially radiation therapy given to the brain. Hair loss is another common side effect.

Steroids   Steroid drugs are used to reduce inflammation and pressure around the brain tumor and can relieve symptoms such as headache and nausea. They are often prescribed before any investigations to confirm the diagnosis of a secondary brain tumor.

At first, steroids for secondary brain cancer are given in high dosages, which can usually be reduced once other treatments such as radiation therapy begin. Among the more common side effects of high dosages of steroids are indigestion, thrush in the mouth, increased appetite and weight gain, muscle weakness, and sleeplessness.

Surgery   Surgery is rarely possible for secondary brain cancer, since there are usually a number of small tumors rather than a single tumor that can be removed. If surgery is an option, the doctor and the patient should consider the patient's general health and fitness in deciding whether the procedure would improve quality of life.

secondary liver cancer   A type of cancer that occurs when malignant cells spread from the original site of cancer through the bloodstream and settle in the liver. It also may be called liver metastasis or cancer recurrence.

The liver is a very important organ in the body, made up of different sections called lobes and surrounded by a membrane called a capsule. It is a near neighbor of several other organs, including the bowel, the diaphragm, and the right kidney. The liver converts food into heat and energy, stores glucose and vitamins, and produces bile to help digest food. The liver also breaks down harmful substances such as alcohol and drugs and produces important proteins needed to help blood clot.

Because the liver is a large organ, it may be able to function even if part of it is affected by cancer.

Symptoms

Secondary liver cancer may not cause any symptoms, or it may cause a number of problems such as pain, nausea, hiccups, ascites, fatigue, anemia, or jaundice.

Pain Secondary liver cancer can stimulate the liver to grow, stretching its capsule and causing mild discomfort or pain below the ribs. The enlarged liver may also press on the nerves that lead to the right shoulder, causing "referred pain" there. Pain can usually be helped with painkillers such as paracetamol or anti-inflammatory drugs such as ibuprofen. Liver pain also responds well to morphine-based drugs. Sometimes steroid drugs can help reduce swelling around the liver, reducing pain. In some cases radiotherapy or chemotherapy may be used to help relieve pain by shrinking the enlarged liver.

Nausea A woman may feel nausea because the enlarged liver causes pressure on the stomach or because toxins are accumulating in the body as a result of liver damage. Nausea can be treated with antinausea drugs. Some women lose their appetite because of the nausea, which may also trigger weight loss.

Hiccoughs Hiccoughs may occur as the enlarged liver presses on the diaphragm, triggering spasms. Women may find that sitting upright and drinking small amounts of liquid frequently are helpful.

Ascites Ascites, a buildup of abdominal fluid, can occur if blood or lymphatic flow through the liver is blocked, causing bloating that may make a woman feel uncomfortable and sometimes breathless. This bloating may develop over weeks or months. Diuretics may help reduce the amount of fluid in the abdomen; insertion of a drain into the abdomen to remove the extra fluid (paracentesis) may be necessary. Paracentesis is usually done with local anesthesia and can be repeated if the fluid builds up again.

Fatigue Many women find that they tire more readily than usual; it may be possible to treat the cause of the tiredness. In some cases, steroid drugs can help to boost energy levels.

Anemia Patients may become anemic for a number of different reasons, including problems with blood clotting. A blood test can identify anemia; in some cases, iron tablets or a blood transfusion can help.

Jaundice Jaundice can occur when the bile duct becomes blocked, tinting the skin and whites of the eyes yellow. In some cases, urine may become darker and stools may become pale. Patients may need to have a stent inserted into the bile duct to drain the bile. Jaundice can cause itching, which may be worse at night. Alcohol can make the itching worse, as can soaps and heavily perfumed products. Antihistamine tablets or cream may help.

Diagnosis

Because secondary liver cancer causes an enlarged liver, the doctor may be able to feel it on examination. Next, blood tests may be ordered since damaged liver cells release certain substances that can be detected in the blood. Blood tests can measure these substances and their results may also indicate how effective any treatment has been.

In most cases a specialist can determine whether the cancer cells in the liver are from the reproductive area. If there is any doubt, a small piece of tissue from the liver is biopsied.

An ultrasound, magnetic resonance imaging, or computed tomography scan can reveal any abnormalities of the liver.

An endoscopic retrograde cholangiopancreatography (ERCP) is used to find out whether the bile duct is blocked. In this procedure, a narrow flexible tube with a lighted end is passed through the mouth and the stomach into the bile duct. A dye is inserted through the tube and a series of X-rays are taken to look at the movement of the dye through the duct.

Treatment

Secondary liver cancer can be treated, although it cannot be cured. The aims are to relieve the patient's symptoms and improve quality of life by slowing the growth of the cancer. Treatments may include chemotherapy, hormone therapy, radiation therapy, or surgery, either alone or in combination.

Chemotherapy If a woman had chemotherapy when her original cancer was first diagnosed, she may receive a similar combination of drugs or different ones.

Hormone therapies   Hormone therapies are typically used to treat cancers that are sensitive to ESTROGEN (estrogen receptor positive). If a woman was already taking a hormone drug such as TAMOXIFEN when secondary liver cancer developed, she may be given a different hormone drug.

Surgery   Rarely, if only a small part of the liver is affected, surgery can be an option. However, in most cases several areas of the liver are affected and surgery is not possible. Liver transplants are not possible for people who have secondary liver cancer.

Thermal ablation   Thermal ablation involves using heat to destroy cancerous cells—a treatment still in its early stages and not widely available. Guided into their position by a scan, needles are inserted into the tumor and heated, causing irreparable damage to the cells.

secondary lung cancer   A type of cancer that occurs when malignant cancer cells spread from the site of an original cancer through the bloodstream to settle in the lungs. This type of spread may also be described as a metastasis or cancer recurrence.

Symptoms

Secondary lung cancer may cause a number of different symptoms ranging from mild to severe, depending on how advanced it is. They may include shortness of breath, cough, pain, pleural effusion, appetite loss, weight loss, and fatigue.

The most common symptom of secondary lung cancer is shortness of breath (dyspnea) or breathing problems. Relaxation techniques can be very helpful in easing breathing, and medicines such as morphine can help ease the feeling of breathlessness and the anxiety that it can cause. If the tumor narrows or blocks the bronchial tubes, a bronchodilator such as albuterol sulfate (Ventolin) can be administered through an inhaler or a nebulizer. If the tumor causes swelling or inflammation, steroid drugs such as dexamethasone or prednisolone can help. Antibiotics may help treat a chest infection.

A cough is another common symptom that may be caused by an infection or by the cancer itself. Cough medicine may control coughing and loosen phlegm; breathing salt water through a nebulizer can also loosen the phlegm, making expelling it easier. If the cough is very difficult to control, a medication such as morphine may help.

The tumor or excessive coughing also may cause pain in the chest, shoulder, or back area. Painkillers such as paracetomol, codeine, or morphine may be used.

Another symptom is PLEURAL EFFUSION, which is a buildup of extra fluid in the pleural space, causing breathlessness. This can be treated by drawing off the extra fluid; drugs also can be injected, which can help to stop fluid accumulation.

Appetite or weight loss may be caused by cancer, symptoms, or side effects of treatment. Nutritional supplements such as high-calorie drinks may help, but meals must not be replaced by these supplements. Secondary lung cancer may also cause fatigue.

Diagnosis

A chest X-ray is usually the first test ordered if secondary lung cancer is suspected. However, if a tumor is small, it may not always show up on an X-ray. If the X-ray findings are not clear, patients may need a scan, such as a computed tomography (CT) scan; if the CT scan result is not clear, a MAGNETIC RESONANCE IMAGING (MRI) scan may be ordered.

If the diagnosis is still uncertain, the doctor may order a biopsy of the lungs. With local anesthesia a tube is inserted through the mouth and down into the lungs so that a small piece of lung tissue can be removed.

Treatment

Secondary lung cancer can be treated, although it cannot be cured. The aims of treatment are to ease symptoms and improve quality of life by slowing the growth of the cancer. Treatments may include CHEMOTHERAPY, HORMONE THERAPY, and radiotherapy, either alone or in combination.

Chemotherapy   Women who had chemotherapy when their original cancer was first treated may be given similar drugs or a different combination.

Hormone therapy   Hormone therapies are usually used to treat cancers that are sensitive to hormones such as estrogen.

Radiation therapy   RADIATION THERAPY is sometimes used to treat secondary lung cancer. It is administered either as a single dose or in divided dosages over a few days.

secondary tumor   A tumor that develops when cancer cells spread beyond their original site to a new site.

See also SECONDARY BONE CANCER; SECONDARY BRAIN CANCER; SECONDARY LIVER CANCER; SECONDARY LUNG CANCER.

selective estrogen-receptor modulators (SERMs) A fairly new group of drugs that cause ESTROGEN-like responses in certain tissues while preventing estrogenlike responses in other parts of the body. Specifically, SERMs block the actions of estrogen in certain tissues by occupying the estrogen receptors on cells. When a SERM is in the estrogen receptor, there is no place for the real estrogen to attach. Although the SERM fit to the estrogen receptor, it does not send messages to the cell nucleus to grow and divide. Three of the best-known SERMs are TAMOXIFEN (Nolvadex), raloxifene (Evista), and toremifene (Fareston).

However, SERMs do send estrogenlike signals when they attach to receptors' bone cells, liver cells, and elsewhere in the body; therefore, SERMs seem to help prevent or slow osteoporosis of postmenopausal women and may help lower cholesterol level. This dual effect—blocking estrogen in some places and imitating estrogen in other places—allows SERMs to have multiple beneficial effects for many women who have cancer.

Tamoxifen

Tamoxifen has been used for more than 20 years and was the first of the SERM antiestrogen medications available. Side effects include hot flashes, vaginal dryness or discharge, irregular periods, nausea, and cataracts. Rare side effects include blood clots and an increased risk of ENDOMETRIAL CANCER. Tamoxifen may be recommended for both pre- and postmenopausal women who have all stages of disease.

Toremifene

Toremifene, a relatively new antiestrogen SERM, has properties and side effects similar to those of

tamoxifen, but unlike tamoxifen, toremifene does not seem to increase the risk of endometrial cancer.

Raloxifene

Raloxifene is an antiestrogen SERM medication that strengthens bones and is U.S. Food and Drug Administration–approved for treating osteoporosis in postmenopausal women. The Study of Tamoxifen and Raloxifene is now comparing the two SERMs in high-risk women.

Side effects are similar to those of tamoxifen, including hot flashes, vaginal changes, and rarely, blood clots, stroke, and pulmonary embolism. Raloxifene does not seem to increase the risk of endometrial cancer.

serous papillary cancer   An aggressive form of cancer that has features identifiable under a microscope. This tumor is usually fast growing and rapidly spreading.

SHARE (Self-Help for Women with Breast or Ovarian Cancer)   A nonprofit organization that offers peer-led support to women who have breast or OVARIAN CANCER and their family and friends. Drawing on their own experiences, cancer survivors help others address the many emotional and practical issues linked to a cancer diagnosis. Services include hotlines, survivor-led support groups, wellness programs, educational forums, outreach programs, and advocacy activities. For contact information, see Appendix I.

smoking   Tobacco is highly addictive and has been linked to 20 percent of all deaths in the United States as a result of its cancer-causing chemicals and the corrosive nature of cigarette smoke on the lungs. Quitting smoking can lower a woman's risk of CERVICAL CANCER or VAGINAL CANCER.

Women who smoke are more likely to have these two types of cancer than those who do not. The reason for this relationship is not known; some experts suspect that smoking causes some abnormal changes in the cells and these cells have a higher likelihood of becoming cancerous. A few studies have found a chemical by-product of nicotine (the addictive drug in cigarettes) in the secretions of the cervix. The poisons in cigarette smoke may also enter the cervix and vagina through the bloodstream.

Moreover, current and past smoking may increase the risk of cervical cancer among women who have been infected with the HUMAN PAPILLO- MAVIRUS (HPV), according to a 2002 NATIONAL CAN- CER INSTITUTE study. In the study of 1,812 women who had tested positive for HPV, former and cur- rent smokers appeared to have an increased risk of cervical cancer when compared with women who never smoked.

The tobacco smoke that a smoker inhales is dif- ferent from the smoke inhaled by those nearby, but it is equally deadly. The major source of passive smoke is the burning of the cigarette rather than what is exhaled by smokers. Both types of smoke contain thousands of similar chemicals, although the concentrations of the chemicals are different. Many of the toxic chemicals in tobacco smoke are found in higher concentrations in the tobacco smoke as it leaves the cigarette compared to inhaled smoke; in some cases, the concentrations are far higher. This smoke is largely produced by the lower-temperature burning of cigarettes between inhalations, and the chemicals are less degraded than in the smokers' inhalations. How- ever many factors, such as room size and airflow, can affect the dilution of the smoke and the result- ing exposures can differ greatly.

Passive exposure to tobacco smoke is very com- mon. Studies conducted in 1991 of the number of nonsmokers in the United States who are exposed to tobacco smoke used a breakdown product of nico- tine, cotinine, in the blood of nonsmokers as a marker for tobacco smoke exposure. They reported that 90 percent of nonsmokers older than age four had measurable levels of cotinine. Because of changes in smoking policies since 1991, the preva- lence of environmental tobacco smoke exposure may have decreased. Measurements made in 1999 of the typical levels of this marker in nonsmokers' blood indicated that levels were substantially lower than levels reported in 1991. Because the typical lev- els of cotinine have decreased, it is also likely that a smaller percentage of people have detectable levels.

Social Security Disability Insurance (SSDI)   A U.S. government social program that pays benefits

to a person who is "insured," meaning that the person worked long enough to be eligible and paid Social Security taxes. A person who becomes dis- abled and expects the condition to continue for at least six months may be eligible for SSDI. Often the government considers cancer that has spread a disability.

Society of Gynecologic Oncologists   A nonprofit international organization made up of obstetricians and gynecologists specializing in gynecologic oncology. The society's purposes are to improve the care of women who have gynecologic cancer, to raise standards of practice in gynecologic oncology, and to encourage ongoing research. For contact information, see Appendix I.

soy products   Foods (such as tofu and miso) that contain proteins and substances called ISOFLAVONES. Isoflavones are a type of PHYTOESTRO- GEN, a type of naturally occurring plant estrogen that may offer some of the benefits of estrogen to women without increasing their risk of cancer. These benefits may include relief from symptoms of menopause and reduced risk of heart disease and bone loss. In addition, soy isoflavones may help prevent some kinds of cancer. However, the effects of soy on cancer are not fully understood, especially on cancer fueled by estrogen; thus, it is not yet possible to determine whether soy helps prevent or promote cancer.

Current advice for eating soy ranges from eating none to eating soy foods (not soy pills and powder) several times a week as a low-fat replacement for animal protein. Patients should seek medical advice regarding soy for their individual needs. Soy can be obtained by eating

- Tofu (a curd made from cooked, pureed soy- beans)
- Miso (a mixture of fermented soybean paste and a grain such as rice or barley)
- Dried soybeans
- Roasted soybeans or nuts (soybeans that are soaked in water and baked)
- Edamame and natto (steamed whole green beans and fermented, cooked whole beans)

- Tempeh (a combination of whole, cooked soy beans and grains cultured with an edible mold)
- Soy milk (the liquid expressed from cooked, pureed soybeans)

The ability of the body to use the nutrients in soy foods varies with the food and the way it is made. In general, soy that has been processed least (such as tofu, tempeh, and mature, green, and roasted soybeans) contains most protein and naturally occurring isoflavones. Soy germ is the source highest in isoflavones.

Isoflavones have become so popular that they are now available as diet supplements. But results of research on the effectiveness and safety of these supplements are contradictory, and for now, no one knows how beneficial or safe it is to use them.

staging   A medical attempt to find out whether a patient's cancer has spread and, if so, to what parts of the body. A doctor stages cancer by studying information obtained during surgery, X-rays and other imaging procedures, and lab tests. Knowing the stage of the disease helps the doctor plan treatment.

Typically, REPRODUCTIVE CANCER stages are numbered from I through IV (IV indicates the most severe); some types of cancer include A and B subcategories.

statistics in reproductive cancer   The usefulness of cancer statistics depends on the ways they are interpreted and used. Cancer statistics are often cited in medical stories and can be helpful in providing a broad perspective; they are less helpful for understanding one person's specific prognosis. Moreover, heredity, ethnicity, reproductive history, lifestyle, and other risk factors all contribute to a woman's overall cancer risk.

A number of terms are important in understanding what statistics mean in relation to REPRODUCTIVE CANCER.

Incidence   The number of new cases of cancer in a specific population group within a set period—usually one year.

Prevalence   The total number of people with cancer or with a particular risk factor for cancer at a particular moment in time in the entire population. For large groups of people, prevalence is estimated by collecting information from a smaller subset of people and then extrapolating that information to the general population.

Morbidity and mortality   *Morbidity* is a state of illness. For instance, experts may comment that smoking is a major cause of morbidity in the United States. *Mortality* pertains to death. The *mortality rate* is the number of people in a population group who die of cancer within a specific period (usually one year). A cancer mortality rate usually is expressed in terms of deaths per 100,000 people.

Prognosis   The prediction of the outcome of a disease, usually including the chances for recovery. Physicians may base a cancer prognosis on statistical precedents; however, an individual's prognosis is affected by many factors, including age and general health, type and stage of cancer, and effectiveness of the particular treatment used. Therefore, although a prognosis may help explain the seriousness of the cancer or guide treatment decisions, it cannot be used to predict cancer outcome for an individual.

Survival rate   *Survival rate* is the number of people who have cancer and survive over a period. Scientists commonly use five-year survival rate as the standard statistical basis for defining when a cancer has been successfully treated. The *five-year survival rate* includes anyone who is living five years after a cancer diagnosis, including those who are cured, those who are in remission, and those who still have cancer and are having treatment.

The *overall five-year survival rate* measures equally all who have ever been diagnosed with a particular cancer; therefore, it may lead to distorted statistics: for example, a 90-year-old woman and a 30-year-old woman who have the same cancer are grouped together. The 90-year-old may die of other causes within the five-year period because of normal life expectancy, and this characteristic can skew the data.

A more statistically accurate view of survival is the *relative five-year survival rate,* which compares a cancer patient's survival rate with the survival rate of the general population, taking into account differences in age, gender, race, and other factors. In this case, the 30-year-old and the 90-year-old are treated as statistically different.

Risk   *Risk* is the chance that an individual will contract a disease. *High-risk* is a term used when the chance of development of cancer is higher than the chance for the general population. For example, women who have HUMAN PAPILLO-MAVIRUS (HPV) have a higher risk of CERVICAL CANCER when compared with women who do not have the virus.

A *risk factor* is anything that has been identified as increasing a person's probability of having a disease. Factors may be controllable or uncontrollable, personal or environmental. For example, risk factors for development of OVARIAN CANCER include having a hereditary predisposition to the disease, such as the *BRCA1* gene (uncontrollable), and contracting HPV by unprotected sex (controllable).

Relative risk is a measure of the extent to which a particular risk factor increases the risk of development of a specific cancer. For example, the risk for ovarian cancer increases by 300 percent for a woman with close relatives who have the disease compared to a woman without a family history. In this example, the relative risk of development of ovarian cancer for those who have a family history is 3, meaning they have three times the risk.

Attributable risk is a measure of the amount of the total incidence of disease that is caused by that risk factor. For example, though the relative risk of breast cancer development for a woman who has the *BRCA1* gene is high, most cases of breast cancer are not caused by the *BRCA1* gene since the prevalance of the *BRCA1* gene is low.

Lifetime risk is the probability of having or dying of cancer during one's lifetime. (See also individual cancers for more information on specific cancer statistics.)

stem cell   A common cell found in BONE MARROW that, in its most primitive state, has the ability to develop into a wide variety of cells. It may be used to help treat women with various REPRODUCTIVE CANCERS. Most stem cells are found in the bone marrow; some stem cells, called peripheral blood stem cells, can be found in the bloodstream. Umbilical cord blood also contains stem cells. Stem cells can divide to form more stem cells, or they can mature into white blood cells, red blood cells, or platelets.

Stem Cell Transplant

High-dose CHEMOTHERAPY can severely damage or destroy a patient's bone marrow so that it is no longer able to produce needed blood cells. A stem cell transplant allows stem cells that are damaged by treatment to be replaced with healthy stem cells that can produce the blood cells the patient needs. Transplantation allows a patient to be treated with high dosages of drugs, radiation, or both. The high dosages destroy normal blood cells in the bone marrow so that later the patient can be given healthy stem cells. New blood cells develop from the transplanted stem cells.

Stem cells may be harvested from the patient (autologous transplant) or from a donor (allogeneic transplant). In an autologous stem cell transplantation, the patient's own stem cells are removed, and the cells are treated to kill any cancer cells. The stem cells are then frozen and stored. After the patient receives high-dose chemotherapy or radiation therapy, the stored stem cells are thawed and returned to the patient. In an allogeneic stem cell transplantation, the patient is given healthy stem cells from a donor (such as a brother, sister, or parent); sometimes the stem cells are from an unrelated donor. Doctors use blood tests to be sure the donor's cells match the patient's cells. In a syngeneic stem cell transplantation, the patient is given stem cells from her healthy identical twin.

Types of Stem Cell Transplants

There are several types of stem cell transplantation:

- *Bone marrow transplantation.* The stem cells are from bone marrow.

- *Peripheral stem cell transplantation.* The stem cells are from peripheral blood.

- *Umbilical cord blood transplantation.* For a child with no donor, stem cells from the blood of an umbilical cord from a newborn may be used; sometimes umbilical cord blood is frozen for later use.

stereotactic radiosurgery   A new technique that focuses high dosages of radiation on a tumor while minimizing radiation delivered to normal tissue. After the location of the tumor is precisely measured by computed tomography or magnetic resonance imaging scan, radiation beams are then aimed from several directions to meet at the tumor. Photon beams from a linear accelerator or X-rays from cobalt 60 are often used; proton beams may also be used. This treatment may be useful for tumors that are in locations where conventional surgery would damage essential tissues or when a patient's condition does not permit conventional surgery.

stomatitis Inflammation of the soft tissues of the mouth that often occurs as a side effect of CHEMOTHERAPY, RADIATION THERAPY, and some types of BIOLOGICAL THERAPY drugs, such as interleukin-2. Stomatitis can cause dry mouth, soreness, burning feelings, swelling, redness, and taste changes. In a cancer patient, symptoms can lead to serious problems of malnutrition, which can further lead to infections. Patients should take medication to ease symptoms and avoid

- Hot, spicy food
- Highly acidic fruits and juices such as tomato or orange
- Carbonated drinks
- Salty food
- Toothpaste or mouthwash containing salt or alcohol

Instead, patients should eat soft, unseasoned food; rinse the mouth and teeth with warm water or a rinse of baking soda and warm water; and use lip balm on the lips.

stress and cancer The complex relationship between cancer and stress is not completely understood. Scientists do know that many types of stress activate the body's endocrine system, which can affect the immune system, although it has not been shown that stress-induced changes in the immune system directly cause cancer.

Some studies have indicated an increased incidence of early cancer death among people who have experienced the recent loss of a spouse or other loved one. However, most cancers have been developing for many years and are diagnosed only

after they have been growing a long time. This fact suggests there cannot always be a link between the death of a loved one and the onset of cancer.

stromal carcinoma, ovarian A fairly unusual type of OVARIAN CANCER that accounts for just 5 percent of all ovarian cancer cases. More than half are found in women older than age 50, but some occur in young girls.

The tumor develops in the connective tissue cells that hold the ovary together and in the cells that produce the female hormones ESTROGEN and progesterone; the two most common types are granulosa cell tumors and Sertoli's and Leydig's cell tumors. Thecomas and fibromas are benign stromal tumors.

Unlike in EPITHELIAL OVARIAN CARCINOMA, 70 percent of the cases of stromal carcinoma are diagnosed in stage I.

Some but not all of these tumors produce female hormones (or less often, male hormones). They can cause vaginal bleeding to resume after menopause or can trigger menstrual periods and breast development in young girls. If male hormones are produced, the tumors can disrupt normal periods and trigger facial and body hair growth.

support groups Groups that give people affected by a condition or illness, such as cancer, an opportunity to meet and discuss ways to cope. Women diagnosed with REPRODUCTIVE CANCER, and their family, face challenges that may lead to feelings of being overwhelmed, afraid, and alone. Cancer support groups can help people affected by this disease feel less alone and can improve their ability to deal with the uncertainties and challenges that cancer causes.

People who have been diagnosed with cancer sometimes find they need help coping with the emotional as well as the practical aspects of their disease. In fact, attention to the emotional burden of reproductive cancer is sometimes part of a patient's treatment plan. Reproductive cancer support groups are designed to provide a confidential atmosphere in which patients or cancer survivors can discuss the challenges that accompany the illness with others who may have experienced the same challenges. Support groups have helped thousands of women cope with similar situations.

Because family and friends also are affected when reproductive cancer touches someone they love, they may need help dealing with family disruptions, financial worries, and changing roles within relationships. To help meet these needs, some support groups are designed for family members of people diagnosed with cancer; other groups encourage families and friends to participate along with patients or cancer survivors.

Several kinds of support groups meet the individual needs of people at all stages of cancer treatment, from diagnosis through aftercare. Some groups are general cancer support groups; more specialized groups work with teens or young adults or with family members. Support groups may be led by a professional, such as a psychiatrist, psychologist, or social worker, or by cancer patients or survivors. In addition, support groups can vary in approach, size, and frequency of their meetings. Many groups are free; some require a fee (insurance may cover the cost).

Locating a Group

Many organizations offer support groups for people diagnosed with cancer and their family members or friends. Oncology health-care workers may have information about support groups, and hospital social service departments can also provide information about cancer support programs. The local office of the AMERICAN CANCER SOCIETY has lists of support groups. Additionally, many newspapers carry a special health supplement containing information about where to find this type of help.

See also LOOK GOOD . . . FEEL BETTER; NATIONAL ASIAN WOMEN'S HEALTH ORGANIZATION; NATIONAL COALITION FOR CANCER SURVIVORSHIP; NATIONAL HOSPICE AND PALLIATIVE CARE ORGANIZATION; NATIONAL LYMPHEDEMA NETWORK; NATIONAL OVARIAN CANCER COALITION; OVARIAN CANCER NATIONAL ALLIANCE; SHARE.

suppressor genes See TUMOR SUPPRESSOR GENES.

Surveillance, Epidemiology, and End Results (SEER) A program of the NATIONAL CANCER INSTITUTE (NCI), that provides the most authoritative

source of information on cancer incidence and survival rates in the United States. The NCI's SEER cancer registry program has been expanded to include more of the racial, ethnic, and socioeconomic diversity of the United States, allowing for better description and tracking of trends in health differences among groups. Methodological studies are seeking better ways to measure socioeconomic factors and determine their relationship to cancer incidence, survival, and mortality rates.

SEER currently collects and publishes cancer incidence and survival data from 14 population-based cancer registries and three supplemental registries covering approximately 26 percent of the U.S. population. Information on more than 3 million in situ and invasive cancer cases is included in the SEER database, and approximately 170,000 new cases are added each year within the SEER coverage areas.

The SEER registries routinely collect data on patient demographics, primary tumor site, stage at diagnosis, first course of treatment, and follow-up. The SEER Program is the only comprehensive source of population-based information in the United States that includes stage of cancer at the time of diagnosis and survival rates within each stage. The mortality data reported by SEER are provided by the National Center for Health Statistics.

Additionally, the NCI supports a growing body of research to examine the environmental, sociocultural, behavioral, and genetic causes of cancer in different populations and apply these discoveries through interventions in clinical and community settings, such as tobacco use, dietary modification, and adherence to better screening.

SEER began collecting data on cases on January 1, 1973, in Connecticut, Iowa, New Mexico, Utah, and Hawaii, and Detroit and San Francisco-Oakland. In 1974–1975, the metropolitan area of Atlanta and the 13-county Seattle-Puget Sound area were added. In 1978, 10 predominantly black rural counties in Georgia were added, followed in 1980 by the addition of American Indians residing in Arizona. Three additional geographic areas participated in the SEER program prior to 1990: New Orleans, Louisiana (1974–1977, rejoined 2001); New Jersey (1979–1989, rejoined 2001); and Puerto Rico (1973–1989). The National Cancer

Institute also funds a cancer registry that, with technical assistance from SEER, collects information on cancer cases among Alaska Native populations residing in Alaska. In 1992, the SEER Program was expanded to increase coverage of minority populations, especially Hispanics, by adding Los Angeles County and four counties in the San Jose-Monterey area south of San Francisco. In 2001, the SEER Program expanded coverage to include Kentucky and Greater California; in addition, New Jersey and Louisiana once again became participants.

Data from the report, and from SEER special studies, are used by NCI and others to design specific research studies to investigate cancer causes. Examples of this research include epidemiologic studies designed to test dietary or hormonal hypotheses suggested by observed incidence and mortality patterns by age, race, sex, and geographic area.

Cancer Statistics Review

This annual database, published in electronic and paperback formats by the SEER program, provides data on cancer incidence, mortality, and patient survival rates for more than 20 different cancers and for all cancers combined. Cancer incidence and survival data represents about 10 percent of the U.S. population are used in the book, along with mortality data from the entire United States. Data are reported by cancer site, age, time period, sex, and race (all races, whites, and blacks). Additional data are presented from registries added to the SEER program in 1992 to increase coverage of minority populations.

The CSR reports and summarizes the key measures of cancer's impact on the U.S. population. The primary statistics reported are the rate at which new cases occur (incidence), the rate of death of cancer (mortality), and the percentage of patients surviving at various points in time after diagnosis.

New additions include the latest data on incidence, mortality, survival, and prevalence rates and probability of having and dying of cancer.

The SEER Cancer Statistics Review (CSR), a report of the most recent cancer incidence, mortality, survival, and prevalence statistics, is published annually by the Cancer Statistics Branch of the NCI. This edition includes incidence, mortality, survival, and prevalence statistics from 1975 through 2001, the most recent year for which data are available.

survival rate   The percentage of patients in a given population who are still alive a specified time after diagnosis with a particular disease. Scientists commonly use five-year survival rate as the standard statistical basis for defining when a reproductive cancer has been successfully treated.

The *five-year survival rate* includes anyone who is living five years after a cancer diagnosis, including those who are cured, those who are in remission, and those who still have cancer and are undergoing treatment.

The *overall five-year survival rate* equally measures everyone who has ever been diagnosed with a particular cancer. Distorted statistics can be produced by this method; for example, a 90-year-old woman and a 30-year-old woman who have the same cancer would be grouped together in this method. If the 90-year-old dies of other causes within the five-year period as a result of normal life expectancy, her death can skew the data.

A more statistically accurate view of survival is the *relative five-year survival rate*, which compares a cancer patient's survival rate with the survival rate of the general population, taking into account differences in age, gender, race, and other factors. In this case, the 30-year-old and the 90-year-old are treated as statistically different.

talcum powder Some cancer experts have suggested that talcum powder that is applied directly to the genital area or on sanitary napkins may be carcinogenic to the ovaries. Indeed, most—but not all—research studies have shown a potential link between talc exposure in the genital area and a slightly increased risk of OVARIAN CANCER.

Talcum powder is produced from talc, which in its natural form may contain asbestos (a known carcinogen). Because of this association with asbestos, all talc products marketed for use in the home have been required to be asbestos free since 1973, including baby powders, body powders, and facial powders.

Studies suggest that talcum powder (including "asbestos-free" talc) may affect the outer layer of the ovaries when applied to the genital area, sanitary napkins, diaphragms, or condoms.

Although all talc products sold for domestic use are required to be free of asbestos, some researchers advise using cornstarch-based rather than talc-based products. Proof of the safety of these newer asbestos-free products will require follow-up studies of women who have used them over a period of many years. There is no evidence at present linking use of cornstarch powders with any female cancers.

tamoxifen (Nolvadex) A drug used for more than 20 years to treat patients who have breast cancer. Tamoxifen is effective against breast cancer in part by interfering with the activity of ESTROGEN, a female HORMONE that promotes the growth of breast cancer cells.

However, tamoxifen also increases the risk of ENDOMETRIAL CANCER, which begins in the lining of the uterus, and uterine SARCOMA, which develops in the muscular wall of the uterus. Like all cancers,

endometrial cancer and uterine sarcoma are potentially life threatening. (Women who have had a hysterectomy and are taking tamoxifen are not at increased risk for these cancers.)

In a 1998 study called the Breast Cancer Prevention Trial (BCPT), women who used tamoxifen had more than twice the probability of development of endometrial cancer of women who used a placebo—the same as the risk of postmenopausal women who used estrogen replacement therapy. This risk is about two cases of endometrial cancer per every 1,000 women who use tamoxifen each year. Most of the endometrial cancers of women who used tamoxifen have been found in the early stages, and treatment has usually been effective. However, for some breast cancer patients in whom endometrial cancer developed while they were taking tamoxifen, the disease was life threatening.

Review of all the clinical trials using tamoxifen confirmed an increased risk of uterine sarcoma as well: in the BCPT, about two cases per 10,000 women who use tamoxifen each year. Research so far suggests that uterine sarcomas are more likely to be diagnosed at later stages than endometrial cancers and may therefore be harder to control and more life threatening.

For these reasons, women who take tamoxifen should have regular pelvic examinations and should be checked promptly if they have any abnormal vaginal bleeding or pelvic pain between scheduled exams.

taxanes A group of drugs that includes paclitaxel (Taxol) and docetaxel (Taxotere), which are used in the treatment of reproductive cancers. Taxanes have a unique way of preventing the growth of cancer cells, affecting cell structures called microtubules that play an important role in cell functions.

In normal cell growth, microtubules are formed when a cell starts dividing. Once the cell stops dividing, the microtubules are broken down or destroyed. Taxanes stop the microtubules from breaking down; cancer cells become so clogged with microtubules that they cannot grow and divide.

tea   Evidence of tea drinking dates back 5,000 years to China and India; where it has been long regarded as an aid to good health. Researchers now are studying tea for possible use in the prevention and treatment of a variety of cancers. Investigators are especially interested in the antioxidants (called catechins) found in tea, which may selectively inhibit the growth of cancer. In animal studies, catechins scavenged oxidants before cell damage occurred, reduced the number and size of tumors, and inhibited the growth of cancer cells. However, results of human studies have proved contradictory, perhaps as a result of such factors as variations in diet, environment, and population. Some studies comparing tea drinkers to non–tea drinkers support the claim that drinking tea prevents cancer; others do not.

The human body constantly produces unstable molecules called oxidants (also known as free radicals). To become stable, oxidants steal electrons from other molecules and, in the process, damage cell proteins and genetic material. This damage may leave the cell vulnerable to cancer. Antioxidants are substances that allow the human body to scavenge and seize oxidants. As other antioxidants do, the catechins found in tea selectively interfere with specific enzyme activities that lead to cancer. They may also target and repair DNA aberrations caused by oxidants.

All varieties of tea are produced from the leaves of a single evergreen plant (*Camellia sinensis*). All tea leaves are picked, rolled, dried, and heated; black tea is produced by an additional process of allowing the leaves to ferment and oxidize. Possibly because it is less processed, green tea contains higher levels of antioxidants than black tea.

Although tea is drunk in different ways and varies in its chemical makeup, one study showed steeping either green or black tea for about five minutes released more than 80 percent of its catechins. Instant iced tea, on the other hand, contains negligible amounts of catechins.

teratocarcinoma   A MIXED GERM CELL TUMOR made up of EMBRYONAL CARCINOMA and TERATOMA.

teratoma   A type of ovarian GERM CELL TUMOR that can be either malignant or benign. The benign form, called a mature teratoma, or dermoid CYST and is by far the most common ovarian germ cell tumor; it usually affects women of reproductive age. The malignant version is called an immature teratoma because its lining resembles skin.

Mature teratomas also contain a variety of other benign tissues that may resemble adult respiratory passages, bone, nervous tissue, teeth, and other tissues.

Immature teratomas occur in girls and young women, usually those younger than 18. These are rare cancers that resemble embryonic or fetal tissues such as connective tissue, respiratory passages, and brain. Tumors that are only mildly immature (grade 1 immature teratoma) and have not spread beyond the ovary are cured by surgical removal of the ovary. However, when they have spread beyond the ovary and/or much of the tumor has a very immature appearance (grade 2 or 3 immature teratomas), CHEMOTHERAPY is recommended in addition to surgical removal of the ovary.

thrombocytopenia   A drop in the number of platelets (blood cells responsible for clotting) that is often a side effect of RADIATION THERAPY or CHEMOTHERAPY. Certain types of cancer also may directly destroy platelets in the blood. Severe cases of thrombocytopenia can have grave consequences if minor injuries result in serious blood loss. The condition can be treated with transfusions of platelets, intravenous gamma globulin, removal of the spleen, and medications to boost the platelet count. When radiation therapy or chemotherapy is stopped, the platelet count should return to normal.

transitional cell carcinoma   A rare type of FALLOPIAN TUBE CANCER.

transvaginal color flow Doppler   A diagnostic device that uses a specialized type of ultrasound instrument to assess blood flow to the ovaries. This test can help detect OVARIAN CANCER, because this malignancy usually increases blood flow. However, several benign conditions can also increase blood flow to the ovaries.

See also CA 125; TRANSVAGINAL ULTRASOUND.

transvaginal ultrasound   An ultrasound test of the ovaries that is performed with the transponder placed inside the vagina instead of outside the body, where it is typically placed for standard ultrasound scans.

Ultrasound devices use sound waves to create an image on a video screen released from a small probe placed into the woman's vagina or on the surface of the abdomen. The sound waves create echoes as they enter the ovaries and other organs, and the probe detects the echoes that bounce back; a computer translates the pattern of echoes into a picture.

Because ovarian tumors and normal ovarian tissue often reflect sound waves differently, this test may be useful in detecting tumors and in determining whether a mass is solid or a fluid-filled cyst. However, although transvaginal sonography can help find a mass in the ovary, it cannot accurately predict which masses are cancers and which are due to benign diseases of the ovary.

In preliminary studies of women at average risk of OVARIAN CANCER, this test did not make any difference in the number of cancer deaths. For this reason, transvaginal sonography is not recommended for ovarian cancer screening for women who do not have known strong risk factors. However, some recent studies found that cancers detected by these tests tend to be somewhat less advanced than cancers of women who did not have screening tests.

See also CA 125.

tumor debulking   Removing the bulk of a tumor to give CHEMOTHERAPY a better chance to treat the cancer. The ultimate aim of debulking is to reduce the tumor at any one site to less than one centimeter.

tumor marker   A substance (also called a biomarker) that can often be detected in higher-than-normal amounts in the blood, urine, or body tissues of some women who have certain types of cancers, including REPRODUCTIVE CANCERS. Tumor markers are produced either by the tumor itself or by the body as a response to the presence of cancer or certain benign conditions. Examples of tumor markers for reproductive cancers include CA 125 and CARCINOEMBRYONIC ANTIGEN (CEA) (OVARIAN CANCER); alpha-fetoprotein (AFP), beta human chorionic gonadotropin (BHCG), and LHH (for GERM CELL TUMORS); and inhibin B (granulose cell tumors).

It can be helpful to measure tumor marker levels—when used with X-rays or other tests—to detect and diagnose some types of cancer. However, tumor marker levels alone are not enough to diagnose cancer, since levels can be high in women who have benign conditions and levels of the markers are not high in every woman who has cancer (especially in the early stages of the disease). Moreover, many tumor markers are not specific to a particular type of cancer; the level of a tumor marker can be raised by more than one type of malignancy.

In addition to their role in cancer diagnosis, some tumor marker levels are measured before treatment to help doctors plan appropriate therapy. In some types of cancer, tumor marker levels reflect the stage of the disease and can be useful in predicting disease response to treatment. Tumor marker levels may also be measured during treatment to monitor a patient's response to treatment; a drop in the level of a tumor marker may indicate that the cancer has responded favorably to therapy, and a rise in the marker level may indicate that the cancer is growing. Finally, measurements of tumor marker levels may be used after treatment as a part of follow-up care to check for recurrence.

Currently, the main uses of tumor markers are to assess a cancer's response to treatment and to check for recurrence. Scientists continue to study these uses of tumor markers as well as their potential role in the early detection and diagnosis of cancer. The patient's doctor can explain the role of tumor markers in detection, diagnosis, or treatment for that person.

CA 125

CA 125 is produced by a variety of cells, but especially by ovarian cancer cells. Studies have shown that many women who have ovarian cancer have high CA 125 levels. Measures of this marker are used primarily to manage treatment for ovarian cancer. In women who have ovarian cancer who are being treated with CHEMOTHERAPY, a falling CA 125 level generally indicates that the cancer is responding to treatment. Rising CA 125 levels during or after treatment, on the other hand, may suggest that the cancer is not responding to therapy or that some cancer cells remain in the body. Doctors may also use CA 125 levels to monitor patients for recurrence of ovarian cancer.

However, not all women who have high CA 125 levels have ovarian cancer. Higher-than-normal CA 125 levels also may be linked to cancers of the uterus or cervix, among others. Noncancerous conditions that can cause high CA 125 levels include endometriosis, pelvic inflammatory disease, peritonitis, pancreatitis, liver disease, and any condition that inflames the tissue that surrounds the lungs and lines the chest cavity. Menstruation and pregnancy can also increase CA 125 level.

Carcinoembryonic Antigen

CEA is normally found in small amounts in the blood of most healthy people, but levels may rise in women who have colon cancer or some benign conditions. A wide variety of other cancers can produce high levels of this tumor marker, including some gynecological cancers as well as cancers of the breast, lung, pancreas, stomach, bladder, kidney, thyroid, or liver.

High CEA levels can also occur in noncancerous conditions, including inflammatory bowel disease, pancreatitis, and liver disease. Tobacco use can also contribute to higher-than-normal levels of CEA.

Alpha-Fetoprotein

AFP is normally produced by a developing fetus. AFP levels begin to decrease soon after birth and are usually undetectable in the blood of healthy adults (except during pregnancy). An elevated level of AFP strongly suggests the presence of germ cell cancer (cancer that begins in the cells that produce eggs) in the ovary. Only rarely do patients who have other types of cancer (such as stomach cancer) have elevated levels of AFP. Noncancerous conditions that can cause high AFP levels include benign liver conditions, such as cirrhosis or hepatitis, ataxia telangiectasia, Wiscott-Aldrich syndrome, and pregnancy.

Human Chorionic Gonadotropin

Human chorionic gonadotropin (HCG) is normally produced by the placenta during pregnancy; it is also used to screen for CHORIOCARCINOMA (a rare cancer of the uterus) in women who are at high risk for the disease. It is also used to monitor the treatment of trophoblastic disease (a rare cancer that develops from an abnormally fertilized egg). High HCG levels may indicate the presence of cancers of the ovary, among others. Pregnancy and marijuana use can also cause elevated HCG levels.

CA 15-3

Although the CA 15-3 marker levels are most useful in following the course of treatment in women diagnosed with advanced breast cancer, cancers of the ovary also may increase CA 15-3 levels. High levels of CA 15-3 may also be associated with noncancerous conditions, such as benign breast or ovarian disease, endometriosis, pelvic inflammatory disease, and hepatitis. Pregnancy and lactation can also cause CA 15-3 levels to rise.

CA 27-29

Similar to the CA 15-3 antigen, CA 27-29 is a marker found in the blood of most breast cancer patients, but it is also present at high levels in uterine or ovarian cancer, among others. First-trimester pregnancy, endometriosis, OVARIAN CYSTS, benign breast disease, kidney disease, and liver disease are noncancerous conditions that can also elevate CA 27-29 levels.

tumor registry An institution that collects and stores data about cancer, diagnosed either in a specific hospital or medical facility (hospital-based registry) or in a defined geographic area (population-based registry). A population-based registry is generally composed of a number of hospital-based registries.

tumors of low malignant potential Also called borderline tumors, this is a class of ovarian tumors that are not likely to invade and spread. However, a tumor of low malignant potential has an intermediate capacity to recur and then spread. Usually, if these tumors recur, they recur very late and usually appear in only one or a few sites. These tumors are more common in younger patients.

tumor suppressor genes Genes that suppress the growth of tumors. These genes have a number of jobs. They may slow down cell division, cause cells to die at the appropriate time, or help repair DNA damage. Tumor suppressor genes are normal genes whose absence can lead to cancer. If a pair of normal tumor suppressor genes are either lost from a cell or inactivated by mutation, their functional absence can cause cancer.

Because genes come in pairs (one inherited from each parent), an inherited defect in one copy will not cause cancer because the other normal copy is still functional. But if the second copy undergoes mutation, the person then may develop cancer because there no longer is any functional copy of the gene. Individuals who inherit an increased risk of developing cancer often are born with one defective copy of a tumor suppressor gene.

Tumor suppressor genes that are linked to reproductive cancers include:

- *BRCA 1* and *BRCA 2:* breast cancer and higher risk of ovarian cancer
- *LKB1:* Also known as STK11, this gene is linked to ovarian cancer
- *MLH1* and *MSH2:* These genes each have been implicated in ovarian and endometrial cancers, among others.
- *MSH6:* Also known as GTBP, this gene has been linked to endometrial cancers, among others.
- *PMS 1* and *2:* These genes (both discovered in 1994), have been linked to ovarian and endometrial cancers, among others.

See also ONCOGENES.

ultrasound guided biopsy   See BIOPSY.

ultrasound scan   A diagnostic technique also called sonography, that uses high-frequency sound waves above the range of human hearing to produce images of structures inside the body.

uterine cancer   Several types of cancer can affect the uterus; the most common is cancer that begins in the lining of the uterus (endometrium), which is called ENDOMETRIAL CANCER. Another cancer that affects the uterus is SARCOMA, a rare uterine cancer that begins in the muscle of the uterus (myometrium) instead of the lining.

Uterine cancer is usually curable when detected early. It is the third most common cancer in women, affecting more than 40,000 women in the United States each year. Most women who have uterine cancer are between the ages of 55 and 70, and 92 percent of women survive this type of cancer when it is detected in its early stages before it spreads; 64 percent of women survive even when it has spread to other parts of the body. The five-year survival rate for women who have uterine cancer is 96 percent.

Different women experience uterine cancer in different ways; even those who have the same type of cancer in the same stage and have the same treatment may have different results. For unknown reasons, the cancer may be eradicated, or it may return or spread.

If uterine cancer does spread, it tends to spread first to pelvic organs and LYMPH NODES nearest the uterus. From there, it may spread to the cervix, vagina, ovaries, lungs, and bones.

The endometrium also may be affected by a pre-cancerous condition called ENDOMETRIAL HYPERPLA-SIA. This overgrowth of cells in the endometrial lining may become malignant if untreated. Women who have endometrial hyperplasia may also experience unusual vaginal bleeding.

Benign Endometrial Conditions

There are some conditions that affect the uterine lining that are not malignant but can cause symptoms similar to those of uterine cancer. One of these conditions is endometriosis—a disorder in which endometrial tissue grows either outside the uterus or within the muscular layer of the uterus. Some women who have this condition may experience cramps and unusual vaginal bleeding.

FIBROID TUMORS are another benign condition that may affect the lining of the uterus. Also called LEIOMYOMAS, these common benign tumors sometimes form in the endometrial muscle. Women who have fibroid tumors may experience unusual bleeding from the vagina and frequent urge to urinate. Fibroid tumors usually require no specific treatment.

Risk Factors

A number of risk factors put certain women at higher likelihood of development of uterine cancer. Being aware of the factors that raise the risk of developing uterine cancer is important, because many can be controlled or modified. A woman may, for example, slightly lower her risk by exercising regularly and eating a healthy DIET. Keeping blood sugar level and blood pressure under control also helps lower the risk of uterine cancer.

Age   Most women who develop uterine cancer are older than age 50; a woman is at higher risk if she is postmenopausal and older than 50.

Endometrial hyperplasia   This condition refers to an increase in the number of normal cells lining the uterus, which may become malignant if untreated. Women who have endometrial hyperplasia may also experience unusual vaginal bleeding.

Estrogen levels Since the incidence of uterine cancer may be related to hormonal changes, any condition that raises ESTROGEN level may put women at increased risk. Estrogen replacement therapy is associated with elevated HORMONE levels. Because women who use ESTROGEN REPLACEMENT THERAPY without additional progesterone have a higher probability of development of uterine cancer, most women who have an intact uterus who need estrogen replacement therapy use a combination of estrogen and progesterone to protect the uterus from cancer. Studies have shown that a woman who receives estrogen supplements after menopause can have a 12 times higher risk of uterine cancer if she does not receive progesterone at the same time.

Obesity Experts believe that being overweight is a very strong risk factor for this cancer. Fatty tissue can produce estrogen, which can promote uterine cancer. Overweight women have uterine cancer twice as often as do women who are not overweight. Most young women who have this type of cancer are obese; it is unusual to have uterine cancer before the age of 45.

Pregnancy Women who have never been pregnant have a higher chance of development of uterine cancer, perhaps because high levels of progestins are produced during pregnancy. If a woman does not ovulate regularly during her reproductive years, the lack of ovulation can upset the delicate balance between the estrogenic hormones that encourage the development of cancer and the progestigenic hormones that protect against cancer.

Irregular periods During a woman's menstrual cycle, there is an interaction between estrogen (which can encourage uterine cancer development) and progesterone (which can protect against uterine cancer). Women who do not ovulate regularly are exposed to high estrogen levels for longer periods. If a woman does not ovulate regularly, this balance is upset and may increase her probability of having uterine cancer.

Early menstruation/late menopause Having a first period at a young age and going through menopause at a late age seem to put women at a slightly higher risk for development of uterine cancer.

Other cancers Women who have had colon, rectal, or breast cancer have a higher chance of uterine cancer.

Race Caucasian women have a higher chance of uterine cancer than do non-Caucasian women. For reasons that are not entirely clear, this type of cancer is approximately twice as common in Caucasians as it is in non-Caucasians.

Tamoxifen This drug, sometimes used to treat breast cancer, may be linked to a higher risk of development of uterine cancer in women who have used it for five or more years. However, although several studies have shown that tamoxifen can significantly increase a woman's risk of uterine cancer, researchers believe that its ability to lower the incidence of breast cancer deaths outweighs the risk of uterine cancer development. A woman who has been receiving tamoxifen does not need routine X-rays or biopsies, but she should be examined by her gynecologist at least once a year (or immediately if irregular bleeding occurs).

High blood pressure High blood pressure has been weakly associated with uterine cancer. It is not very clear whether high blood pressure alone is responsible for increasing the risk of uterine cancer, or whether the risk is related to the finding that these women are also generally obese.

Diabetes Women who have diabetes have twice the risk of uterine cancer of women who do not have diabetes. However, many women who have diabetes are also overweight, and experts are not sure how much of the increased risk in women who have diabetes is due to the diabetic condition and how much is due to overweight.

Hereditary nonpolyposis colorectal cancer (Lynch syndrome II) HEREDITARY NONPOLYPOSIS COLORECTAL CANCER is the most common type of hereditary uterine cancer syndrome, in which multiple family members can have cancers that begin in the colon, uterus, small intestine, kidney system, or ovaries.

Symptoms

When uterine cancer develops, it is almost always linked with unexpected vaginal bleeding—often in a postmenopausal woman. The vaginal bleeding may appear watery at first, with a small amount of blood; eventually, the bleeding may appear less watery and more bloody. Other symptoms include pain during urination, pain during sex, or pelvic pain. Because symptoms of uterine cancer can also be caused by less serious problems, a woman should discuss them with her doctor.

Diagnosis

Currently, there are no screening tests for uterine cancer that are recommended for routine use other than yearly pelvic exams by a gynecologist or other primary care doctor. To determine the cause of any symptoms, a doctor performs a careful physical exam to check for any lumps or changes in the shape of the uterus, feeling the vagina, uterus, ovaries, bladder, and rectum. The doctor may also perform one or more of the following tests.

Pap test A PAP TEST is performed during a pelvic exam. Using a wooden spatula or small brush, the doctor takes a sample of cells from the cervix and upper vagina and examines them for abnormalities. However, the Pap test is used primarily to detect CERVICAL CANCER; because cancer of the endometrium begins inside the uterus, it is not usually revealed by a Pap test. The Pap test does not detect most uterine cancers. For this reason, the doctor may also do an endometrial biopsy or D&C (dilation and curettage) or similar test to remove pieces of the lining of the uterus (see later discussion).

Endometrial biopsy The only way to produce a definitive diagnosis of endometrial cancer is to perform an endometrial BIOPSY. During the biopsy, a doctor removes some tissue from the inner endometrial lining by inserting a thin plastic tube through the vagina and cervix into the uterus. The procedure usually results in a brief period of endometrial cramping. The tissue specimen is then examined under a microscope by a pathologist. A formal report is given to the doctor and patient within several days.

Although most uterine cancers occur in postmenopausal women, some cases develop in younger women. In these premenopausal women, a uterine biopsy should be obtained if menstrual periods are very heavy or irregular. Irregular bleeding may be due to lack of regular ovulation but also

can be caused by the development of cancerous or precancerous uterine changes.

Dilation and curettage If the cervical canal is very narrow or a sample of tissue cannot be obtained by an endometrial biopsy, the doctor may need to perform a D&C of the endometrial cavity. This procedure is usually performed in an operating room with the patient under general anesthesia. During a D&C, the opening of the cervix is stretched with a spoon-shaped instrument and the walls of the uterus are gently scraped to remove any growths. This tissue is then checked for cancer cells. Afterward, the woman may experience mild cramps and vaginal bleeding for a few days. In order to check for tumors, a lighted scope may be inserted into the endometrial cavity during the D&C (a procedure called HYSTEROSCOPY).

Staging When endometrial cancer is diagnosed, the doctor needs to know the stage of the cancer, which is based on the size of the tumor, the number of lymph nodes involved, and the extent of spread of the cancer to other organs. The most common staging system for uterine cancer is a system developed by the International Federation of Gynecology and Obstetrics in which the numerals from 0 (the earliest stage) to IV (the most advanced stage) represent the different stages of the cancer.

Stage I: The cancer is only in the body of the uterus.
Stage IA: The cancer is only in the endometrium.
Stage IB: The cancer has spread less than halfway through the myometrium.
Stage IC: The cancer has spread halfway through the myometrium.
Stage II: The cancer has spread from the uterus to the cervix.
Stage IIA: The cancer is in the body of the uterus and the endocervical glands.
Stage IIB: The cancer is in the body of the uterus and the cervical stroma.
Stage III: The cancer has spread outside the body of the uterus but has not left the pelvic area.
Stage IIIA: The cancer has spread to the serosa of the uterus, or the adnexa, or there are no cancer cells in peritoneal fluid.
Stage IIIB: The cancer has spread to the vagina.
Stage IIIC: The cancer has spread to the lymph nodes near the uterus.

Stage IV: The cancer has spread to the mucosa of the bladder or the rectum, the lymph nodes in the groin, or other organs such as the lungs or the bones.

Stage IVA: The cancer has spread to the mucosa or inner lining of the rectum or bladder.

Stage IVB: The cancer has spread to the lymph nodes in the groin area and/or other organs such as the lungs or bones.

Treatment

The treatment choices for each woman depend on the size and location of the tumor, the results of lab tests, and the stage or extent of the disease. A doctor also considers the woman's age and general health in determining a treatment plan.

Women whose uterine cancer recurs may be treated with CHEMOTHERAPY or HORMONAL THERAPY as well as RADIATION THERAPY. These treatments are frequently used to relieve pain, nausea, and abnormal bowel function.

Surgery Surgery is the most common treatment for cancer of the endometrium. After the diagnosis of a cancer, surgery should be performed relatively soon (generally within one or two weeks). Several different types of surgery can be performed to treat uterine cancer: simple abdominal or vaginal HYSTERECTOMY, radical hysterectomy, or bilateral SALPINGO-OOPHORECTOMY.

In a *simple hysterectomy,* the uterus (including the cervix) is removed during a one- to three-hour operation, typically followed by a three- or four-day hospital stay. An abdominal hysterectomy is performed through an incision that runs from about the pubic bone to the navel. In a vaginal hysterectomy, the uterus is removed through the vagina. Samples of lymph nodes in the area are usually taken during surgery to determine whether they include cancerous cells. (The lymph nodes are small, bean-shaped structures found throughout the body that produce and store infection-fighting cells but may also contain cancer cells.)

A *radical hysterectomy* is performed when the cancer has spread to the cervix or the tissues beside the uterus; this operation is very uncommonly used for uterine cancer. In this surgery the entire uterus is removed along with the tissues beside the uterus and the upper part of the vagina beside the cervix.

A radical hysterectomy is performed through an abdominal incision. Women who have a radical hysterectomy also have a sample of nearby lymph nodes taken at the same time.

More recently, some gynecologic oncologists have been performing uterine cancer surgery laparoscopically. The advantages of this approach are that smaller incisions are used and the hospitalization and recovery periods are shorter.

In a *bilateral salpingo-oophorectomy,* both fallopian tubes, and the ovaries are removed. In nearly all cases of uterine cancer, the fallopian tubes and ovaries are removed. It is important to remove the ovaries during surgery because they are an area where uterine cancer may spread. Lymph nodes from the pelvic and lower aortic areas often are removed to look for spread of the cancer, since this is the most common route of spread.

After hysterectomy, additional treatment with radiation therapy and/or chemotherapy is required in some cases in which spread of disease outside the uterus has been found or is suspected.

Radiation therapy The goal of radiation therapy is to kill cancer cells by using X-rays. This treatment can shrink a tumor before surgery, treat a tumor without surgery, or remove any remaining cancer cells after surgery. Radiation therapy can also be used if the cancer has spread to distant organs, such as the brain or bones, to reduce pain or other symptoms.

External radiation may be directed at the body by a machine or may be directed from a very small container of radioactive material placed directly into or near the tumor (called internal radiation or brachytherapy). Some patients receive both kinds of radiation therapy.

If a patient is having external beam radiation therapy of the pelvic area for uterine cancer, treatment is given in an outpatient department of a hospital or clinic five days a week for four to six weeks. At the end of treatment, an extra boost of radiation is sometimes directed at a smaller area where the tumor first developed.

The radiation oncologist may also choose to use internal radiation therapy over several weeks at the doctor's office. In most cases, the internal radiation is placed either after the external radiation or when the vagina has healed after the surgery. In these situations the implant is placed against the skin at the top of the vagina. If the radiation oncologist chooses to use standard dose delivery (low-dose-rate brachytherapy), the implant is placed in the hospital. This implant is temporary; when it is removed, no radioactivity is left in the body.

Chemotherapy Anticancer drugs are used when the cancer can no longer be treated with local treatments alone. Chemotherapy can also be given after surgery for patients who have a high risk for distant spread. The goal of chemotherapy in this setting is to kill any cells that may have spread before the tumor was surgically removed.

Chemotherapy is given in cycles. A woman who has uterine cancer receives chemotherapy treatment for a certain length of time, then has a rest period, after which treatment begins again. Common endometrial cancer chemotherapy drugs include cisplatin (Platinol or carboplatin), ADRIAMYCIN, and paclitaxel (Taxol). Potential side effects depend on the kind of drug. Common side effects of chemotherapy include nausea and vomiting, HAIR LOSS, CONSTIPATION or DIARRHEA, and FATIGUE. Other serious side effects that may occur as a consequence of a decrease in blood cell counts include infection and bleeding.

Hormonal therapy In hormonal therapy, drugs are used to prevent malignant cells from getting the hormones they need to grow. Response to hormone therapy can be predicted by factors such as tumor grade, presence of progesterone receptors, and (if the cancer has recurred) interval from the first treatment to recurrence.

Hormonal therapy may be used as a treatment if surgery is not possible. Or hormones may often be used to treat precancerous changes, helping the uterus shed the endometrial lining along with the precancerous changes. Sometimes, hormonal therapy may shrink or completely kill the uterine cancer.

Hormonal therapy is usually administered in the form of a progestin tablet that is taken daily for a period of time, or by injection. Several progestin drugs and regimens have been studied for the treatment of advanced or recurrent uterine cancer. Research suggests that the response rate of uterine adenocarcinomas to progestin therapy ranges from 10 percent to 50 percent. Well- and moderately differentiated tumors respond more frequently to progesterone therapy than do poorly differentiated carcinomas.

Uterine cancers are known to be dependent on estrogen for growth; women who have high levels of estrogen are at risk for the development of uterine cancer. The main sources of estrogen are the ovary and conversion of other hormones into estrogen. In postmenopausal women, the conversion of testosterone into estrogen in fat tissue by the aromatase enzyme is an important source of estrogen; experts believe that inhibiting this conversion may be an effective manner of treating uterine cancers.

Several such agents that competitively inhibit or inactivate the enzymes needed for the conversion of testosterone to estrogen have been developed. Estrogen antagonist aromatase inhibitors (such as tamoxifen) are being evaluated for endometrial cancer. Tamoxifen inhibits the growth of estrogen-receptor-positive breast cancers; when used for patients who have recurrent or advanced endometrial cancer, it can produce occasional durable responses and a significant incidence of disease stabilization. The objective response rate to tamoxifen in several studies is between 20 percent and 60 percent, with occasional long-term survivors. Although tamoxifen may be of some benefit to the occasional patient who has advanced or recurrent endometrial cancer, those for whom initial hormonal therapy with progestin has failed are unlikely to respond to estrogen.

After Treatment

Many women who have endometrial cancer feel tired for a period after treatment is finished. Such fatigue can interfere with daily life. It is important for the doctor to check a woman's red blood count, since anemia may be the cause of the lack of energy of some patients. In some cases, a blood transfusion may be necessary, or medications may be prescribed that increase the red blood cell count. Some people do not want to eat or exercise when they are tired. However, unhealthy diet and limited exercise can make the condition worse.

Prevention

There are certain changes a woman can make in her lifestyle to lessen her risk of endometrial cancer. These include the following factors.

Diet Studies have shown that eating foods that contain less fat may help prevent endometrial cancer. Consuming a plant-based diet low in fat, high in fiber, and rich in whole grains, vegetables, fruit, and legumes (especially soybeans) may reduce the risk of endometrial cancer, according to recent studies. This type of diet may partly explain the lower rates of uterine cancer in Asian countries compared with those in the United States. As with breast and ovarian cancers, rates for endometrial cancer are lower in Japan, China, and other Asian countries than they are in the United States and Europe. Eating of less fiber and SOY PRODUCTS and more fat may explain the increase in uterine cancer found among Asians who have migrated to the West.

In recent years, researchers have focused on possible dietary factors that may influence these differences—especially the possibility that dietary fat intake increases the risk of endometrial cancer. In one study, energy intake from fat but not from other sources was positively associated with endometrial cancer. Among women who consumed most dietary fat, the risk was 1.6 times greater than that of those who consumed least fat. However, women who consumed the most fiber from cereals, vegetables, and fruit had a 29 percent to 46 percent reduction in cancer risk when compared to those who ate the least fiber. In addition, several groups of PHYTOESTROGEN-rich foods (such as legumes, tofu, and other soy products) were linked to a lower risk of endometrial cancer. Phytoestrogens are plant compounds that have effects similar to those of the hormone estrogen. Women who ate the highest amount of foods rich in these compounds had a 54 percent reduction in cancer risk, compared with those who consumed the least. Phytoestrogens compete with estrogen for cell-receptor binding sites. In doing so, they help control the level of estrogen circulating in the blood. Phytoestrogens' "antiestrogen effect" may block the development of endometrial cancer by reducing hormonal activities that cause endometrial cells to proliferate uncontrollably.

Other factors that may decrease the risk of uterine cancer include the following:

- *Pregnancy.* Child birth may lower a woman's chance of having endometrial cancer.
- *Body weight.* Exercise that results in significant weight loss can lower a woman's risk of endometrial cancer.
- *Birth control pills.* Use of birth control pills with estrogens and/or progestins during childbearing years can lower a woman's risk of both endometrial and ovarian cancer.
- *Estrogen replacement therapy.* Use of estrogen after the childbearing years can significantly lower a woman's risk of endometrial cancer and offers other benefits. It may prevent hot flashes, thinning of the vagina, and osteoporosis.

uterine sarcoma One of two general types of UTERINE CANCER, uterine sarcoma is a very rare type of reproductive cancer. In this condition, cancer cells begin growing in the muscles of the uterus. (Cancers that start in connective tissues, such as muscle, fat, bone, and fibrous tissue are called sarcomas.) Most uterine sarcomas fall into one of three categories, which are based on the type of cell from which they develop:

- *Endometrial stromal sarcomas* develop in the supporting connective tissue (stroma) of the endometrium; they are the rarest uterine sarcomas.
- *Uterine leiomyosarcomas* begin in the muscular wall of the uterus; they are the second most common type of uterine sarcoma.
- *Uterine carcinosarcomas* (also known as malignant mixed mesodermal tumors or malignant mixed müllerian tumors) begin in the endometrium and have features of both sarcomas and carcinomas. The most common of the sarcomas, these tumors are usually classified with uterine sarcomas; however, some doctors believe they are more closely related to carcinomas.

The other general type of uterine cancer is uterine carcinoma, which begins in the tissues lining the surface of an organ. More than 95 percent of cancers of the uterus are carcinomas, which develop from cells of the uterine lining. Carcinomas of the cervix are called cervical carcinomas (CERVICAL CANCER), and carcinomas that develop from the cells lining the upper part of the uterus are called endometrial carcinomas (ENDOMETRIAL CANCER).

The AMERICAN CANCER SOCIETY estimates that about 40,320 women in the United States are diagnosed with uterine cancer per year; only about 1 or 2 percent of these cancers are uterine sarcomas.

If uterine sarcoma spreads outside the uterus, cancer cells may be found in nearby lymph nodes, nerves, or blood vessels. If the cancer has reached the lymph nodes, cancer cells may have spread to other lymph nodes and other organs, such as the lungs, liver, and bones.

Risk Factors

Currently, there is little insight into the exact causes of uterine sarcoma, but a few risk factors have been uncovered.

Pelvic radiation   Between 10 percent and 25 percent of uterine sarcoma malignancies occur in women who received pelvic radiation five to 25 years earlier for benign bleeding. As in other cancers of its type, risk factors for uterine cancer include diabetes, hypertension, obesity, and high estrogen levels.

Age   Middle-aged and older women are more likely than younger women to have uterine sarcomas. The disease is most commonly diagnosed after menopause.

Race   African-American women are more likely than Caucasians or Asian Americans to have uterine sarcomas.

Hormonal risk factors   Uterine sarcomas develop more often in women who have hormonal risk factors, such as obesity, estrogen replacement therapy, infertility, diabetes, late onset of menstruation or late onset of menopause, or treatment with TAMOXIFEN.

Symptoms

There are few symptoms in the early stages. When symptoms do appear, the most common is bleeding after menopause or bleeding at times other than during menstruation. Other symptoms may include abnormal discharge without any visible blood, or pelvic pain. Although these symptoms may be caused by other conditions or problems, they should be evaluated by a doctor.

Diagnosis

If there are signs of uterine sarcoma, a doctor conducts a pelvic examination to feel for any lumps or changes in the shapes of the pelvic organs. The doctor may then do a PAP TEST to check cells on the cervix. However, because uterine sarcoma begins inside the uterus, this cancer is not usually visible on a Pap test result. Next, the doctor may perform a dilation and curettage (D&C) to stretch the cervix and remove tissue from the uterine lining to check for cancer cells.

Staging

If sarcoma of the uterus has been diagnosed, more tests are done to find out whether the cancer has spread from the uterus to other parts of the body. A doctor needs to know the stage of the disease to plan treatment. The following stages are used to describe sarcoma of the uterus.

Stage I: Cancer is found only in the main part of the uterus (it is not found in the cervix).
Stage II: Cancer cells have spread to the cervix.
Stage III: Cancer cells have spread outside the uterus but have not spread outside the pelvis.
Stage IV: Cancer cells have spread beyond the pelvis, to other body parts, or into the lining of the bladder or rectum.

Treatment

The prognosis and treatment choice depend on the stage of the sarcoma and the patient's general state of health.

Surgery is the most common treatment for cancer of the uterus. During surgery, the cancer is removed along with the uterus, fallopian tubes, ovaries, and some lymph nodes in the pelvis and around the aorta (the main vessel in which blood passes away from the heart). The operation is called a total abdominal HYSTERECTOMY, bilateral SALPINGO-OOPHORECTOMY, and lymphadenectomy.

In addition, patients may have RADIATION THERAPY to kill cancer cells and shrink tumors, CHEMOTHERAPY, and/or HORMONE THERAPY. The exact type of treatment of sarcoma of the uterus used depends on the stage and cell type of the disease and on the patient's age and overall condition.

vaccines against cancer A form of BIOLOGICAL THERAPY that encourages a cancer patient's immune system to recognize and destroy cancer cells. Unlike vaccines against infectious diseases that work by teaching the body's immune defenses to recognize invading viruses and bacteria, cancer vaccines are designed to be injected after the disease is diagnosed, rather than before it develops. Cancer vaccines given when a tumor is small may be able to eradicate the cancer.

The immune system is constantly scanning the body for foreign invaders, but because cancer cells originate in the body, they are usually not detected by the immune system. In a cancer vaccine, tumor cells would be removed, marked as "foreign" by adding a special gene, and then injected beneath the skin along with an immunostimulant (such as interleukin-2). This process stimulates the immune system react as if it has just been newly infected with cancer, so that it will destroy this "new" antigen. Scientists hope such a vaccine would help the body recognize cancer, rejecting tumors and preventing cancer recurrence.

Early cancer vaccine studies primarily involved melanoma patients, but scientists today are testing the vaccines for many other types of cancer. Scientists in California and Germany have successfully used an oral vaccine to stop cancerous tumor growth in animals by choking off the tumor's blood supply. Researchers first targeted a protein produced in new blood vessels (vascular endothelial growth factor [VEGF] receptor 2), one of several substances that trigger new blood vessel growth (a process called angiogenesis). New blood vessel growth is critical to allow cancerous tumors to grow and spread. When researchers administered genetically engineered bacteria that contained a gene to express the VEGF receptor 2 protein, they triggered the animals' immune system to fight off the mild infection from the bacteria—and in the process, kill the protein that spurs new blood vessel growth to the tumors.

HPV Vaccine

Although most types of cancer are caused primarily by genetic mutations and environmental factors, virtually all cases of CERVICAL CANCER are caused by a sexually transmitted virus—the HUMAN PAPILLOMAVIRUS (HPV).

Scientists have achieved dramatic results with an HPV vaccine study, leading some experts to hope that the disease may someday be cured. They also hope it may help prevent many cases of the more rare VAGINAL CANCER, which is also linked to HPV.

In the study, the HPV vaccine prevented HPV infection in every woman who had injections. Although it remains unclear how long the protection may last, researchers say a vaccine could reach the market by 2007. A vaccine for cervical cancer is urgently sought because the disease strikes about 450,000 women worldwide each year, killing about half of them. In the United States, where the PAP TEST is widely used to screen for this cancer, it still develops in about 15,000 women annually and kills about a third of them.

The new vaccine is aimed at the viral strain type 16 that is responsible for about half the cases of cervical cancer. It was tested on women between the ages of 16 and 23 at 16 sites around the United States in an 18-month study led by Merck & Co. and the University of Washington. (Merck developed the vaccine and funded the research.)

Of 768 women who had vaccine injections, none showed type 16 infections or precancerous tissue. Of 765 who had dummy injections, 41 had persistent infections and nine had precancerous tissue. Women who were vaccinated produced up to almost 60 times the concentration of virus-fighting antibodies noted in naturally infected women. Although some researchers were worried that the cervical mucous membrane would interfere with these antibodies, that did not occur.

However, because cervical cancer is caused by multiple strains of HPV, it is not clear whether the disease can ever be wiped out completely. In addition, scientists do not know whether the antibodies persist for more than five years, as would be important in assuring lifetime protection.

Still, scientists hope that a vaccine targeting multiple viral strains encompassing the vast share of cases might be available fairly quickly. Such a vaccine could also stop other problems caused by the virus, including genital warts in both men and women and rare forms of penile, anal, vaginal, and oral cancer. The vaccine could also be given to men to prevent them from infecting their partners.

vaginal adenosis A condition in which some of the cells lining the vagina change and resemble those found in glands of the lower uterus or upper uterine lining (endometrium). Normally, the vagina is lined by flat cells called squamous cells, but in about 40 percent of women who have already entered puberty, the vagina may contain one or more areas where the vagina is lined instead with these unusual cells.

Vaginal adenosis occurs in nearly all women exposed during fetal development to a drug known as DIETHYLSTILBESTROL (DES). Although adenosis increases the risk of development of CLEAR CELL CARCINOMA, this cancer is still extremely rare, and the risk that a woman with adenosis not exposed to DES will have clear cell carcinoma is extremely low. Nonetheless, many doctors recommend especially careful screening for these women.

vaginal cancer A rare type of cancer that begins in the vagina. Vaginal cancer represents only about 3 percent of cancers of the female reproductive system. It usually occurs among elderly women who have abnormal bleeding. About 2,000 new cases of vaginal cancer are diagnosed each year in the United States, and about 800 women die.

Types of Vaginal Cancer

There are several types of vaginal cancer; the most common (between 85 percent and 90 percent) of vaginal cancers are SQUAMOUS CELL CARCINOMAS. These cancers begin in the epithelial lining of the vagina and tend to occur in the upper area of the vagina near the cervix. Vaginal squamous cell carcinomas develop over a period of many years, beginning with precancerous changes called VAGINAL INTRAEPITHELIAL NEOPLASIA (VAIN).

Verrucous carcinoma is a rare type of squamous cell carcinoma that tends to grow slowly, usually toward the inside of the vagina, and often appears as cauliflowerlike lumps. Compared with other squamous cell carcinomas, it is much less likely to invade deeply through the vaginal wall or spread to other organs. This type of vaginal cancer has a relatively good prognosis.

About 5 to 10 percent of vaginal cancers are *ADENOCARCINOMAS*. The usual type of vaginal adenocarcinoma typically develops in girls and women between the ages of 12 and 30. One type, called clear cell adenocarcinoma, occurs more often in young women who were exposed to DIETHYLSTILBESTROL (DES) before birth. In the past some pregnant women were given DES to prevent miscarriage. The drug became available during the late 1940s and was banned in the United States in 1971.

Malignant melanoma is a cancer that develops from pigment-producing cells called melanocytes. Although these cancers usually appear on sun-exposed areas of the skin, they may occasionally form on the vagina. They make up 2 to 3 percent of all vaginal cancers. Melanoma tends to affect the lower or outer portion of the vagina and show considerable variation in size, color, and growth pattern.

Another 2 to 3 percent of vaginal cancers are *SARCOMAS*. These cancers form deep in the wall of the vagina and occur as one of several types. The most common is LEIOMYOSARCOMA, which typically affects women older than 50. Leiomyosarcomas resemble the involuntary muscle cells of the vaginal wall.

RHABDOMYOSARCOMA is a childhood cancer usually diagnosed before the age of three. Its cells resemble voluntary muscle cells—tissue not normally found in the vaginal wall.

Cancers that begin in the vagina are less common than cancers that start in other organs (such as the uterus) and then spread into the vagina.

Risk Factors

Scientists have found that certain risk factors make a woman more likely to have vaginal cancer, although many women who have vaginal cancer have no apparent risk factors.

Age   Age is a risk factor for squamous cell carcinoma; about half of women are 60 years old or older when they are diagnosed. Most cases of the disease are diagnosed in women between the ages of 50 and 70.

Diethylstilbestrol   About one of every 1,000 women whose mother took DES during pregnancy has clear cell adenocarcinoma of the vagina or cervix. Clear cell adenocarcinomas are more common in the vagina than in the cervix. Although about 99.9 percent of "DES daughters" do not contract this cancer, the risk appears to be greatest in those whose mother took the drug during the first 16 weeks of pregnancy.

The average age at diagnosis is 19 years; most DES daughters are now between 30 and 60 years old, so the number of new cases of cervical and vaginal clear cell adenocarcinomas that are DES-related has been decreasing during the past two decades. However, this type of cancer has recently been found in a woman in her early 40s, and doctors still do not know exactly how long women remain at risk for DES-related cancers.

Although DES daughters have an increased risk of clear cell carcinomas, about 40 percent of women who have this cancer have no known exposure to DES or related medications. Some mothers of these patients may have taken DES but did not recall the name of the drug. It is clear, however, that DES exposure is not required for the development of clear cell carcinoma as cases of the disease were diagnosed before DES was invented.

Vaginal adenosis   In vaginal adenosis, some of the cells lining the vagina change. Normally, the vagina is lined by flat cells called squamous cells, but in about 40 percent of women who have already entered puberty, the vagina may contain one or more areas where the vagina is lined instead by cells that resemble those in glands of the lower uterus or upper uterine lining (endometrium). It occurs in nearly all women exposed to DES during fetal development. Although having adenosis increases the risk of development of clear cell carcinoma, this cancer is extremely rare. The risk that a woman who has adenosis but was not exposed to DES will have clear cell carcinoma is extremely low. Nonetheless, many doctors recommend especially careful screening of these women.

Human papillomavirus (HPV) infection   A group of more than 70 types of viruses that cause warts in different parts of the body. Some types cause common warts on the hands and feet; other types can infect the genital organs and the anal area. These HPV types are passed from one person to another during sexual contact. When HPVs infect the skin of the external genital organs and anal area, or internal genital organs such as the vagina or cervix, they often cause raised bumpy warts. These may be barely visible or may be several inches across. In infections of the vagina or cervix, a warty growth may not always be visible, but the virus can still cause abnormal cell growth that increases the risk of squamous cell cancer.

Certain types of sexual behavior increase a woman's risk of HPV infection, including beginning sex at an early age, having many sexual partners, having sex with a person who has had many partners, and having unprotected sex at any age.

HPV infection does not always produce warts or other symptoms, so a person may be infected with, and pass on, HPV without knowing it. Condoms cannot protect against infection with HPV, because the virus can be passed from person to person by skin-to-skin contact with any HPV-infected area of the body, such as skin of the genitals or the anal area. The absence of visible warts cannot be used to decide whether caution is warranted, since HPV can be passed to another person even when there are no visible warts or other symptoms. HPV can be present for years with no symptoms. Prevention of HPV infection reduces vaginal cancer risk, but since not all vaginal cancers are caused by HPV infections, this approach does not entirely prevent the disease.

Cervical cancer   Having CERVICAL CANCER or cervical precancerous conditions, such as cervical intraepithelial neoplasia or cervical DYSPLASIA, increases a woman's risk of vaginal squamous cell cancer. Cervical and vaginal cancer have similar risk factors (such as HPV infection). Some studies suggest that women whose cervical cancers were treated with radiation therapy have an increased risk of vaginal cancer, possibly because the radiation damaged the deoxyribonucleic acid of vaginal cells. However, other studies have not supported this conclusion and the issue remains unresolved.

Vaginal irritation Occasionally, loosening pelvic ligaments may cause the uterus to sag into the vagina or even extend outside the vagina. This condition (called uterine prolapse) can be treated by surgery or by use of a pessary (a device to keep the uterus in place). Some studies suggest that long-term irritation of the vagina by pessary use may slightly increase the risk of squamous cell vaginal cancer. However, this association is extremely rare, and no studies have conclusively proved that pessaries actually cause vaginal cancer.

Tobacco use Smoking may also increase a woman's risk of vaginal cancer, particularly for younger women, as it does for cervical cancer.

Symptoms

Up to 90 percent of women who have with invasive vaginal cancer have at least one symptom—most typically, abnormal vaginal bleeding (often after intercourse). Other signs and symptoms include an abnormal vaginal discharge, a mass that can be felt, pain during sex, painful urination, constipation, or continuous pelvic pain. Because a number of harmless conditions (such as infections) can produce similar symptoms, reporting any symptoms to a doctor promptly is important.

Diagnosis

If vaginal cancer is suspected, there are several tests that may be needed to reach a diagnosis, including colposcopy and biopsy.

In a colposcopy, an instrument with binocular magnifying lenses is used to scan the walls of the vagina as well as the cervix. If a suspicious area is found, the doctor performs a BIOPSY. In this procedure, the physician may numb the area with a local anesthetic and remove a small piece of tissue for lab analysis.

Staging

Evaluation of the spread of vaginal cancer involves a general physical exam, a PELVIC EXAMINATION, imaging tests (such as intravenous pyelogram, barium enema, and chest X-ray), and in some cases endoscopic tests such as cystoscopy and proctoscopy.

Vaginal cancer is staged by using a system created by the INTERNATIONAL FEDERATION OF GYNECOLOGY AND OBSTETRICS, called the FIGO system. An alternative system is recommended by the American Joint Committee on Cancer and the International Union against Cancer, called the tumor-node-metastasis (TNM) system. Nearly all gynecologic oncologists prefer the FIGO system, which is summarized as follows:

- *Stage 0:* In this stage, cancer cells are limited to the vaginal lining and have not spread to other layers of the vagina. Cancers of this stage cannot spread to other parts of the body. Stage 0 vaginal cancer is also called carcinoma in situ or vaginal intraepithelial neoplasia 3 (VAIN 3).

- *Stage I:* The cancer has invaded the vaginal lining but is confined to the vaginal mucosa.

- *Stage II:* The cancer has spread to the connective tissues beside the vagina but has not spread to the wall of the pelvis or to other organs.

- *Stage III:* Cancer extends to the wall of the pelvis and/ or has spread to a lymph node on the same side as the tumor.

- *Stage IV:* Cancer has invaded the bladder or rectum and/or spread beyond the pelvic region.

- *Stage IVA:* Cancer has spread to neighboring organs beside the vagina (such as the bladder or rectum), and/or has spread beyond the pelvis, and/or has spread to lymph nodes on both sides of the pelvis.

- *Stage IVB:* Cancer has spread to distant organs such as the lungs.

- *Recurrent:* The cancer has returned despite treatment. Vaginal cancer usually recurs near the vagina but may also recur in distant locations.

Treatment

Treatments are available for all patients who have cancer of the vagina, including surgery, RADIATION THERAPY, and CHEMOTHERAPY. Surgery is the most common treatment of all stages of cancer of the vagina; it may involve laser surgery or wide local excision.

Surgery In laser surgery, which is most useful for precancerous conditions, a narrow beam of light is used to kill cancer cells. Wide local excision is a procedure designed to remove the cancerous cells and some of the tissue around them. A patient may need to have skin grafts to repair the vagina after the cancer has been removed.

A VAGINECTOMY, in which the vagina is removed, may be performed if the cancer is not advanced. When the cancer has spread outside the vagina, vaginectomy may be combined with surgery to remove the uterus, ovaries, and fallopian tubes (radical HYSTERECTOMY). During these operations, lymph nodes in the pelvis may also be removed (lymph node dissection).

If the cancer has spread outside the vagina and the other female organs, the doctor also may remove the lower colon, rectum, or bladder (depending on where the cancer has spread) along with the cervix, uterus, and vagina (exenteration). A patient may need skin grafts and plastic surgery to create an artificial vagina after these operations.

If the cancer has recurred and spread beyond the reproductive organs, a surgeon may remove the cervix, uterus, lower colon, rectum, or bladder, depending on where the cancer has spread.

However, surgery is not the mainstay of treatment for this type of cancer. It is primarily performed only for small tumors that are confined to the vaginal mucosa only. The standard treatment for vaginal cancer is radiation.

Radiation therapy and chemotherapy Radiation treatments may be used alone or after surgery. Chemotherapy may be used after surgery, either as an intravenous treatment or as a topical medication inserted directly into the vagina itself (intravaginal chemotherapy).

Prevention

The best way to reduce the risk of vaginal cancer is to avoid known risk factors whenever possible, including infection with HPV and smoking. But since the disease can occur in women who have no known risk factors, there is no apparent way to prevent this disease completely.

Experts believe most vaginal squamous cell cancers develop from precancerous changes that may be present for years before a true cancer forms. Finding these precancers with an annual regular PAP TEST can prevent the lesions from evolving into a true cancer.

The American Cancer Society recommends that all women begin cervical cancer screening about three years after they begin having vaginal intercourse—but no later than age 21. Screening with the regular Pap test should be done every year or every two years using the newer liquid-based Pap test.

Beginning at age 30, women who have had three consecutive normal Pap test results may be screened every two to three years with either the conventional (regular) or the liquid-based Pap test. However, women who have certain risk factors such as DES exposure before birth, human immunodeficiency virus (HIV) infection, or a weakened immune system as a result of organ transplantation, chemotherapy or long-term steroid use should continue to be screened annually.

Another reasonable option for women older than age 30 is to be screened every three years (but not more frequently) with either the conventional or the liquid-based Pap test, plus the HPV DNA test.

Women 70 years of age or older who have had three or more consecutive normal Pap test results and no abnormal Pap test results in the last 10 years may choose to stop having cervical cancer screenings. Women who have a history of cervical cancer, DES exposure before birth, HIV infection, or a weakened immune system should continue to have screening as long as they are in good health.

Women who have had a total HYSTERECTOMY (removal of the uterus and cervix) may choose to stop having Pap smears unless the surgery was a treatment for cancer or precancer. Women who have had a hysterectomy without removal of the cervix should continue to follow the guidelines.

In the Future

Researchers are currently studying the use of photodynamic therapy in the treatment of vaginal cancer. In this procedure, a chemical that makes cancer cells very sensitive to certain types of colors of light is injected. A light of this color is then focused on an area of the vagina where the cells exist, killing many of them. In preliminary studies, this approach appears promising as a treatment for VAIN and early vaginal cancers.

vaginal hysterectomy   See HYSTERECTOMY.

vaginal intraepithelial neoplasia (VAIN)   Precancerous changes that appear in the vagina as a precursor to vaginal squamous cell carcinoma. Many women who have VAIN may also have a similar condition involving their cervix called cervical intraepithelial neoplasia (CIN). If CIN is found by a PAP TEST, a colposcopy is used to examine the cervix, the vagina, and at times, the vulva thoroughly.

Diagnosis

The exact location of VAIN within the vagina is determined by viewing the vaginal lining with a colposcope, an instrument that has binocular magnifying lenses. A biopsy confirms the diagnosis.

Treatment

Because low-grade VAIN often disappears without treatment, some doctors treat only intermediate-grade or high-grade VAIN. They recommend periodic Pap tests (and colposcopy as needed) for low-grade VAIN and reserve treatment for cases that have persisted for some time. However, this approach is controversial. A wide local excision or partial VAGINECTOMY is rarely performed but may be needed to rule out an invasive cancer may be employed or after other treatments have failed.

These lesions can be treated in several ways, including LASER SURGERY, loop electroexcision procedure, or topical chemotherapy.

Laser surgery   In laser surgery, the colposcopist focuses a beam of high-energy light to vaporize the abnormal tissue. This is a very effective treatment, especially with large lesions, but the doctor must be sure that the largest lesion has been biopsied and that there is no concern about invasive cancer.

Loop electrosurgical excision procedure   A thin wire heated by electric current is used to remove vaginal lesions. This may be useful for treating small lesions or for ruling out the possibility of an invasive cancer.

Topical chemotherapy   Topical CHEMOTHERAPY, a chemotherapy drug called FLUOROURACIL (5-FU) is applied directly to the lining of the vagina. There are several disadvantages of topical chemotherapy: it must be repeated weekly for about 10 weeks or given nightly for one to two weeks, and it may cause severe vaginal and vulvar irritation. Also, it may be less effective than surgical removal or laser vaporization.

See also VAGINAL CANCER.

vaginal pelvic exam   See PELVIC EXAMINATION.

vaginectomy   A surgical procedure in which the vagina is removed. This procedure may be performed as a way of treating advanced VAGINAL CANCER. When cancer has spread outside the vagina, vaginectomy may be combined with surgery to remove the uterus, ovaries, and fallopian tubes (radical HYSTERECTOMY). During these operations, LYMPH NODES in the pelvis may also be removed (LYMPH NODE DISSECTION).

vesicant   An intravenous CHEMOTHERAPY drug capable of damaging tissue and causing pain and swelling if it leaks into the skin. Many chemotherapy drugs cause local tissue damage if they leak out of the vein. These include the following:

- Anthracyclines (daunorubicin, doxorubicin [ADRIAMYCIN], epirubicin, idarubicin)
- antibiotics (bleomycin, mitomycin, actinomycin)
- mustards (mustine)
- vinca alkaloids (vincristine, vinblastine, vindesine)
- others (etoposide, tenoposide, amsacrine, mitoxantrone)

vomiting   See NAUSEA.

vulvar cancer   A type of cancer that may appear on any part of the external reproductive system but most often affects the inner edges of the labia majora or the labia minora. (The vulva is the outer part of the female genitalia, including the labia and clitoris.) Less often, cancer occurs on the clitoris or in Bartholin's glands (the small mucus-producing glands on each side of the vaginal opening).

Vulvar cancer accounts for about 4 percent of cancers of the female reproductive organs, and less than 1 percent of all cancers in women; it occurs most often in women older than age 60; 3,970 cancers of the vulva are diagnosed in the United States each year, with about 850 deaths. Most women who have vulvar cancer are older than age 50, but this type of malignancy is becoming more common in women younger than age 40.

When vulvar cancer is detected early, it is highly curable; the overall five-year survival rate when the lymph nodes are not involved is 90 percent. In the United States, half of all vulvar cancers are found when they are very small (less than two centimeters). However, the rate drops to between 30 and 55 percent if cancer has spread to the lymph nodes. Within this range, the chance of survival is influenced by the number of involved lymph nodes; women who have many involved lymph nodes have a less favorable prognosis.

Types of Vulvar Cancer

Squamous cell carcinoma   More than 90 percent of cancers of the vulva are squamous cell carcinomas: cancers that begin in squamous cells, the main cell type of the skin. This type of cancer usually forms over many years and is usually preceded by precancerous tissue changes called DYSPLASIA or VULVAR INTRAEPITHELIAL NEOPLASIA (VIN). *Intraepithelial* means that the precancerous cells are confined to the epithelium (the surface layer of the vulvar skin). VIN is often divided into three categories—VIN1, VIN2, and VIN3; as the numbers increase, the closer to true cancer the condition becomes. Not all women who have VIN have vulvar cancer, but since it is not possible to predict which women will have a malignancy, treatment of women who have VIN is very important.

A slow-growing subtype of squamous cell carcinoma, called verrucous carcinoma, resembles a large wart (in fact, a biopsy is required to distinguish them). It tends to have a good prognosis.

Melanoma   The second most common type of vulvar cancer (about 4 percent) is melanoma, which develops from the pigment-producing cells that determine the skin's color. Between 5 and 8 percent of melanomas in women occur on the vulva (usually on the labia minora and clitoris).

Adenocarcinoma   A small percentage of vulvar cancers develop from Bartholin's glands; they are called ADENOCARCINOMAS. Bartholin's glands, found at the opening of the vagina, produce a mucuslike lubricating fluid. Although most Bartholin's gland cancers are adenocarcinomas, some (particularly those that develop from the ducts of the gland) may be either transitional cell carcinomas or squamous cell carcinomas. Adenocarcinomas can also form in the sweat glands of the vulvar skin, although quite rarely.

Paget's disease of the vulva is a condition in which adenocarcinoma cells are found in the vulvar skin. Between 20 and 25 percent of vulvar Paget's disease patients also have an invasive adenocarcinoma of a Bartholin's gland or sweat gland. In the remaining 75 to 80 percent, the malignant cells are found only in the skin's top layer and do not involve the tissues below that layer. Since a tumor in the Bartholin's gland is easily mistaken for a cyst, delay in obtaining an accurate diagnosis is common.

Sarcoma   Less than 2 percent of vulvar cancers are SARCOMAS—tumors of the connective tissues below the skin that tend to grow rapidly. Unlike other cancers of the vulva, vulvar sarcomas can occur at any age, including in childhood.

Basal cell carcinoma   Basal cell carcinoma, the most common cancer of sun-exposed areas of the skin, occurs very rarely on the vulva.

Symptoms

Symptoms of vulvar cancer include itching in the vulvar area, burning pain or discomfort, a sore on the vulva, or changes in skin color. Squamous cell vulvar cancer may appear as a raised red, pink, or white nodule, with itching, pain, bleeding, vaginal discharge, and painful urination. Malignant melanoma of the vulva usually appears as a pigmented, ulcerated growth. Other types of vulvar cancer may appear as a distinct mass of tissue, sore and scaly areas, or cauliflowerlike growths that resemble warts.

Risk Factors

Experts do not know a great deal about the risk factors in vulvar cancer, although sexually transmitted diseases are believed to play a part in many cases.

Human papillomavirus (HPV)   HPV, which causes genital warts, is an important factor in most CERVICAL CANCER and may play a role in vulvar cancer as well.

Other gynecologic cancers   A history of other reproductive cancers places a woman at increased risk for vulvar cancer. In fact, nearly one-third of all women diagnosed with vulvar cancer had in situ or squamous cancer of the cervix at least five years before.

Vulvar irritation   Chronic vulvar irritation, including a history of inflammation, itching, burning, shrinkage, and thickening of vulvar tissues, increases the risk of vulvar cancer.

Diabetes   A few studies have suggested that diabetes is linked with an increased risk of vulvar cancer.

Smoking   Smoking cigarettes is a risk factor for this disease.

Caffeine   Drinking more than two cups of coffee a day has been linked to a development of this type of cancer.

Advanced age   Women older than age 70 are at increased risk of development of this type of cancer.

Careers   Women who work as maids or in laundries, dry cleaning, or other garment services appear to have a higher risk for vulvar cancer.

Obesity   Some experts believe that obese women who have extra moisture and warmth in the genital area are predisposed to vulvar cancer.

Diagnosis

If vulvar cancer is suspected, a doctor may first look at the vulva and feel for any lumps. This examination may be followed by a biopsy in which a doctor numbs the area and then removes a small piece of vulvar tissue for lab analysis. If local anesthesia is used, a woman may feel some pressure during the biopsy but usually no pain. This test is often done in a doctor's office.

Treatment

Treatment for vulvar cancer depends on its stage and the patient's general health. The primary treatment is surgery to remove the affected area. A wide local excision is a surgical procedure designed

to remove the cancer and some of the normal tissue around it; a radical local excision takes out the cancer and a larger portion of normal tissue. Lymph nodes may also be removed.

Alternatively, the surgeon may use a laser to burn off a minimal amount of tissue or a scalpel to remove more of the tissue, depending on the severity of the cancer. Surgery to remove all or part of the vulva is called a VULVECTOMY. A skinning vulvectomy removes only the skin of the vulva that contains the cancer; a partial vulvectomy removes a portion of the vulva, and a simple vulvectomy removes the entire vulva, but no lymph nodes. A vulvectomy may require skin grafts from other areas of the body to cover the wound.

If the cancer has spread outside the vulva and the other reproductive organs, the doctor may also remove the lower colon, rectum, or bladder, depending on where the cancer has spread, along with the cervix, uterus, and vagina.

Surgery may be followed by chemotherapy and radiation therapy to kill additional cancer cells; sometimes, radiation therapy is administered before surgery to shrink the tumor before operating.

Prevention

Regular examinations are necessary to detect precancerous conditions that can be treated before the cancer becomes invasive. Since some vulvar cancer is a type of skin cancer, the American Cancer Society also recommends self-examination of the vulva with a mirror.

vulvar intraepithelial neoplasia (VIN)   This benign condition of the vulva can sometimes be a precancerous condition. Not all women who have VIN will have VULVAR CANCER, but since it is not possible to predict which women will have a malignancy, treatment of women who have VIN is very important. Like cervical intraepithelial neoplasia, VIN is considered to be a CARCINOMA IN SITU (precancer); the term *intraepithelial* indicates that the precancerous cells are confined to the epithelium (the surface layer of the vulvar skin).

Risk Factors

Experts suspect that herpes simplex virus type II and the HUMAN PAPILLOMAVIRUS (HPV) may trigger the cellular changes that lead to cancer. When a woman's immune system breaks down, she is more likely to be susceptible to the malignant effects of viral infections.

Diagnosis

A routine PELVIC EXAMINATION can identify VIN. If a doctor notes abnormal areas, of the vulva a biopsy with local anesthesia to remove suspect tissue can be done. VIN is often divided into three categories—VIN1, VIN2, and VIN3; as the numbers increase, the closer to true cancer the condition becomes.

Treatment

The type of treatment for this precancerous condition depends on the extent and location of the abnormal tissue.

Minor VIN If the abnormal tissue is contained in one area, surgical removal of the tissue is sufficient. Topical CHEMOTHERAPY with 5-FLUOROURACIL is no longer used because it creates large, painful sores. Laser surgery with general anesthesia requires only a short hospital stay and has high cure rates; the pain is most severe four to five days after surgery. For the first two years after surgery, patients should have a colposcopy and PAP TEST every three to four months.

Extensive VIN For VIN that involves several areas of the vulva, a skinning VULVECTOMY is usually preferred because it offers high cure rates and a normal appearance after surgery. In this procedure, the doctor removes the vulvar skin and replaces it with a skin graft, saving the clitoris. Alternatively, a laser vulvectomy can be used, to preclude the need for skin grafts; it can be done on an outpatient basis. The cure rate and appearance are similar to those produced by a skinning vulvectomy, with fewer problems after surgery.

Interferon is being used as an experimental treatment for VIN, especially in cases associated with HPV infection.

vulvar self-examination A woman should examine her own vulva once a month, to better identify changes or warning signs. The vulva is the external portion of the female reproductive organs that surrounds the vaginal opening. It includes the vestibule, the hymen, the urethral opening, the vaginal lips (labia minora and majora) and the clitoris, the mons pubis and the perineum. When performing a self-exam, the woman should identify the color of the vulvar tissue, noting whether the area is a healthy pink color or if the skin is becoming white or reddened. As each section is examined, the woman should watch for skin texture, noting sores, splitting skin, lumps, CYSTS, or scaly tissue. Any areas of special sensitivity should be identified, along with any unusual discharge, odor, or bleeding.

A self-exam should be performed during or after a bath, using a mirror to make viewing easier. A flashlight also can help make some areas more readily visible.

See also VULVAR CANCER.

vulvectomy An operation to remove all or part of the vulva as treatment for VULVAR CANCER. A wide local excision is a surgical procedure designed to remove the cancer and some of the normal vulvar tissue around it; a radical local excision takes out the cancer and a larger portion of normal tissue. Lymph nodes also may be removed. A skinning vulvectomy takes out only the skin of the vulva that contains the cancer, a partial vulvectomy takes out a portion of the vulva, and a simple vulvectomy removes the entire vulva. A vulvectomy may require skin grafts from other areas of the body to cover the wound.

Alternatively, the surgeon may use a laser to burn off a minimal amount of tissue or a scalpel to remove more of the tissue, depending on the severity of the cancer.

If the cancer has spread outside the vulva and the other reproductive organs, the doctor also may remove the lower colon, rectum, or bladder, depending on where the cancer has spread, along with the cervix, uterus, and vagina.

warning signs in reproductive cancer Although some REPRODUCTIVE CANCERS occur without any warning signs, there are a number of symptoms that may indicate the presence of cancer.

Bleeding

Bleeding is the number one symptom for many types of reproductive cancers in women. Women in their childbearing years, and particularly in the years before menopause, sometimes experience bleeding between menstrual periods. Women may experience bleeding after menopause as well. These incidents can happen as a result of minor trauma, such as sexual intercourse or douching, but if a woman has more than two or three such cycles it can be a sign of cancer and should be reported to a doctor. UTERINE CANCER is the most common of all gynecologic cancers, but fortunately most uterine cancers have an obvious warning sign: abnormal bleeding. ENDOMETRIAL HYPERPLASIA, which can be a precursor to uterine cancer, also causes abnormal bleeding. CERVICAL CANCER, VAGINAL CANCER, and (more rarely) OVARIAN CANCER can also have bleeding as a symptom. Cancer of the fallopian tubes is rare; bleeding is one of the main symptoms of this malignancy as well.

Occasionally, endometrial hyperplasia or uterine cancer can cause extraheavy menstrual periods. Any sudden change in periods that continues for more than one or two cycles should be reported. Although not usually a sign of cancer, sudden heavy bleeding that requires a change of sanitary protection more than once per hour, that happens more than once, or that lasts more than 24 hours should be reported.

Noncancerous causes of bleeding include fibroid tumors, polyps, inflammation of the cervix, thyroid problems, bleeding disorders, and the use of hormones such as birth controll pills.

Pelvic Pain

Pelvic pain is defined as abdominal pain below the level of the naval. Because the female reproductive system is fairly crowded in the pelvic area, tumors can press on other structures and cause pain that occurs during certain movements or during sexual intercourse. Persistent pelvic pain of unknown cause, including pain with intercourse, should always be reported to a doctor. (Cramps associated with menstrual periods are not a warning sign of cancer.)

Noncancerous causes of pelvic pain include ovulation, benign cysts or tumors, pelvic inflammatory disease, endometriosis, diverticulitis, ulcerative colitis, and appendicitis.

Gastrointestinal Disturbances

Tumors or swelling pressing on the digestive system can cause symptoms such as constipation, diarrhea, nausea, indigestion, gas, or a constant feeling of fullness, regardless of the last meal. Although, most sources of digestive discomfort occur within that system (intestines, colon, and so on), any of the symptoms described that lasts for more than two or three weeks should be reported to a doctor.

Urinary Problems

Because of the proximity of the female reproductive system to the bladder and urethra, tumors or swelling can cause symptoms similar to those of urinary tract infections, including burning or pain with urination, urgency, difficulty in urinating, and bladder spasms.

Abdominal Swelling

One of the primary symptoms of ovarian cancer is abdominal bloating or swelling. Sometimes this can be part of the normal premenstrual period, but if the symptom persists, it should be reported to a doctor.

Vulvar or Vaginal Changes

Color changes or lumps, bumps, sores, or thickening in the vulva or vagina should be reported to a doctor. Vulvar or vaginal itching, burning, bleeding, or unusual discharge could also be a sign of cancer or precancerous changes. Round bumps on the vulva, vagina, or cervix are most often benign cysts, but a doctor should check them to be sure.

Low Back Pain

Low back pain can sometimes signal ovarian or uterine cancer. There are many noncancerous conditions that cause low back pain.

warts, genital   See HUMAN PAPILLOMAVIRUS.

wine and cancer   There are many biologically active plant-based chemicals in wine. Some scientists believe that particular compounds called polyphenols found in red wine (such as catechins and resveratrol) may have antioxidant or anticancer properties.

Polyphenols are antioxidant compounds found in the skin and seeds of grapes, which are dissolved by alcohol produced by the fermentation process. Red wine contains more polyphenols than white wine because when white wine is made, the skins are removed after the grapes are crushed. The phenols in red wine include catechin, gallic acid, and epicatechin.

Polyphenols have been found to have ANTIOXIDANT properties; that means they can protect cells from damage caused by molecules known as FREE RADICALS. These free radicals can damage important parts of cells (including proteins, membranes, and DNA), and that damage may lead to cancer. Research on the antioxidants found in red wine has shown that they may help inhibit the development of certain cancers.

Resveratrol is a type of polyphenol that is produced as part of a plant's defense system in response to an invading fungus, stress, injury, infection, or ultraviolet irradiation. Red wine contains high levels of the antioxidant resveratrol, as do grapes, raspberries, peanuts, and other plants. Resveratrol has been shown to reduce tumor incidence in animals by affecting one or more stages of cancer development and has been shown to inhibit growth of many types of cancer cells in culture. It also appears to reduce inflammation and activation of a protein produced by the body's immune system when it is under attack. This protein affects cancer cell growth and metastasis.

However, it is still too early to draw conclusions about the association between red wine consumption and cancer in women. Consumption of large amounts of alcoholic beverages may increase the risk of some cancers; there is growing evidence that the health benefits of red wine are related to its nonalcoholic components.

Women's Cancer Network   An interactive Web site dedicated to informing women around the world about REPRODUCTIVE CANCERS and to enable them to be their own health advocates. The network's goal is to help women who have cancer, and their family, to understand more about the disease, learn about treatment options, and gain access to new or experimental therapies. The network was established by the GYNECOLOGIC CANCER FOUNDATION and CANCERSOURCE with an unrestricted educational grant provided by Bristol-Myers Squibb Oncology. For contact information, see Appendix I.

yolk sac tumor This second most common malignant ovarian GERM CELL TUMOR occurs in childhood, adolescence, and in women younger than age 30). The growth can be either a pure germ cell tumor or a component of a mixed germ cell tumor, almost always a unilateral solid or solid and cystic tumor. This highly malignant tumor is resistant to radiation therapy but responds to combination CHEMOTHERAPY.

APPENDIXES

APPENDIX I
HELPFUL ORGANIZATIONS

ADVOCACY

Gynecologic Cancer Foundation
401 North Michigan Avenue
Chicago, IL 60611
(312) 644-6610
http://www.wcn.org

A nonprofit organization established by the Society of Gynecologic Oncologists to raise funds to support philanthropic programs to benefit women who have or who are at risk for developing a gynecologic cancer.

National Patient Advocate Foundation
753 Thimble Shoals Boulevard
Suite A
Newport News, VA 23606
(757) 873-0438; (800)532-5274
http://www.npaf.org

A national health care reform network that supports legislation to enable cancer survivors to obtain insurance funding for medical care and participation in clinical trials. Services include referrals, information education, advocacy, and health insurance assistance.

AFRICAN-AMERICAN ISSUES

See RACIAL ISSUES IN CANCER.

AIRLINE TRANSPORTATION (FREE)

Air Care Alliance
1515 East 71st Street
Suite 312
Tulsa, OK 74136
(918) 745-0384
(888) 260-9707 (toll-free)
http://www.aircareall.org/

The Air Care Alliance (ACA) is a nationwide league of humanitarian flying organizations dedicated to community service. The ACA has member groups whose activities involve health care, patient transport, and related kinds of public benefit flying.

AIRLIFELINE
50 Fullerton Court
Suite 200
Sacramento, CA 95825
(916) 641-7800
(877) AIRLIFE (toll-free)
http://www.airlifeline.org

The organization provides transportation to and from medical destinations for patients in financial need to destinations within 1,000 air miles of any departure point in the United States.

Corporate Angel Network
Westchester County Airport, Building 1
White Plains, NY 10604
(914) 328-1313
(866) 328-1313 (toll-free)
http://www.corpangelnetwork.org

Corporate Angel Network finds free air transportation (on corporate planes) for cancer patients who need medical attention. Patients must be ambulatory.

National Patient Air Transport Hotline
P.O. Box 1940
Manassas, VA 22110-0804
(800) 296-1217
http://www.npath.org

National Patient Air Transport Hotline is a clearinghouse for patients who cannot afford travel for medical care.

ALASKA-NATIVE ISSUES

See RACIAL ISSUES IN CANCER.

ALTERNATIVE HEALTH

Office of Cancer Complementary and Alternative Medicine
National Cancer Institute, NIH
Executive Boulevard North
Suite 102
Bethesda, MD 20892
(800) 4CANCER
http://www.cancer.gov/cam

The Office of Cancer Complementary and Alternative Medicine (OCCAM) was established in 1998 to enhance the activities of the National Cancer Institute in the arena of complementary and alternative medicine. The OCCAM's goal is to increase the amount of high-quality cancer research and information about the use of complementary and alternative modalities.

APPEARANCE

Look Good . . . Feel Better
CTFA Foundation
1101 17th Street NW
Washington, DC 20036
(202) 331-1770
(800) 395-5665 (toll-free)

ASIAN ISSUES

See RACIAL ISSUES IN CANCER.

BONE MARROW TRANSPLANT

Blood & Marrow Transplant Information Network
2900 Skokie Valley Road
Suite B
Highland Park, IL 60035
(847) 433-3313

(888) 597-7674 (toll-free)
http://www.marrow.org

A nonprofit organization that provides publications and support services to bone marrow, peripheral blood stem cell, and cord blood transplant patients and survivors. Services include a quarterly patients' newsletter *(Blood & Marrow Transplant Newsletter),* a resource directory, a "patient-to-survivor" telephone link, and a 157-page book describing physical and emotional aspects of marrow and stem cell transplantation. A second book, *Mira's Month* ($5), helps prepare young children for their parent's transplant. Additional public resources are a directory of transplant centers, which includes information on types and number of transplants performed and diseases treated, and an attorney list, to help resolve insurance problems.

Bone Marrow Foundation
70 East 55th Street, 20th Floor
New York, NY 10022
(212) 838-3029
(800) 365-1336 (toll-free)
http://www.bonemarrow.org

The foundation provides eligible transplant candidates with financial assistance to defray the cost of ancillary services needed to ensure proper care during the transplant procedure, as well as in pre- and post-transplant treatment phases.

Bone Marrow Transplant Family Support Network
P.O. Box 845
Avon, CT 06001
(800) 826-9376 (toll-free)

A national telephone support network for patients and their families. Services include referrals, bone marrow transplant information, counseling, children's services, and health insurance information. The network answers questions raised by the person calling and connects newly diagnosed patients with recovered bone marrow transplant (BMT) patients of the same age or who have the same diagnosis, stage of disease, and other common characteristics.

National Bone Marrow Transplant Link
20411 West 12 Mile Road
Suite 108

Southfield, MI 48076
(800) LINK-BMT (800-546-5268, toll free)
http://www.comnet.org

National Bone Marrow Transplant Link funds research and acts as a national clearinghouse for a variety of bone marrow transplant issues. Services include patient advocacy, referrals, and an excellent resource guide on bone marrow transplant (BMT).

National Marrow Donor Program
3001 Broadway Street NE
Suite 500
Minneapolis, MN 55413-1753
(800) MARROW2 (800-627-7692, toll free)
(888) 999-6743 (Office of Patient Advocacy)
http://www.marrow-donor.org

The National Marrow Donor Program maintains a registry of bone marrow donors, provides information about how to become a donor, and organizes donor recruitment drives.

BRCA1/BRCA2 ISSUES

See GENETICS.

CANCER

AMC Cancer Research Center–Cancer Information and Counseling Line
1600 Pierce Street
Denver, CO 80214
(303) 233-6501
(800) 525-3777 (toll free)
(800) 321-1557 (toll free)
http://www.amc.org

A nonprofit research institute dedicated to the prevention of cancer. Services include providing up-to-date facts about all aspects of cancer as well as the latest information on cancer prevention, detection, diagnosis, treatment, and rehabilitation, including the Physicians' Data Query (PDQ), a database of research studies and treatment protocols from the nation's cancer centers. Also provided is personal assistance from counselors trained and experienced in dealing with the fear, confusion, conflicts, and other problems often

associated with the disease. All staff members are paid professionals with degrees in counseling or related health areas. The service mails out thousands of free brochures and other literature every year and helps put callers in touch with cancer-related resources in their communities. In addition, the organization funds research.

American Cancer Society (ACS)
1599 Clifton Road, NE
Atlanta, GA 30329-4251
(800) 227-2345
http://www.cancer.org

Dedicated to eliminating cancer as a major health problem through research, education, and service, the American Cancer Society (ACS) is a nationwide, community-based organization with chartered divisions in every state plus Washington, D.C., and Puerto Rico. Services include a variety of programs, such as Reach to Recovery, Cansurmount, I Can Cope, Road to Recovery, Man to Man, International Association of Laryngectomees, Look Good . . . Feel Better, and Resources, Information, and Guidance (RIG). ACS also operates Hope Lodges (temporary housing) in selected areas.

American Joint Committee on Cancer
633 North Saint Clair
Chicago, IL 60611
(312) 202-5290

An organization established in 1959 to publish systems of classification of cancer, including staging and end results reporting, for doctors to use in selecting most effective treatment, determining prognosis, and evaluating cancer control measures. The organization includes six founding organizations, four sponsoring organizations, and seven liaison organizations. Membership is reserved for those organizations whose missions or goals are consistent with or complementary to those of the American Joint Committee on Cancer.

Association of Cancer Online Resources
173 Duane Street
Suite 3A
New York, NY 10013
(212) 226-5525
http://www.acor.org

The association provides access to numerous cancer-specific mailing lists to patients and their families. These currently include 99 electronic mailing lists and a variety of unique Web sites, specifically designed to be public online support groups and provide information and community to tens of thousands of patients, caregivers, or others looking for answers about cancer and related disorders.

Cancer Care
275 Seventh Avenue
New York, NY 10001
(212) 712-8080
(800) 813-HOPE (4673, toll free)
http://www.cancercare.org

A national nonprofit agency offering a range of free support services to cancer patients and their families. Services include professional individual and group counseling, bereavement counseling, on-line support and counseling, educational programs, workshops, teleconferences, financial assistance, and referrals. Services are offered at all stages of the disease, to patients and to families. Supplementary financial assistance is awarded for home care, transportation, and pain medication. The funds are limited to cancer treatment in the New York, New Jersey, and Connecticut region only. There are African-American and Hispanic Outreach programs, as well. Review the Web site for detailed program information and on-line services; Cancer Care has offices in New Jersey, Connecticut, and Long Island.

Cancer Hope Network
Two North Road
Chester, NJ 07930
(877) 467-3638 (877-HOPENET)
http://www.cancerhopenetwork.org

Cancer Hope Network is a nonprofit organization that provides free and confidential one-on-one support to cancer patients and their families. Services include volunteer training programs, peer support for individuals and families, and a toll-free information number. The network matches cancer patients and/or family members with trained volunteers who have themselves under-gone and recovered from a similar cancer experience. Through the matching process, Cancer Hope Network strives to provide support and hope.

Cancer Information and Counseling Line
1600 Pierce Street
Denver, CO 80214
(800) 525-3777
http://www.amc.org

A toll-free telephone service that is part of the psychosocial program of the AMC Cancer Research Center. Professional counselors provide up-to-date medical information, emotional support through short-term counseling, and resource referrals to callers nationwide between the hours of 8:30 a.m. and 5:00 p.m. MST. Individuals may also submit questions about cancer and request resources via e-mail.

Cancer Information Service
9000 Rockville Pike
Building 31, Room 10A16
Bethesda, MD 20892
(301) 402-5874
(800) 4-CANCER (9:00 a.m.–4:30 p.m. local time,
   Monday through Friday)
(800) 332-8615 (TTY)
http://www.icic.nci.nih.gov

The service is a nationwide network founded by the National Cancer Institute (NCI). Calls are routed to local Career Information Service (CIS) offices, where trained cancer information specialists answer virtually any question on cancer. More than 100 free pamphlets are offered. In addition to answering callers' questions, the CIS is committed to increasing the public's awareness through outreach. The CIS Outreach Coordinator is available to groups to help them set up their own education programs.

Cancer Net
31 Center Drive, MSC 2580
Building 31, Room 10A03
Bethesda, MD 20892-2580
(301) 435-3848
http://www.cancernet.nci.nih.gov

A Web site providing cancer information from the National Cancer Institute that offers a wide range of cancer information, including details on treatment options, clinical trials, reduction of cancer risk, and ways of coping with cancer. Resources on support groups, financial assistance, and educational materials are also available.

Cancer Research Institute
681 Fifth Avenue
New York, NY 10022-4209
(212) 688-7515
http://www.cancerresearch.org

A nonprofit organization that funds research projects and scientists across the country. Services include publication of The Cancer Research Institute Help Book and information on clinical trials using immunological treatments.

Cancer Survivors Network
American Cancer Society (ACS)
1599 Clifton Road, NE
Atlanta, GA 30329-4251
(877) 333-4673
http://www.cancer.org

Both a telephone and an Internet-based service for cancer survivors, families, caregivers, and friends. The telephone component gives survivors and families access to prerecorded discussions. The Web-based component offers live on-line chat sessions, virtual support groups, prerecorded talk shows, and personal stories. Cancer Survivors Network is supported by the American Cancer Society.

Cancervive
11636 Chayote Street
Suite 500
Los Angeles, CA 90049
(310) 203-9232
(800) 4-TO-CURE (toll free)
http://www.cancervive.org

Assists cancer survivors to face and overcome the challenges of "life after cancer." Services include support groups, educational materials, insurance information and assistance, and advocacy for cancer survivors.

Exceptional Cancer Patient (EcaP)
522 Jackson Park Drive
Meadville, PA 16335
(814) 337-8192
http://www.ecap-online.org

Exceptional Cancer Patient, Inc. (EcaP), offers programs and services to cancer patients, people who have terminal illness, and health professionals.

Information and Referral Network
http://www.ir-net.com/index.html

Information and Referral Network provides a place where people who need help can find information and referral services and other community resources. The network is a kind of "one-stop" shopping center for human services.

International Cancer Alliance for Research and Education
4853 Cordell Avenue
Suite 206
Bethesda, MD 20814
(800) ICA-RE61
(301) 654-7933
http://www.icare.org/frontpage.htm

A nonprofit organization that provides high-quality cancer information to patients and their doctors. The International Cancer Alliance for Research and Education (ICARE) has developed several unique patient-centered programs through an extensive process of collection, evaluation, and dissemination of information, putting the cancer patient in contact with top physicians and scientists around the world. This organization is operated by a network of people: scientists, clinicians, caring staff, and lay volunteers, many of whom are patients.

International Union against Cancer
3 rue du Conseil General
1205 Geneva
Switzerland
http://www.uicc.org

The objectives of the International Union against Cancer (IUCC) are to advance scientific and medical knowledge in research, diagnosis, treatment, and prevention of cancer and to promote all other aspects of the campaign against cancer throughout the world. It emphasizes professional and public education. IUCC is a nongovernmental, independent association of more than 290 member organizations in about 85 countries. Members include voluntary cancer leagues and societies, cancer research and/or treatment centers, and, in some countries, ministries of health.

SHARE (Self-Help for Women with Breast or Ovarian Cancer)
1501 Broadway
Suite 704A
New York, NY 10036
(212) 719-0364
(866)891-2392 (toll-free)
http://www.sharecancersupport.org

Support group offering programs led by cancer survivors who draw on their experiences to help individuals face breast or ovarian cancer.

CAREGIVERS

National Alliance for Caregiving
4720 Montgomery Lane, Fifth Floor
Bethesda, MD 20814
http://www.caregiving.org

Provides support, information, reviews of books and videos about caregiving issues, links to organizations that focus on different aspects of caregiving, and Tips for Family Caregivers.

National Family Caregivers Association (NFCA)
10400 Connecticut Avenue
Suite 500
Kensington, MD 20895-3944
(301) 942-6430
(800) 896-3650 (toll free)
http://www.nfcacares.org

National Family Caregivers Association provides educational and emotional support for family caregivers. Services include advocacy; and individual, family, group, peer, and bereavement counseling.

Well Spouse Foundation
P.O. Box 30093
Elkins Park, PA 19027
(800) 838-0879
http://www.wellspouse.org

A membership organization that provides emotional support and information to the "well spouse" or the caregiver of the chronically ill. Services include a newsletter, local support groups, round robin letter writing, an annual weekend conference, and bereavement counseling.

CERVICAL CANCER

National Breast and Cervical Cancer Early Detection Program
CDC/DCPC
4770 Buford Highway, NE
MS K64
Atlanta, GA 30341
(888) 842-6355
http://www.cdc.gov/cancer/nbccedp/index.htm

A government program that works in states, U.S. territories, and tribal organizations to ensure that women who have little or no insurance have access to lifesaving cancer screening, diagnostic, and treatment services. As of 2004, the program had provided four million breast and cervical cancer screening services to more than 1.75 million uninsured and underinsured women.

National Cervical Cancer Coalition
16501 Sherman Way
Suite #110
Van Nuys, CA 91406
(800) 685-5531 (toll free)
(818) 909-3849
http://www.nccc-online.org

A coalition of women, patients' family members, caregivers, women's groups, scientists, labs, corporations, hospitals, and organizations interested in educating the public about cervical cancer prevention, new screening and treatment options, screening and follow-up programs, human papilomavirus (HPV), and the Pap test. The National Cervical Cancer Coalition emphasizes outreach support to women and family members battling cancer.

CHEMOTHERAPY

CHEMOcare
231 North Avenue
Westfield, NJ 07090

(800) 552-4366 (toll free)
(908) 233-1103
http://www.chemocare.com

The program and Web site sponsored by the Scott Hamilton Cancer Alliance for Research Education and Survivorship (CARES) initiative are designed to provide the latest information about chemotherapy, management of side effects, and living well during treatment to patients and their families.

Chemotherapy Foundation
183 Madison Avenue
Suite 302
New York, NY 10016
(212) 213-9292
http://www.neoplastics.mssm.edu/
    sympbrochure.html

A public foundation established in 1968, dedicated to the control, cure, and prevention of cancer through innovative medical therapies including chemotherapy, chemoimmunotherapy, chemohormonal therapy, chemoprevention, and biotechnologies. The foundation is also dedicated to the education of physicians, patients, and the public through educational literature and sponsors selected basic and clinical research initiatives at six major New York City metropolitan medical centers.

CLINICAL TRIALS

Cancer Liaison Program (CLP)
Food and Drug Administration (FDA Room 9-
    49CFH-12)
5600 Fishers Lane
Rockville, MD 20857
(888) INFO-FDA (toll free)
http://www.fda.gov/oashi/cancer/cancer.html

As a division of the FDA, the Cancer Liaison Program works directly with cancer patients and advocacy programs to provide information on the FDA drug approval process, cancer clinical trials, and access to investigational therapies when entering into an existing clinical trial is not possible.

Coalition of National Cancer Cooperative Groups
1818 Market Street, #1100
Philadelphia, PA 19103

(877) 520-4457
http://www.ca-coalition.org

The Coalition of National Cancer Cooperative Groups, Inc., is the premier U.S. network of cancer clinical trials specialists. Services include a variety of programs and information for physicians, payers, patient advocate groups, and patients designed to improve the clinical trials process.

DEATH AND DYING

See also HOSPICE.

Partnership for Caring
1620 I Street, NW
Suite 202
Washington, DC 20006
(202) 296-8071
(800) 989-9455 (toll free)
http://www.partnershipforcaring.org

An advocacy and research organization that protects the rights of dying patients by providing information to help people prepare for end-of-life decisions. Services include referrals, guest speakers, counseling, legal assistance, patient advocacy, pain management, volunteer services, hospice care, and distribution of advance directives, including living wills, durable power of attorney, and explanatory guidelines appropriate to state of residence. The group also offers publications, videos, and audios related to advance care planning and end-of-life issues.

Widowed Persons Service
NY Service Program for Older People, Inc. (SPOP)
188 West 88th Street
New York, NY 10024
(212) 787-7120 ext 139
(212) 721-6279
http://www.spop.org

SPOP's Widowed Persons Service, cosponsored by the American Association of Retired Persons, serves widows, men, and women of all ages, offering peer support and information to the newly widowed.

ENDOMETRIAL CANCER

See UTERINE CANCER.

FATIGUE

CancerFatigue.org
http://www.cancerfatigue.org

Web site of the Oncology Nursing Society that explains why fatigue occurs and offers practical advice for coping with it.

FINANCIAL AID

Bone Marrow Foundation
70 East 55th Street, 20th Floor
New York, NY 10022
(212) 838-3029
(800) 365-1336 (toll free)
http://www.bonemarrow.org

Provides eligible transplant candidates with financial assistance limited to helping defray the cost of ancillary services needed to ensure proper care during the transplant procedure, as well as in the pre- and post-transplant treatment phases.

Cancer Fund of America
2901 Breezewood Lane
Knoxville, TN 37921-1009
(865) 938-5281
http://www.cfoa.org

Cancer Fund of America is dedicated to providing direct aid in the form of goods to financially indigent patients.

Corporate Angel Network
Westchester County Airport, Building 1
White Plains, NY 10604
(914) 328-1313
http://www.corpangelneetwork.org

Corporate Angel Network finds free air transportation (on corporate planes) for cancer patients who need medical attention. Patients must be ambulatory.

Ensure Health Connection
P.O. Box 29139
Shawnee, KS 66201
(800) 986-8501 (toll free)
http://www.ensure.com

The organization provides coupons and valuable information to people who are in need of the nutritional supplement Ensure. Ensure donates their product to food banks, where a person in need may be able to receive a free supply when available.

Hill-Burton Free Hospital Care
5600 Fishers Lane
Rockville, MD 20857
(800) 638-0742 (toll free)
(301) 443-5656
http://www.hrsa.gov/osp/dfcr/

The Hill-Burton program is run by the U.S. government to arrange for certain medical facilities or hospitals to provide free or low-cost care. For information, call the hotline or access the program through the Web site (click on "Obtaining Free Care").

Medicine Program
P.O. Box 520
Doniphan, AL 63935
(573) 996-7300
http://www.themedicineprogram.com

The program provides free prescription medicine to those who qualify; a $5.00 processing fee is required for each medication requested.

Mission of Hope Cancer Fund
802 First Street
Jackson, MI 49023
(517) 782-4643
(888) 544-6423 (toll free)
http://www.cancerfund.org

A nonprofit organization established by a cancer survivor to help cancer patients and their families who have specific financial needs. The goal is to help relieve some of the extra financial burdens of cancer patients and their families who are dealing with cancer treatment and recovery. Services include information, counseling, housing, financial assistance, and assistance for medications.

National Association of Hospital Hospitality
4915 Auburn Avenue
Bethesda, MD 20814

(800) 542-9730 (toll free)
http://www.nahhh.org

A nonprofit corporation that serves facilities that provide lodging and other supportive services to patients and their families when confronted with medical emergencies. Services include referrals and housing and lodging facilities.

National Breast and Cervical Cancer Early Detection Program

CDC/DCPC
4770 Buford Highway, NE
MS K64
Atlanta, GA 30341
(888) 842-6355
http://www.cdc.gov/cancer/nbccedp/index.htm

A U.S. government program that works in states, U.S. territories, and tribal organizations to ensure that women who have little or no insurance have access to lifesaving cancer screening, diagnostic, and treatment services. The program had provided breast and cervical cancer screening services to more than 1.5 million uninsured and underinsured women.

National Patient Air Transport Hotline

P.O. Box 1940
Manassas, VA 22110-0804
(800) 296-1217 (toll free)
http://www.npath.org

A clearinghouse for patients who cannot afford travel for medical care.

Patient Advocate Foundation (PAF)

753 Thimble Shoals Boulevard
Suite B
Newport News, VA 23606
(757) 873-6668
(800) 532-5274 (toll free)
http://www.patientadvocate.org

Patient Advocate Foundation helps cancer patients deal with insurance coverage, payment for managed care treatment, and understanding of managed care. Services include specializing in mediation, negotiation, and education on behalf of patients experiencing the following issues: preauthorization, coding and billing, insurance appeal process, expedited appeal process, debt crisis, job retention, access to pharmaceutical agents, access to chemotherapy, access to medical devices, access to surgical procedures, and expedited applications for Social Security, Medicare, Medicaid, and other agencies.

GENETICS

FORCE: Facing Our Risk of Cancer Empowered

934 North University Drive, PMB #213
Coral Springs, FL 33071
(954) 255-8732
http://www.facingourrisk.org

Nonprofit organization for women at high risk of reproductive cancers as a result of family history and genetic status, and for members of families who may have a BRCA mutation.

National Society of Genetic Counselors

233 Canterbury Drive
Wallingford, PA 19086-6617
(610) 872-7608
http://www.nsgc.org/

The National Society of Genetic Counselors promotes the genetic counseling profession as a recognized and integral part of health care delivery, education, research, and public policy. Services include referrals, educational programs, and genetic screening.

GOVERNMENT AGENCIES

Cancer Liaison Program (CLP)

Food and Drug Administration (FDA Room 9-49CFH-12)
5600 Fishers Lane
Rockville, MD 20857
(888) INFO-FDA (toll free)
http://www.fda.gov

As a division of the FDA, the Cancer Liaison Program works directly with cancer patients and advocacy programs to provide information on the FDA drug approval process, cancer clinical trials, and access to investigational therapies when entry into an existing clinical trial is not possible.

Centers for Disease Control and Prevention, Division of Cancer Prevention and Control (DCPC)

4770 Buford Highway, NE
MS K-64
Atlanta, GA 30341-3717
(770) 488-4751
(800) 311-3435 (toll free)
http://www.cdc.gov/cancer

The Division of Cancer Prevention and Control of the Centers for Disease Control serves as a leader for nationwide cancer prevention and control and as a partner with state health agencies and other key groups.

National Cancer Institute

Building 31, Room 10A03
31 Center Drive, MSC 2580
Bethesda, MD 20892-2580
(301) 435-3848
(800) 422-6237 (toll free)
http://www.cancer.gov

The National Cancer Institute (NCI) is the U.S. federal government's principal agency for cancer research. Services include a comprehensive database, called the Physician's Data Query (PDQ), which contains peer-reviewed summaries and the most current information on cancer treatment, screening, prevention, genetics, and supportive care. NCI also maintains a registry of cancer clinical trials being conducted worldwide and directories of physicians, professionals who provide genetic services, and organizations that provide care to people with cancer.

National Center for Complementary and Alternative Medicine

NCCAM Clearinghouse
P.O. Box 7923
Gaithersburg, MD 20893-7923
(301) 519-3153
(866) 464-3615 (TTY)
(888) 644-6226 (toll free)
http://www.nccam.nih.gov

The National Center for Complementary and Alternative Medicine (NCCAM) supports rigorous research on complementary and alternative medicine (CAM), trains researchers in CAM, and disseminates information to the public and professionals on which CAM modalities work, which do not, and why. Services include a toll-free telephone line, information packages, fact sheets, a newsletter, referrals, meetings and workshops, and treatment information.

Social Security Administration (SSA)

Office of Public Inquiries
6401 Security Boulevard, Room 4-C-5 Annex
Baltimore, MD 21235
(800) 772-1213 (toll free)
http://www.ssa.gov

The Social Security Administration is the U.S. government agency that runs the Social Security program. It also provides information about retirement and disability benefits, Supplemental Security Income (SSI), and Medicare (the government program that pays for the medical care of the elderly). Services include a toll-free number, referrals, financial assistance, and education.

GYNECOLOGIC CANCERS

Gynecologic Cancer Foundation

401 North Michigan Avenue
Chicago, IL 60611
(312) 644-6610
http://www.wcn.org/gcf

The foundation was established by the Society of Gynecologic Oncologists (SGO) in 1991 as a not-for-profit charitable organization to raise funds to support philanthropic programs to benefit women who have, or who are at risk for development of, a gynecologic cancer.

HISPANIC ISSUES

See RACIAL ISSUES IN CANCER.

HOME CARE

See also HOSPICE.

Visiting Nurse Association of America (VNAA)

11 Beacon Street
Suite 910

Boston, MA 02108
(617) 523-4042
(800) 426-2547 (toll free)

Visiting Nurses Association of America provides information on all aspects of home health care, including general nursing; physical, occupational, and speech therapy; medical social service; home health aide and homemaker services; nutritional counseling; and hospice care. Callers are referred to a local visiting nurse service. Services include educational information, referrals, home care, and hospice care.

HOSPICE

Hospice Education Institute
3 Unity Square
P.O. Box 98
Machiasport, ME 04655-0098
(207) 255-8800
http://www.hospiceworld.org

An independent, nonprofit organization serving the public and health care professionals with information and education about the many facets of caring for the dying and the bereaved. Services include a toll-free information and referral service (HospiceLink), regional seminars, professional education, advice, and assistance.

HospiceLink
Hospice Education Institute
190 Westbrook Road
Essex, CT 06426
(800) 331-1620 (toll free)
(203) 767-1620

A service offered by the Hospice Education Institute that maintains a computerized directory of all hospice and palliative care programs in the United States. The toll-free telephone number provides referrals to hospice and palliative care programs and general information about the principles and practices of good hospice and palliative care.

National Hospice and Palliative Care Organization
1700 Diagonal Road
Suite 625
Alexandria, VA 22314

(703) 837-1500
http://www.nhpco.org

The National Hospice and Palliative Care Organization provides information and referrals to nationwide hospice programs via a toll-free phone number. Services include referrals, patient advocacy, research, public engagement, and professional education.

National Hospice Foundation
1700 Diagonal Road
Suite 625
Alexandria, VA 22314
(703) 516-4928
http://www.nhpco.org

A charitable organization created in 1992 to broaden understanding of hospice through research and education, expanding America's vision for end-of-life care. In doing so, it engages and informs the public about the high-quality end-of-life care that hospice provides.

HOUSING (TEMPORARY)

American Cancer Society (ACS)
1599 Clifton Road, NE
Atlanta, GA 30329-4251
(800) 227-2345
http://www.cancer.org

The American Cancer Society operates Hope Lodges (temporary housing) in selected areas.

National Association of Hospital Hospitality Houses, Inc.
P.O. Box 18087
Asheville, NC 28814-0087
(828) 253-1188
(800) 542-9730 (toll free)

A nonprofit corporation serving facilities that provide lodging and other supportive services to patients and their families when confronted with medical emergencies.

INFERTILITY

Fertile Hope
P.O. Box 624
New York, NY 10014

(888) 994-HOPE
http://www.fertilehope.org

Fertile Hope is a national nonprofit organization that addresses the reproductive needs of cancer patients and survivors. Services include raising of awareness, education, financial assistance, research, and support.

LATINA ISSUES

See RACIAL ISSUES IN CANCER.

LEGAL ISSUES

Cancer Legal Resource Center
919 South Albany Street
Los Angeles, CA 90019-0015
(213) 736-1455
http://www.wlcdr.org/clrc.html

The center provides information for cancer patients about their legal rights and the legal issues they face while battling cancer. It has access to a panel of volunteer attorneys and other professionals who are willing to assist people with cancer.

LESBIAN/GAY GROUPS

Mary-Helen Mautner Project for Lesbians with Cancer
1707 I Street, NW
Washington, DC 20036
(202) 332-5536
http://www.mautnerproject.org

To provide direct services, education, information, and advocacy.

NATIVE AMERICAN ISSUES

See RACIAL ISSUES IN CANCER.

OVARIAN CANCER

FORCE: Facing Our Risk of Cancer Empowered
934 North University Drive, PMB #213
Coral Springs, FL 33071
(954) 255-8732
http://www.facingourrisk.org

A nonprofit organization for women at high risk of having ovarian or breast cancer as a result of their family history and genetic status, and for members of families who may have a BRCA mutation.

Gilda Radner Familial Ovarian Cancer Registry
Roswell Park Cancer Institute
Elm and Carlton Streets
Buffalo, NY 14263-0001
(716) 845-4503
http://www.ovariancancer.com/contact.asp

An international registry of families in whom two or more relatives have ovarian cancer. In addition to ovarian cancer research, the registry offers a HELPLINE, education, and peer support for women at high risk of ovarian cancer.

Lynne Cohen Foundation for Ovarian Cancer Research
P.O. Box 7128
Santa Monica, CA 90406-7128
(877) OVARY-11
http://www.lynnecohenfoundation.org

An organization that supports groundbreaking research to improve the survival rate of women who have ovarian cancer.

National Ovarian Cancer Association
620 University Avenue
Toronto, M5G 2L7
Canada
(416) 971-9800
(877) 413-7970
http://www.ovariancanada.org

A Canadian organization dedicated to overcoming ovarian cancer, supporting women living with the disease, building awareness in the general public, encouraging research into early detection, improved treatment, and, ultimately, a cure.

National Ovarian Cancer Coalition
500 NE Spanish River Boulevard
Suite 14
Boca Raton, FL 33431
(561) 393-0005
(888)-OVARIAN
http://www.ovarian.org/pages.asp?page=
   CONTACT%20NOCC

The first comprehensive U.S. organization focused on providing awareness of and education about ovarian cancer.

Ovarian Cancer Canada

600 West 10th Avenue, Second Floor
Vancouver, BC V5Z 4E6
Canada
(604) 877-6187
(800) 749-9310
http://www.ovariancancercanada.ca

A Canadian group dedicated to education, information, support, and fund raising.

Ovarian Cancer Research Fund

One Pennsylvania Plaza
Suite 1610
New York, NY 10119
(800) 873-9569
http://www.ocrf.org

A fund dedicated to creating early diagnostic treatment programs and research into finding a cure for ovarian cancer.

PAIN

American Chronic Pain Association (ACPA)

P.O. Box 850
Rocklin, CA 95677
(800) 533-3231 (toll free)
http://www.theacpa.org

A self-help organization that offers educational material and peer support to help people combat chronic pain. Services include referrals to pain control facilities, publications on managing daily pain, and support groups.

American Pain Society

4700 West Lake Avenue
Glenview, IL 60025
(847) 375-4715
http://www.ampainsoc.org

A multidisciplinary educational and scientific organization dedicated to serving people in pain. Members research and treat pain and act as advocates for people who have pain. Services include the Pain Facilities Directory, which lists information on more than 500 specialized pain treatment centers across the United States (usually a part or a program of a hospital, clinic, or medical care complex), counseling for pain, referrals, and education programs.

National Chronic Pain Outreach Association

P.O. Box 274
Millboro, VA 24460
(540) 862-9437
http://www.chronicpain.org

A nonprofit organization whose purpose is to lessen the suffering of people who have chronic pain by educating pain sufferers, health care professionals, and the public about chronic pain and its management.

PROFESSIONAL GROUPS

American Association for Cancer Education (AACE)

9500 Euclid Avenue (R30)
Cleveland, OH 44195
(216) 444-9827
http://www.aaceonline.com/index.asp

A professional organization of educators in many disciplines who are working to improve cancer education, advance cancer prevention, expedite early cancer detection, promote individualized therapy, and develop rehabilitation programs for cancer patients. AACE includes members of the faculties of schools of medicine, dentistry, osteopathy, education, pharmacy, nursing, public health, and social work. The association encourages projects for the training of paramedical personnel and educational programs for the general public, populations at risk, and cancer patients.

American College of Obstetricians and Gynecologists

409 12th Street SW
P.O. Box 96920
Washington, DC 20090-6920
(202) 863-2518
http://www.acog.org

American College of Radiology

1891 Preston White Drive
Reston, VA 20191

(703) 648-8912
(703) 648-8900
(800) 227-5463 (toll free)
http://www.acr.org

A medical professional organization designed to advance the science of radiology, improve radiologic service to the patient, study the economic aspects of the practice of radiology, and encourage improved and continuing education for radiologists and members of allied professional fields.

American Society for Colposcopy and Cervical Pathology

20 West Washington Street
Suite 1
Hagerstown, MD 21740
(301) 733-3640
(800) 787-7227 (toll free)
http://www.asccp.org

A nonprofit organization of health care professionals committed to improving health care through the study, prevention, diagnosis, and management of lower genital tract disorders.

American Society of Clinical Oncology

1900 Duke Street
Suite 200
Alexandria, VA 22314
(703) 299-0150
http://www.asco.org

An organization that represents more than 10,000 cancer professionals worldwide and offers scientific and educational programs and other initiatives intended to foster the exchange of information about cancer. Services include ASCO OnLine, which offers services for both professionals and people with cancer, including extensive information on its patient page.

Association of Community Cancer Centers

11600 Nebel Street
Suite 201
Rockville, MD 20852-2557
(301) 984-9496 ext. 200
http://www.accc-cancer.org

Organization that helps oncology professionals adapt to the complex challenges of program man-

agement, ACCC is the leading oncology policy organization for the cancer care team.

Gay and Lesbian Medical Association

(415) 255-4547
http://www.glma.org

The association works to combat homophobia within the medical profession and society, to promote high-quality health care for human immunodeficiency virus (HIV)–positive people, to foster a professional climate in which diverse members can achieve their full potential, and to support members challenged by discrimination on the basis of sexual orientation.

Gynecologic Cancer Foundation

401 North Michigan Avenue
Chicago, IL 60611
(312) 644-6610
http://www.wcn.org

A nonprofit organization established by the Society of Gynecologic Oncologists to raise funds to support philanthropic programs to benefit women who have, or who are at risk for development of, a gynecologic cancer.

National Society of Genetic Counselors

233 Canterbury Drive
Wallingford, PA 19086-6617
(610) 872-7608
http://www.nsgc.org/

The National Society of Genetic Counselors promotes the genetic counseling profession as a recognized and integral part of health care delivery, education, research, and public policy. Services include referrals, educational programs, and genetic screening.

Oncology Nursing Society (ONS)

125 Enterprise Drive
Pittsburgh PA 15275
(866) 257-4ONS
http://www.ons.org

A professional organization of more than 30,000 registered nurses and other health-care providers dedicated to excellence in patient care, education, research, and administration in oncology nursing.

The largest professional oncology association in the world, ONS was established in 1975; it has grown to include more than 218 chapters and 32 special interest groups. It provides information to nurses around the world and plays an active role in advocacy activities at the local, state, national, and international levels.

Society of Gynecologic Nurse Oncologists
6024 Welch Avenue
Ft. Worth, TX 76133
(800) 446-3180
http://www.sgno.org

An international organization of nurses and health professionals dedicated to the advancement of patient care, education, and research in the field of gynecologic oncology and women's health care.

Society of Gynecologic Oncologists
401 North Michigan Avenue
Chicago, IL 60611
(312) 644-6610
http://www.sgo.org

A nonprofit international organization of obstetricians and gynecologists specializing in gynecologic oncology dedicated to improving the care of gynecologic cancer patients, raising standards, and encouraging ongoing research. The group also offers a referral service.

RACIAL ISSUES IN CANCER

Indian Health Service
The Reyes Building
801 Thompson Avenue
Suite 400
Rockville, MD 20852-1627
(301) 443-1083
http://www.ihs.gov

An agency within the U.S. Department of Health and Human Services responsible for providing federal health services to Native Americans and Alaska Natives. The Indian Health Service currently provides health services to approximately 1.5 million Native Americans and Alaska Natives who are members of more than 557 federally recognized tribes in 35 states.

Intercultural Cancer Council
PMB-C
1720 Dryden
Houston, TX 77030
(713) 798-4617

The council promotes policies, programs, partnerships, and research to eliminate the unequal burden of cancer among racial and ethnic minorities and medically underserved populations in the United States and its associated territories. The Intercultural Cancer Council works in partnership with both federal and private agencies and institutions.

National Asian & Pacific Islanders Cancer Survivorship & Advocacy Network
450 Sutter Street
Suite 600
San Francisco, CA 94108
(415) 954-9988 or (202) 466-7772
http://www.apiahf.org

The network gives personal, empathetic support to Asian and Pacific Islander cancer survivors and their families and friends.

National Asian Women's Health Organization
250 Montgomery Street
Suite 900
San Francisco, CA 94104
(415) 989-9747
http://www.nawho.org

Organization founded in 1993 to achieve health equity for Asian Americans. NAWHO tries to raise awareness about the health needs of Asian Americans through research and education, support Asian Americans as decision makers through leadership development and advocacy, and strengthen systems serving Asian Americans.

Through its programs, NAWHO is increasing knowledge of breast and cervical cancers, training violence prevention advocates, expanding access to immunizations, changing attitudes about reproductive health care, and breaking the stigma around depression and mental health.

National Black Leadership Initiative on Cancer
(312) 996-8046
(800) 724-1185 (toll free)

http://www.uic.edu/UI-Service/programs/
   UIC168.html

An organization that is working to create cancer awareness in the African-American community by training individuals to form coalitions throughout the United States.

National Black Women's Health Imperative
600 Pennsylvania Avenue, SE
Suite 310
Washington, DC 20003
(202) 548-4000
http://www.blackwomenshealth.org

A group that aims to improve the health of black women through self-help and empowerment.

National Latina Health Organization
3507 International Boulevard
Oakland, CA 94601
(510) 534-1362
http://www.atinahealth.org

An organization that is working for bilingual access to high-quality health care and the empowerment of Latinas through education.

Native American Cancer Research
3022 South Nova Road
Pine, CO 80470
(303) 838-9359
http://members.aol.com/natamcan/aboutnac.htm

The goals of Native American Cancer Research (NACR) are to reduce Native American cancer incidence and mortality rates and to increase the cancer survival rate among Native Americans. To accomplish these goals, NACR implements programs of cancer primary prevention, secondary prevention, risk reduction, screening (early detection), education, training, research, diagnoses, control, treatment, support, quality of life, and/or studies of cancer among Native Americans. NACR projects and studies are primarily supported by federal agencies and national organizations.

Native CIRCLE: The American Indian/Alaska Native Cancer Information Resource Center and Learning Exchange
Charlton 6, Room 282
200 First Street SW

Rochester, MN 55905
(877) 372-1617
http://www.mayo.edu/nativecircle/native.html

The purpose of Native CIRCLE is to stimulate, develop, maintain, and disseminate culturally appropriate cancer information materials for American Indian/Alaska Native educators, healthcare leaders, and students.

RADIATION THERAPY

American College of Radiology
1891 Preston White Drive
Reston, VA 20191
(703) 648-8912
(703) 648-8900
(800) 227-5463 (toll free)
http://www.acr.org

A medical professional organization designed to advance the science of radiology, improve radiologic service to the patient, study the economic aspects of the practice of radiology, and encourage improved and continuing education for radiologists and members of allied professional fields.

RESEARCH

American Institute for Cancer Research (AICR)
1759 R Street, NW
Washington, DC 20009
(202) 328-7744
(800) 843-8114
http://www.aicr.org

A national cancer organization that focuses exclusively on the relationship between nutrition and cancer. The institute supports research in the area of nutrition and cancer treatment and cancer prevention. Services include a wide array of education materials for consumers to help them lower their cancer risk through diet. The AICR nutrition toll-free hot line allows consumers to speak personally with a registered dietitian about dietary concerns.

Cancer Research Foundation of America
1600 Duke Street
Suite 110
Alexandria, VA 22314

(703) 836-4412
(800) 227-2732 (800-227-CRFA; toll free)
http://www.preventcancer.org

The Cancer Research Foundation of America is a nonprofit organization dedicated to cancer prevention through research and education. Services include peer-reviewed research grants and fellowships and development of educational programs that focus on prevention and early detection, including free newsletters, brochures, videos, public service announcements, and CD-ROMs.

Cancer Research Institute
681 Fifth Avenue
New York, NY 10022-4209
(212) 688-7515
http://www.cancerresearch.org

European Organisation for Research and Treatment of Cancer
Avenue Mounierlaan, 83/11
Brussel 1200 Brussels
Belgium
http://www.eortc.be/

SUPPORT GROUPS (GENERAL)

Cancer Care Connection (CCC)
3 Innovation Way
Suite 210
Newark, DE 19711
(302) 266-8050
(866) 266-7008 (toll free)
http://www.cancercareconnection.org

A nonprofit agency that provides information, referrals, and compassionate listening to people affected by cancer through a free phone service. Services include providing referrals for services ranging from local solutions to global cancer information via a specially designed searchable database as well as referrals to physician locator services and to clinical trial principal investigators. Services are offered in Delaware, southern Pennsylvania, southern New Jersey, and northern Maryland.

Center for Attitudinal Healing
33 Buchanan Drive
Sausalito, CA 94965

(415) 331-6161
http://www.healingcenter.org

The Center for Attitudinal Healing is an agency that provides nonsectarian spiritual and emotional support.

Comfort Connection
269 East Main Street
Newark, DE 19711
(302) 455-1501

The Comfort Connection is committed to improving overall well-being and making life a little more peaceful through new services aimed at supporting the mind, body, and soul. Services include massage therapy, relaxation for stress management (including muscle relaxation, guided imagery, meditation, and problem-solving tactics), counseling, nutrition support, cosmetic services, and volunteer services.

Gilda's Club Worldwide
322 Eighth Avenue
Suite 1402
New York, NY 10001
(800) GILDA-4-U
http://www.gildasclub.org

Group Room Radio Talk Show
Vital Options TeleSupport Cancer Network
15821 Ventura Blvd.
Suite 645
Encino, CA 91436
(818) 788-5225
(800) GRP-ROOM (toll free)
http://www.vitaloptions.org

A weekly syndicated call-in cancer talk show that links patients, survivors, and health-care professionals. Services include using communication technology, counseling, and support for patients and their families and friends and providing referrals.

Gynecologic Cancer Foundation
401 North Michigan Avenue
Chicago, IL 60611
(312) 644-6610
http://www.wcn.org

A nonprofit organization established by the Society of Gynecologic Oncologists to raise funds to support philanthropic programs to benefit women who have, or who are at risk for development of, a gynecologic cancer.

Make Today Count

1235 East Cherokee
Springfield, MO 65804
(800) 432-2273

Make Today Count is an organization that draws together people with life-threatening illnesses for "mutual support." Services include cancer counseling and general counseling

National Association of Hospital Hospitality Houses, Inc.

P.O. Box 18087
Asheville, NC 28814-0087
(828) 253-1188
(800) 542-9730 (toll free)

A nonprofit corporation that serves facilities that provide lodging and other supportive services to patients and their families when confronted with medical emergencies. Services include referrals, housing and lodging facilities, and volunteer services.

R.A. Bloch Cancer Foundation

4435 Main Street
Kansas City, MO 64111
(816) 932-8453
(800) 433-0464
http://www.blochcancer.org

The foundation provides a toll-free hotline that matches newly diagnosed patients with someone who has survived the same cancer. It also offers free information lists of multidisciplinary second-opinion centers. Services include the Cancer Hotline, home volunteers who have similar diagnoses to clients', support groups, and educational and special interest presentations.

Wellness Community

35 East 7th Street
Suite 412
Cincinnati, OH 45202
(513) 421-7111
(888) 793-WELL (toll free)
http://www.wellness-community.org

The Wellness Community provides free psychosocial support to people who are fighting to recover from cancer. There are 20 Wellness Community facilities nationwide. Services are related to counseling, support groups, networking groups, educational information, nutritional information, volunteer services, and survivor concerns.

Well Spouse Foundation

P.O. Box 30093
Elkins Park, PA 19027
(800) 838-0879 (toll free)
http://www.wellspouse.org

A membership organization that provides emotional support and information to the "well spouse" or the caregiver of the chronically ill. Services include a newsletter, local support groups, round robin letter writing, an annual weekend conference, and bereavement counseling.

SURVIVORS

National Coalition for Cancer Survivorship

1010 Wayne Avenue
Suite 770
Silver Spring, MD 20910
(301) 650-9127
(877) NCCS-YES (toll free)
http://www.canceradvocacy.org

The National Coalition for Cancer Survivorship (NCCS) is a survivor-led organization working on behalf of all cancer survivors. NCCS's mission is to ensure high-quality cancer care for all Americans. Services include referrals, information education, and advocacy.

Well Spouse Foundation

P.O. Box 30093
Elkins Park, PA 19027
(800) 838-0879 (toll free)
http://www.wellspouse.org

A membership organization that provides emotional support and information to the "well spouse" or the caregiver of the chronically ill. Services include a newsletter, local support groups, round robin letter writing, an annual weekend conference, and bereavement counseling.

TEENS/YOUNG ADULTS

Planet CANCER
1804 East 39th Street
Austin, TX 78722
(512) 481-9010
http://www.planetcancer.org

Planet Cancer is an international network of young adults (between ages 18 and 35) who have cancer who support each other in communities online and face to face. Services include peer support; a Planet Cancer Forum, in which patients communicate directly with each other; advocacy; Adventure Therapy, an outdoor expedition for young adults.

Ulman Cancer Fund for Young Adults
PMB # 505
4725 Dorsey Hall Drive, Suite A
Ellicott City, MD 21042
(410) 964-0202
(888) 393-FUND (toll free)
http://www.ulmanfund.org

The fund was established to provide support programs, education, and resources, free of charge, to benefit young adults, their families, and their friends, who are affected by cancer and to promote awareness and prevention. Services include support groups, a guidebook *("No Way, It Can't Be": A Young Adult Faces Cancer)*, a nationwide skin protection campaign, and a scholarship program.

UTERINE FIBROIDS/CANCER

National Uterine Fibroids Foundation
P.O. Box 9688
Colorado Springs, CO 80932-0688
(719) 633.3454
http://www.nuff.org

The National Uterine Fibroids Foundation (NUFF) is a nonprofit public benefit corporation organized to engage in charitable, educational, and scientific activities related to the care and treatment of women who have uterine fibroids or related conditions of the reproductive system.

WOMEN'S ISSUES

National Women's Health Information Center (NWHIC)
8550 Arlington Boulevard
Suite 300
Fairfax, VA 22031
(800) 994-9662 (toll free)
http://www.4woman.org

Web site and toll-free call center supported by the Office on Women's Health in the U.S. Department of Health and Human Services, which provides free reliable health information for women everywhere.

APPENDIX II
CANCER CENTERS

ALABAMA

University of Alabama at Birmingham Comprehensive Cancer Center*
1824 Sixth Avenue South
Birmingham, AL 35294-3300
(205) 975-8222
(800) UAB-0933 ([800] 822-0933)
http://www.ccc.uab.edu/

ARIZONA

Arizona Cancer Center*
The University of Arizona
1515 North Campbell Avenue
P.O. Box 245024
Tucson, AZ 85724
(520) 626-2900 (New Patient Registration Line)
(800) 622-2673 ([800] 622-COPE)
http://www.azcc.arizona.edu/

CALIFORNIA

Burnham Institute
10010 North Torrey Pines Road
La Jolla, CA 92037
(858) 646-3400 (Cancer Center)

Chao Family Comprehensive Cancer Center*
University of California at Irvine
Building 23, Route 81
101 The City Drive
Orange, CA 92868
(714) 456-8200
http://www.ucihs.uci.edu/cancer/

City of Hope*
Cancer Center and Beckman Research Institute
1500 East Duarte Road
Duarte, CA 91010-3000
(626) 359-8111
(800) 826-4673 ([800] 826-HOPE)
http://www.cityofhope.org/
E-mail: becomingapatient@coh.org

Jonsson Comprehensive Cancer Center at UCLA*
8-684 Factor Building
UCLA Box 951781
Los Angeles, CA 90095-1781
(310) 825-5268
http://www.cancer.mednet.ucla.edu/
E-mail: jcccinfo@mednet.ucla.edu

Salk Institute
10010 North Torrey Pines Road
La Jolla, CA 92037
(858) 453-4100 x.1386 (Cancer Center)

UC Davis Cancer Center
University of California, Davis
4501 X Street, Suite 3003
Sacramento, CA 95817
(916) 734-5800 (Clinical Cancer Center)

University of California, San Diego Cancer Center*
9500 Gilman Drive
La Jolla, CA 92093-0658
(858) 534-7600
http://cancer.ucsd.edu

University of California, San Francisco Comprehensive Cancer Center*
Box 0128, UCSF
2340 Sutter Street

---

*Comprehensive cancer centers
**Clinical cancer centers

San Francisco, CA 94143-0128
(415) 476-2201 (general information)
(800) 888-8664 (cancer referral line)
http://cc.ucsf.edu/
E-mail: cceditor@cc.ucsf.edu

USC/Norris Comprehensive Cancer Center and Hospital*
1441 Eastlake Avenue
Los Angeles, CA 90033-0804
(323) 865-3000
(800) 872-2273 ([800] USC-CARE)
http://ccnt.hsc.usc.edu/
E-mail: cainfo@ccnt.hsc.usc.edu (For general information)

COLORADO

University of Colorado Cancer Center*
Box F-704
1665 North Ursula Street
Aurora, CO 80010
(720) 848-0300
(800) 473-2288 (cancer referral line)
http://uch.uchsc.edu/uccc/

CONNECTICUT

Yale Cancer Center*
Yale University School of Medicine
333 Cedar Street
P.O. Box 208028
New Haven, CT 06520-8028
(203) 785-4095 (administrative offices)
http://www.info.med.yale.edu/ycc/

DISTRICT OF COLUMBIA

Lombardi Cancer Center*
Georgetown University Medical Center
3800 Reservoir Road, NW
Washington, DC 20007
(202) 784-4000
http://lombardi.georgetown.edu/

FLORIDA

H. Lee Moffitt Cancer Center & Research Institute at The University of South Florida*
12902 Magnolia Drive
Tampa, FL 33612-9497

(813) 972-4673 ([813] 972-HOPE)
http://www.moffitt.usf.edu/

HAWAII

Cancer Research Center of Hawaii**
1236 Lauhala Street
Honolulu, HI 96813
(808) 586-3010
http://www.hawaii.edu/crch/

ILLINOIS

Robert H. Lurie Comprehensive Cancer Center*
Northwestern University
Olson Pavilion 8250
710 North Fairbanks Court
Chicago, IL 60611-3013
(312) 908-5250
http://www.lurie.nwu.edu/
E-mail: s-markman@northwestern.edu

University of Chicago Cancer Research Center*
Mail Code 9015
5758 South Maryland Avenue
Chicago, IL 60637-1470
(773) 702-9200
(888) 824-0200 (new patients)
http://www-uccrc.uchicago.edu/
E-mail: aholub@mcis.bsd.uchicago.edu

INDIANA

Indiana University Cancer Center**
535 Barnhill Drive
Indianapolis, IN 46202-5289
(317) 278-4822
(888) 600-4822
http://iucc.iu.edu

Purdue University Cancer Center
Hansen Life Sciences Research Building
South University Street
West Lafayette, Indiana 47907-1524
(765) 494-9129 (Cancer Center)

IOWA

Holden Comprehensive Cancer Center at The University of Iowa*
5970-Z JPP

200 Hawkins Drive
Iowa City, IA 52242-1009
(800) 777-8442 (patient referral)
(800) 237-1225 (general information)
http://www.uihealthcare.com/
  DeptsClinicalServices/CancerCenter
E-mail: Cancer-Center@uiowa.edu

MAINE

Jackson Laboratory
600 Main Street
Bar Harbor, ME 04609-0800
(207) 288-6041 (Cancer Center)

MARYLAND

Johns Hopkins Oncology Center*
Weinberg Building
401 North Broadway
Baltimore, MD 21231-2410
(410) 502-1033 (information)
http://www.hopkinskimmelcancercenter.org

**Sidney Kimmel Comprehensive Cancer
  Center at Johns Hopkins**
North Wolfe Street, Room l57
Baltimore, Maryland 21287-8943
(410) 955-8822 (Comprehensive Cancer Center)

MASSACHUSETTS

Center for Cancer Research
Massachusetts Institute of Technology
77 Massachusetts Avenue, Room E17-110
Cambridge, MA 02139-4307
(617) 253-8511 (Cancer Center)

Dana-Farber Cancer Institute*
44 Binney Street
Boston, MA 02115
(617) 632-3000 (ask for patient information)
http://www.dana-farber.org/

MICHIGAN

Barbara Ann Karmanos Cancer Institute*
Operating the Meyer L. Prentis Comprehensive
  Cancer Center of Metropolitan Detroit
Wertz Clinical Center
4100 John R Street
Detroit, MI 48201-1379

(800) 527-6266 ([800] KARMANOS)
http://www.karmanos.org/
E-mail: info@karmanos.org

**University of Michigan Comprehensive
  Cancer Center***
1500 East Medical Center Drive
Ann Arbor, MI 48109
(800) 865-1125
http://www.cancer.med.umich.edu/
E-mail: wwwcancer@umich.edu

MINNESOTA

Mayo Clinic Cancer Center*
200 First Street, SW.
Rochester, MN 55905
(507) 284-2111 (appointment information desk)
http://www.mayo.edu/cancercenter/

University of Minnesota Cancer Center*
Box 806 Mayo
420 Delaware Street, SE.
Minneapolis, MN 55455
(612) 624-8484
http://www.cancer.umn.edu/

MISSOURI

Siteman Cancer Center**
Barnes-Jewish Hospital and Washington
  University School of Medicine
Box 8100
660 South Euclid
St. Louis, MO 63110-1093
(314) 747-7222
(800) 600-3606
http://www.siteman.wustl.edu/
E-mail: info@ccadmin.wustl.edu

NEBRASKA

UNMC Eppley Cancer Center**
University of Nebraska Medical Center
986805 Nebraska Medical Center
Omaha, NE 68198-6805
(402) 559-4238
http://www.unmc.edu/cancercenter/

NEW HAMPSHIRE

Norris Cotton Cancer Center*
Dartmouth-Hitchcock Medical Center

One Medical Center Drive
Lebanon, NH 03756-0002
(603) 650-6300 (administration)
(800) 639-6918 (cancer help line)
http://www.dartmouth.edu/dms/nccc
E-mail: cancerhelp@dartmouth.edu

NEW JERSEY

Cancer Institute of New Jersey**
Robert Wood Johnson Medical School
195 Little Albany Street
New Brunswick, NJ 08901
(732) 235-2465 ([732] 235-CINJ)
http://cinj.umdnj.edu

NEW YORK

**Albert Einstein Comprehensive Cancer
   Center***
Albert Einstein College of Medicine
1300 Morris Park Avenue
Bronx, NY 10461
(718) 430-2302
http://www.aecom.yu.edu/cancer
E-mail: aeccc@aecom.yu.edu

Herbert Irving Comprehensive Cancer Center*
Columbia Presbyterian Center
New York-Presbyterian Hospital
PH 18, Room 200
622 West 168th Street
New York, NY 10032
(212) 305-9327 (office of administration)
http://www.ccc.columbia.edu/

Kaplan Comprehensive Cancer Center*
New York University School of Medicine
550 First Avenue
New York, NY 10016
(212) 263-6485
http://www.nyucancerinstitute.org/

Memorial Sloan-Kettering Cancer Center*
1275 York Avenue
New York, NY 10021
(800) 525-2225
http://www.mskcc.org/

Roswell Park Cancer Institute*
Elm and Carlton Streets
Buffalo, NY 14263-0001

(800) 767-9355 ([800] ROSWELL)
http://www.roswellpark.org/

NORTH CAROLINA

**Comprehensive Cancer Center of Wake
   Forest University***
Wake Forest University Baptist Medical Center
Medical Center Boulevard
Winston-Salem, NC 27157-1082
(336) 716-4464
http://www.bgsm.edu/cancer/

Duke Comprehensive Cancer Center*
Duke University Medical Center
Box 3843
301 MSRB
Durham, NC 27710
(919) 684-3377
http://www.cancer.duke.edu

**UNC Lineberger Comprehensive Cancer
   Center***
School of Medicine
University of North Carolina at Chapel Hill
Campus Box 7295
Chapel Hill, NC 27599-7295
(919) 966-3036
http://cancer.med.unc.edu/
E-mail: dgs@med.unc.edu

OHIO

Ireland Cancer Center*
University Hospitals of Cleveland
11100 Euclid Avenue
Cleveland, OH 44106-5065
(216) 844-5432
(800) 641-2422
http://www.irelandcancercenter.org
E-mail: info@irelandcancercenter.org

**Ohio State University Comprehensive
   Cancer Center***
The Arthur G. James Cancer Hospital and
Richard J. Solove Research Institute, Suite 519
300 West 10th Avenue
Columbus, OH 43210-1240
(800) 293-5066 (The James Line)
http://www.jamesline.com
E-mail: cancerinfo@jamesline.com

OREGON

Oregon Cancer Center**
Oregon Health Sciences University
CR145
3181 Southwest Sam Jackson Park Road
Portland, OR 97201-3098
(503) 494-1617
http://www.ohsu.edu/oci/

PENNSYLVANIA

Fox Chase Cancer Center*
7701 Burholme Avenue
Philadelphia, PA 19111
(215) 728-2570 (to schedule an appointment)
(888) 369-2427 ([888] FOX CHASE)
http://www.fccc.edu/
E-mail: info@fccc.edu

Kimmel Cancer Center**
Thomas Jefferson University
Bluemle Life Sciences Building
233 South 10th Street
Philadelphia, PA 19107-5541
(215) 503-4500
(800) 533-3669 ([800] JEFF-NOW) (Jefferson
    Cancer Network)
(800) 654-5984 (TDD)
http://www.kcc.tju.edu/

University of Pennsylvania Cancer Center*
15th Floor, Penn Tower
3400 Spruce Street
Philadelphia, PA 19104-4283
(215) 662-4000 (main)
(800) 789-7366 ([800] 789-PENN
    referral/schedule an appointment)
http://www.oncolink.upenn.edu/

University of Pittsburgh Cancer Institute*
Suite 206
Iroquois Building
3600 Forbes Avenue
Pittsburgh, PA 15213-3489
(800) 237-4724 ([800] 237-4PCI)
http://www.upci.upmc.edu/
E-mail: PCI-INFO@msx.upmc.edu

Wistar Institute
3601 Spruce Street

Philadelphia, PA 19104-4268
(215) 898-3926 (Cancer Center)

TENNESSEE

St. Jude Children's Research Hospital**
332 North Lauderdale Street
Memphis, TN 38105-2794
(901) 495-3300
http://www2.stjude.org

Vanderbilt-Ingram Cancer Center*
Vanderbilt University
649 The Preston Building
Nashville, TN 37232-6838
(615) 936-1782
(615) 936-5847
(800) 811-8480 (Clinical trial or treatment option
    information)
(888) 488-4089 (all other calls)
http://www.vicc.org/

TEXAS

San Antonio Cancer Institute*
8122 Datapoint Drive
San Antonio, TX 78229-3264
(210) 616-5590
http://www.ccc.saci.org/

**University of Texas M. D. Anderson Cancer
    Center***
1515 Holcombe Boulevard
Houston, TX 77030
(713) 792-6161
(800) 392-1611
http://www.mdanderson.org/

UTAH

Huntsman Cancer Institute**
University of Utah
2000 Circle of Hope
Salt Lake City, UT 84112
(801) 585-0303
(877) 585-0303
http://www.hci.utah.edu/

VERMONT

Vermont Cancer Center*
University of Vermont
Medical Alumni Building

Burlington, VT 05401
(802) 656-4414
http://www.vermontcancer.org
E-mail: vcc@uvm.edu

VIRGINIA

Cancer Center at the University of Virginia**
University of Virginia Health System
Box 800334
Charlottesville, VA 22908
(804) 924-9333
(800) 223-9173
http://www.med.virginia.edu/medcntr/cancer/
home.html

Massey Cancer Center**
Virginia Commonwealth University
401 College Street
Post Office Box 980037
Richmond, VA 23298-0037
(804) 828-0450
http://www.vcu.edu/mcc/

WASHINGTON

Fred Hutchinson Cancer Research Center*
LA-205
Post Office Box 19024
1100 Fairview Avenue North
Seattle, WA 98109-1024
(206) 288-1024
(800) 804-8824 (appointments and medical
referral—Seattle Cancer Care Alliance)
http://www.fhcrc.org/
E-mail: hutchdoc@seattlecca.org (patient
information)

WISCONSIN

University of Wisconsin Comprehensive Cancer Center*
600 Highland Avenue, K5/601
Madison, WI 53792-6164
(608) 263-8600
(608) 262-5223 (Cancer Connect)
(800) 622-8922 (Cancer Connect)
http://www.cancer.wisc.edu
E-mail: uwccc@uwcc.wisc.edu/

APPENDIX III
CLINICAL TRIALS IN GYNECOLOGICAL CANCER

CERVICAL CANCER

DIAGNOSTIC STUDY OF COMPUTED TOMOGRAPHY AND MAGNETIC RESONANCE IMAGING IN THE PRETREATMENT EVALUATION OF PATIENTS WITH INVASIVE CERVICAL CANCER

This diagnostic trial will determine the effectiveness of MRI and CT scans in evaluating invasive cervical cancer before treatment of patients. Patients will undergo MRI and CT scans and then may undergo surgery within six weeks. Quality of life will be assessed at one month and a year, and patients will receive follow-up evaluations every three months for two years.

DIAGNOSTIC STUDY OF FLUDEOXYGLUCOSE F 18 POSITRON EMISSION TOMOGRAPHY IN PATIENTS WITH PRIMARY OR RECURRENT CERVICAL CANCER UNDERGOING SURGERY

This clinical trial will study the effectiveness of fludeoxyglucose F 18 PET scan in diagnosing primary or recurrent cervical cancer in patients who are undergoing surgery.

No more than two weeks before surgery, patients with primary cervical cancer will receive an infusion of fludeoxyglucose F 18 followed by PET scanning and CT scans of the abdomen and pelvis. These patients will then undergo hysterectomy and lymphadenectomy. Patients with recurrent cervical cancer will undergo PET scanning and CT scans of the chest, abdomen, and pelvis before surgery. Tissue removed during the two diagnostic procedures will be evaluated.

PHASE I STUDY OF EXTENDED FIELD RADIOTHERAPY, CISPLATIN, AND TOPOTECAN IN PATIENTS WITH LOCALLY ADVANCED CERVICAL CANCER

This Phase I trial will study the effectiveness of combining radiation therapy with chemotherapy in treating patients who have locally advanced cervical cancer. Patients will undergo radiation therapy to the pelvis five days a week for five to six weeks. They will also receive an infusion of cisplatin and topotecan by mouth once a week for six weeks. Patients will be evaluated every three months for two years, every six months for three years, and once a year thereafter.

PHASE I STUDY OF IMMUNIZATION WITH ALTERNATING LIPIDATED HUMAN PAPILLOMAVIRUS 16 E7 (HPV-16 E7) PEPTIDE VACCINE AND DENDRITIC CELL-HPV-16 E7 PEPTIDE VACCINE IN PATIENTS WITH RECURRENT OR PERSISTENT CERVICAL CANCER

This Phase I trial will study the effectiveness of vaccine therapy in treating patients with recurrent or persistent cervical cancer that cannot be treated with surgery or radiation therapy. White blood cells will be collected in weeks 1 and 5 and treated in the laboratory to make part of the vaccine. Patients will receive injections of one vaccine in weeks 1 and 3 and injections of a second vaccine in weeks 2 and 4. Treatment may be repeated six weeks after the end of the first course. Patients will be evaluated at one week.

PHASE I STUDY OF PHOTODYNAMIC THERAPY WITH LUTETIUM TEXAPHYRIN IN PATIENTS WITH GRADE II OR III CERVICAL INTRAEPITHELIAL NEOPLASIA

This Phase I trial will study the effectiveness of photodynamic therapy with lutetium texaphyrin in treating patients who have cervical intraepithelial neoplasia. Photodynamic therapy uses light and drugs such as lutetium texaphyrin that make abnormal cells more sensitive to light and may kill abnormal cells in the cervix and prevent the development of cervical cancer.

Patients will receive an infusion of lutetium texaphyrin followed by laser light to the cervix, followed by a procedure in which a heated wire is used to remove the abnormal tissue from the cervix. Patients will receive follow-up evaluations at 48 hours, once a week for a month, and at four months.

PHASE I/II STUDY OF DOXORUBICIN HCL LIPOSOME AND CARBOPLATIN IN PATIENTS WITH GYNECOLOGICAL TUMORS

This Phase I/II trial will study the effectiveness of combining liposomal doxorubicin with carboplatin in treating patients who have gynecologic cancer. Patients will receive an infusion of liposomal doxorubicin followed by an infusion of carboplatin once every four weeks for six courses. Patients will be evaluated at four through six weeks and every three months thereafter.

PHASE I/II STUDY OF EXTENDED FIELD RADIOTHERAPY WITH CONCURRENT PACLITAXEL AND CISPLATIN CHEMOTHERAPY IN PATIENTS WITH PREVIOUSLY UNTREATED CARCINOMA OF THE CERVIX METASTATIC TO THE PARA-AORTIC LYMPH NODES

This Phase I/II trial will study the effectiveness of radiation therapy plus paclitaxel and cisplatin in treating patients whose cancer of the cervix has spread to the lymph nodes in the pelvis and abdomen. Paclitaxel and cisplatin may increase the effectiveness of radiation therapy by making the tumor cells more sensitive to the radiation.

Patients will receive radiation therapy to the lymph nodes in the pelvis and abdomen once a day for five weeks. They will also receive infusions of paclitaxel and cisplatin once a week for six weeks. Patients will be evaluated every three months for two years, every six months for three years, and once a year thereafter.

PHASE I/II STUDY OF EXTERNAL BEAM RADIOTHERAPY AND BRACHYTHERAPY CONCURRENTLY WITH CELECOXIB, FLUOROURACIL, AND CISPLATIN IN PATIENTS WITH LOCALLY ADVANCED CERVICAL CANCER

This Phase I/II trial will study the effectiveness of radiation therapy plus celecoxib, fluorouracil, and cisplatin in treating patients who have locally advanced cervical cancer.

Patients will undergo external-beam radiation to the pelvis five days a week for five weeks. Patients will then undergo internal radiation. While undergoing radiation therapy, they will also receive an infusion of cisplatin followed by a four-day continuous infusion of fluorouracil in weeks 1, 4, and 7. Beginning on day 1, patients will receive celecoxib by mouth twice a day for one year. Patients will be evaluated every three months for two years, every four months for one year, every six months for two years, and once a year thereafter.

PHASE I/II STUDY OF EXTERNAL BEAM RADIOTHERAPY, INTRACAVITARY BRACHYTHERAPY, AND CISPLATIN WITH OR WITHOUT AMIFOSTINE IN PATIENTS WITH PARA-AORTIC OR HIGH COMMON ILIAC LYMPH NODE–POSITIVE CARCINOMA OF THE UTERINE CERVIX

This Phase I/II trial will study the effectiveness of combining chemotherapy and radiation therapy in treating patients who have stage IIIB or stage IVA cancer of the cervix.

Patients will undergo radiation therapy for up to 10 weeks. At the same time, patients will also receive an infusion of cisplatin once a week for six weeks. Some patients will repeat this treatment with the addition of an infusion of amifostine once a day for up to eight weeks. Patients will receive follow-up evaluations every three months for two years, every four months for one year, every six months for two years, and then once a year thereafter.

PHASE I/II STUDY OF RADIOTHERAPY COMBINED WITH PACLITAXEL AND CISPLATIN IN PATIENTS WITH STAGE IB2, IIA, IIB, IIIB, OR IVA INVASIVE CARCINOMA OF THE CERVIX

This Phase I/II trial will study the effectiveness of radiation therapy to the pelvis plus paclitaxel and cisplatin in treating patients who have cervical cancer.

Patients will receive external-beam radiation therapy to the pelvis five days a week for five weeks, plus internal radiation therapy. At the same time, patients will receive infusions of paclitaxel and cisplatin once a week for six weeks. Patients will receive follow-up evaluations every three months for two years, every six months for three years, and once a year thereafter.

PHASE II ADJUVANT STUDY OF THE RECOMBINANT VACCINIA VIRUS VACCINE EXPRESSING THE HUMAN PAPILLOMAVIRUS 16, 18, E6 AND E7 IN EARLY CERVICAL CANCER

This Phase II trial will study the effectiveness of vaccine therapy made from human papillomavirus plus surgery in treating patients with early cervical cancer. Vaccines made from human papillomavirus may make the body build an immune response to and kill cervical cancer cells. Combining vaccine therapy with surgery may be a more effective treatment for cervical cancer.

Patients will receive two vaccinations of human papillomavirus at least four weeks apart, one vaccination before and one after surgery. Patients will receive follow-up evaluations every three months for two years, every six months for three years, and once a year thereafter.

PHASE II PILOT STUDY OF GEFITINIB IN PATIENTS WITH OVARIAN EPITHELIAL CANCER OR CERVICAL CANCER

This Phase II trial will study the effectiveness of gefitinib in treating patients who have ovarian epithelial cancer or cervical cancer. Biological therapies such as gefitinib may interfere with the growth of the tumor cells and slow the growth of ovarian epithelial cancer or cervical cancer. Comparing results of diagnostic procedures performed before, during, and after treatment with gefitinib may help doctors predict a patient's response to treatment and help plan the most effective treatment.

Patients will receive gefitinib by mouth once a day for as long as benefit is shown. Patients will undergo biopsies of the sentinel lymph node and areas of normal skin at the start of the study and after four weeks of treatment. Patients will be evaluated once a month.

PHASE II PILOT STUDY OF HUMAN PAPILLOMAVIRUS 16 (HPV16) E6 AND E7 PEPTIDE VACCINES IN PATIENTS WITH ADVANCED OR RECURRENT CARCINOMA OF THE CERVIX OR OTHER TUMORS CARRYING HPV-16

This Phase II trial will study the effectiveness of human papillomavirus vaccine therapy in treating patients who have advanced or recurrent cancer of the cervix, vagina, penis, anus, esophagus, or head and neck. Vaccines made from certain human papillomaviruses may be able to help the body to kill more tumor cells.

Peripheral stem cells will be collected and treated in the laboratory to make the vaccine. Patients will receive vaccinations in weeks 1, 3, 7, and 11. Treatment may be repeated for as long as benefit is shown. Patients will receive a follow-up evaluation one month after the final vaccination.

PHASE II PILOT STUDY OF NONMYELOABLATIVE ALLOGENEIC PERIPHERAL BLOOD STEM CELL TRANSPLANTATION WITH FLUDARABINE AND LOW-DOSE TOTAL BODY IRRADIATION FOLLOWED BY CYCLOSPORINE AND MYCOPHENOLATE MOFETIL FOLLOWED BY DONOR LYMPHOCYTE INFUSION IN PATIENTS WITH RECURRENT METASTATIC OR LOCALLY ADVANCED HUMAN PAPILLOMAVIRUS–ASSOCIATED CERVICAL OR VAGINAL CARCINOMA

This Phase II trial is designed to study the effectiveness of donor peripheral stem cell transplantation plus chemotherapy and total-body irradiation followed by donor white blood cell infusion in treating patients who have recurrent metastatic or locally advanced cancer of the cervix or vagina that is associated with human papillomavirus. Donor peripheral stem cell transplantation and donor white blood cell infusions may be able to replace immune cells that were destroyed by chemotherapy or radiation therapy used to kill tumor cells. Sometimes the transplanted cells are rejected by the body's normal tissues. Mycophenolate mofetil and cyclosporine may prevent this from happening.

Patients will receive infusions of fludarabine on days 1 through 3, plus total-body irradiation and an infusion of donor peripheral stem cells on day 5. Patients will also receive cyclosporine twice a day by infusion on days 4 and 5, and by mouth on days 6 through 61. They will receive mycophenolate mofetil by mouth twice a day on days 5 through 32. Some patients may receive donor white blood cell infusions on day 61 and then every 65 days for up to four doses. Patients will be evaluated once a week for three months, once a month for six months, every six months for two years, and once a year for five years.

PHASE II RANDOMIZED CHEMOPREVENTION STUDY OF TOPICAL IMIQUIMOD PRECEDING LOCAL ABLATIVE OR EXCISIONAL THERAPY IN PATIENTS WITH RECURRENT OR HIGH-GRADE CERVICAL INTRAEPITHELIAL NEOPLASIA

This randomized Phase II trial is designed to study the effectiveness of applying topical imiquimod before abnormal cervical cells are removed in preventing cervical cancer in patients who have recurrent or persistent cervical neoplasia. Applying topical imiquimod before abnormal cervical cells are removed may be effective in preventing cervical cancer.

Patients will be randomly assigned to one of two groups. Patients in group one will undergo therapy to remove the abnormal cervical cells, and patients in group two will receive topical imiquimod applied to the cervix twice a week for a total of five doses. Within three to four weeks following the last application of imiquimod, patients will have the abnormal cervical cells removed as in group one. Quality of life will be assessed periodically and patients will be evaluated periodically for five years.

PHASE II RANDOMIZED STUDY OF SGN-00101 IN PATIENTS WITH GRADE III CERVICAL INTRAEPITHELIAL NEOPLASIA

This randomized Phase II trial is designed to study the effectiveness of vaccine therapy in preventing cervical cancer in patients who have cervical

intraepithelial neoplasia. Vaccines made from antigens may make the body build an immune response to kill abnormal cervical cells and may be effective in preventing cervical cancer.

Patients will be randomly assigned to one of two groups. Patients in group one will receive an injection of the vaccine once every four weeks for three vaccinations. Patients in group two will receive standard care. At week 15, all patients will undergo a colposcopy. Patients will be evaluated at 4.5 months, every three months for a year, every six months for two years, and once a year thereafter.

PHASE II STUDY OF ANTINEOPLASTONS A10 AND AS2-1 IN PATIENTS WITH STAGE IV CARCINOMA OF THE UTERINE CERVIX AND/OR VULVA

This Phase II trial will study the effectiveness of antineoplaston therapy in treating patients with stage IV cancer of the cervix and/or vulva. Antineoplastons are naturally occurring substances found in urine that may inhibit the growth of cancer cells.

Patients will receive infusions of antineoplastons six times a day. Treatment may be repeated for as long as benefit is shown. Patients will be evaluated every two months for a year and then every three months for a year.

PHASE II STUDY OF BEVACIZUMAB IN PATIENTS WITH PERSISTENT OR RECURRENT SQUAMOUS CELL CARCINOMA OF THE CERVIX

This Phase II trial is designed to study the effectiveness of bevacizumab in treating patients who have persistent or recurrent cancer of the cervix. Monoclonal antibodies such as bevacizumab can locate tumor cells and either kill them or deliver tumor-killing substances to them without harming normal cells.

Patients will receive an infusion of bevacizumab every three weeks for as long as benefit is shown. Patients will be evaluated every three months for two years, every six months for three years, and once a year thereafter.

PHASE II STUDY OF CAPECITABINE IN PATIENTS WITH ADVANCED, PERSISTENT, OR RECURRENT SQUAMOUS CELL CARCINOMA OF THE CERVIX

This Phase II trial is designed to study the effectiveness of capecitabine in treating patients who have advanced, persistent, or recurrent cervical cancer.

Patients will receive capecitabine by mouth twice a day for two weeks. Treatment may be repeated every three weeks for as long as benefit is shown. Patients will be evaluated every three months for two years, every six months for three years, and once a year thereafter.

PHASE II STUDY OF CAPECITABINE IN PATIENTS WITH PERSISTENT OR RECURRENT NON–SQUAMOUS CELL CARCINOMA OF THE CERVIX

This Phase II trial is designed to study the effectiveness of capecitabine in treating patients who have persistent or recurrent cervical cancer.

Patients will receive capecitabine by mouth twice a day for two weeks. Treatment may be repeated every three weeks for as long as benefit is shown. Patients will be evaluated every three months for two years, every six months for three years, and once a year thereafter.

PHASE II STUDY OF DOCETAXEL IN PATIENTS WITH PERSISTENT OR RECURRENT SQUAMOUS CELL CARCINOMA OF THE CERVIX

This Phase II trial is designed to study the effectiveness of docetaxel in treating patients who have persistent or recurrent cervical cancer.

Patients will receive a one-hour infusion of docetaxel every three weeks for as long as benefit is shown. Patients will be evaluated every three months for two years, every six months for three years, and once a year thereafter.

PHASE II STUDY OF DOXORUBICIN HCL LIPOSOME IN PATIENTS WITH PERSISTENT OR RECURRENT SQUAMOUS CELL CARCINOMA OF THE CERVIX

This Phase II trial is designed to study the effectiveness of liposomal doxorubicin in treating patients who have persistent or recurrent cancer of the cervix.

Patients will receive an infusion of liposomal doxorubicin every four weeks for as long as benefit is shown. Patients will be evaluated every three months for two years, every six months for three years, and once a year thereafter.

PHASE II STUDY OF DX-8951F IN WOMEN WITH ADVANCED OR RECURRENT SQUAMOUS CELL CARCINOMA OF THE CERVIX

This Phase II trial is designed to study the effectiveness of DX-8951f in treating women who have advanced or recurrent cancer of the cervix.

Patients will receive an infusion of DX-8951f once a day for five days. Treatment may be repeated every three weeks for as long as benefit is shown. Patients will be evaluated every three months.

PHASE II STUDY OF ERLOTINIB IN PATIENTS WITH PERSISTENT OR RECURRENT SQUAMOUS CELL CARCINOMA OF THE CERVIX

This Phase II trial is designed to study the effectiveness of erlotinib in treating patients who have persistent or recurrent cancer of the cervix. Biological therapies such as erlotinib may interfere with the growth of tumor cells and slow the growth of the tumor.

Patients will receive erlotinib by mouth once a day. Treatment may continue for as long as benefit is shown. Patients will be evaluated every three months for two years, every six months for three years, and once a year thereafter.

PHASE II STUDY OF TOPOTECAN AND PACLITAXEL IN PATIENTS WITH RECURRENT OR METASTATIC CANCER OF THE CERVIX

This Phase II trial is designed to study the effectiveness of topotecan and paclitaxel in treating patients who have recurrent or metastatic cancer of the cervix. Patients will receive infusions of paclitaxel on day 1 and infusions of topotecan on days 1 through 5. Filgrastim will be given on days 6 through 14. Treatment may be repeated every three weeks for as long as benefit is shown. Patients will receive follow-up evaluations every three weeks.

PHASE II STUDY OF WHOLE BODY HYPERTHERMIA COMBINED WITH DOXORUBICIN HCL LIPOSOME AND FLUOROURACIL IN PATIENTS WITH METASTATIC BREAST, OVARIAN, ENDOMETRIAL, OR CERVICAL CANCER

This Phase II trial is designed to study the effectiveness of fluorouracil and liposomal doxorubicin combined with systemic hyperthermia in treating patients with metastatic breast, ovarian, endometrial, or cervical cancer.

Hyperthermia therapy kills tumor cells by heating them to several degrees above body temperature. Drugs used in chemotherapy use different ways to stop tumor cells from dividing so they stop growing or die. Combining chemotherapy with hyperthermia may kill more tumor cells.

Patients will receive a 24-hour continuous infusion of fluorouracil on days 1 through 5 followed by an infusion of liposomal doxorubicin on day 6. One day later, patients will receive up to four six-hour hyperthermia treatments. Treatment may be repeated every four or five weeks for four courses. Some patients may receive further chemotherapy without hyperthermia. Patients will be evaluated at four weeks and every six months for a year.

PHASE III RANDOMIZED STUDY OF CISPLATIN ONLY VERSUS CISPLATIN PLUS TOPOTECAN VERSUS METHOTREXATE, VINBLASTINE, DOXORUBICIN, AND CISPLATIN IN PATIENTS WITH STAGE IVB, RECURRENT, OR PERSISTENT CARCINOMA OF THE CERVIX

This randomized Phase III trial is designed to compare the effectiveness of three different chemotherapy regimens in treating patients with stage IVB, recurrent, or persistent cervical cancer.

Patients will be randomly assigned to one of two groups. Patients in the first group will receive an infusion of cisplatin once every three weeks. Patients in the second group will receive an infusion of cisplatin on day 1 plus an infusion of topotecan on days 1, 2, and 3. Treatment may be repeated every three weeks. Treatment for patients in both groups may continue for six courses. Quality of life will be assessed periodically, and patients will be evaluated every three months for two years, every six months for three years, and then once a year thereafter.

PHASE III RANDOMIZED STUDY OF NEOADJUVANT CISPLATIN-BASED CHEMOTHERAPY FOLLOWED BY RADICAL HYSTERECTOMY VERSUS STANDARD THERAPY WITH CONCURRENT RADIOTHERAPY AND CISPLATIN-BASED

CHEMOTHERAPY IN PATIENTS WITH STAGE IB2, IIA, OR IIB CERVICAL CANCER

This randomized Phase III trial is designed to compare the effectiveness of chemotherapy followed by radical hysterectomy with that of chemotherapy plus radiation therapy in treating patients who have stage IB or stage II cervical cancer. It is not yet known whether chemotherapy is more effective followed by surgery or combined with radiation therapy in treating cervical cancer.

Patients will be randomly assigned to one of two groups. Patients in group one will receive chemotherapy every three weeks for at least three courses. Within six weeks after course three, patients will undergo surgery to remove the uterus, pelvic lymph nodes, and surrounding tissue. Some patients may then undergo radiation therapy five days a week for five to six weeks. Patients in group two will undergo radiation therapy as in group one. At the same time they will receive chemotherapy once a week for six weeks. Treatment in both groups will continue for as long as benefit is shown. Quality of life will be assessed periodically. Patients will be evaluated every three months for a year, every six months for four years, and once a year thereafter.

PHASE III RANDOMIZED STUDY OF OCTREOTIDE FOR PREVENTION OF ACUTE DIARRHEA IN PATIENTS RECEIVING RADIOTHERAPY TO THE PELVIS

This randomized Phase III trial is designed to determine the effectiveness of octreotide in preventing diarrhea in patients who are undergoing radiation therapy to the pelvis. It is not yet known whether octreotide is an effective treatment for diarrhea in such patients.

No more than four days after beginning radiation therapy, patients will be randomly assigned to one of two groups. Patients in group one will receive an injection of short-acting octreotide on day 1 and an injection of long-acting octreotide on days 2 and 29. Patients in group two will receive an injection of a placebo as in group one. Treatment in both groups may continue for as long as benefit is shown. Patients will complete questionnaires periodically. They will be evaluated once a week for four weeks, at a year, and at two years.

PHASE III RANDOMIZED STUDY OF ONDANSETRON WITH OR WITHOUT DEXAMETHASONE AS PROPHYLAXIS FOR RADIATION-INDUCED EMESIS IN PATIENTS RECEIVING UPPER ABDOMINAL RADIOTHERAPY

This randomized Phase III trial is designed to compare the effectiveness of ondansetron with or without dexamethasone in preventing vomiting in patients with cancer who are receiving radiation therapy to the upper abdomen. Antiemetic drugs may help to reduce or prevent vomiting in such patients. It is not yet known if ondansetron is more effective with or without dexamethasone.

Patients will be randomly assigned to one of two groups; all patients will receive radiation therapy. Patients in group one will receive ondansetron by mouth twice a day and dexamethasone by mouth once a day for five to seven days. Patients in group two will receive ondansetron by mouth twice a day and a placebo once a day for five to seven days. Quality of life will be assessed periodically. Patients will be evaluated at one month.

PHASE III RANDOMIZED STUDY OF RADICAL HYSTERECTOMY AND TAILORED CHEMORADIOTHERAPY VERSUS PRIMARY CHEMORADIOTHERAPY IN PATIENTS WITH STAGE IB2 CARCINOMA OF THE CERVIX

This randomized Phase III trial is designed to compare the effectiveness of different regimens of radiation therapy, chemotherapy, and surgery in treating patients who have primary stage I cancer of the cervix.

Patients will be randomly assigned to one of two groups. Patients in group one will undergo laparotomy. Some patients will then undergo surgery to remove the uterus, cervix, and lymph nodes in the pelvis. These patients will then undergo internal radiation and external-beam radiation to the pelvis five days a week for four to six weeks and receive a one-hour infusion of cisplatin once a week for five to six weeks. Other patients will receive internal radiation alone, external-beam radiation alone, or no further treatment. Patients in group two will undergo radiation therapy and chemotherapy alone as in group one. Quality of life will be assessed periodically. Patients will be evaluated every three

months for two years, every six months for three years, and once a year thereafter.

PHASE III RANDOMIZED STUDY OF RADIOTHERAPY AND CISPLATIN WITH OR WITHOUT EPOETIN ALFA IN PATIENTS WITH CERVICAL CANCER AND ANEMIA

This randomized Phase III trial is designed to study the effectiveness of epoetin alfa in treating anemia in patients who have cervical cancer.

Patients will be randomly assigned to one of two groups. Patients in group one will receive internal and external radiation therapy three to five days a week for up to seven weeks. At the same time, they will receive an infusion of cisplatin once a week for up to six weeks. Patients in group two will receive the same treatment as in group one plus an injection of epoetin alfa once a week for up to seven weeks. Quality of life will be assessed periodically in both groups. Patients will be evaluated every three months for two years, every six months for three years, and once a year thereafter.

PHASE IV RANDOMIZED STUDY OF EPOETIN BETA FOR ANEMIA MANAGEMENT IN PATIENTS WITH STAGE IIB, III, OR IVA CERVICAL CANCER TREATED WITH CISPLATIN AND RADIOTHERAPY

This randomized Phase IV trial is designed to determine the effectiveness of epoetin beta in treating anemia in patients who are receiving cisplatin and radiation therapy for stage IIB, stage III, or stage IVA cervical cancer. Epoetin beta may stimulate red blood cell production to prevent or control anemia in patients treated with chemotherapy and radiation therapy.

Patients will be randomly assigned to one of two groups. Patients in group one will undergo radiation therapy five days a week for six weeks. They will also undergo internal radiation. Beginning on day 1 of radiation therapy, patients will receive an infusion of cisplatin once a week for six weeks. They will also receive injections of epoetin beta three times a week beginning two weeks before radiation therapy and continuing for eight weeks. Patients in group two will undergo radiation therapy and internal radiation and receive cisplatin as in group one. Quality of life will be assessed periodically. Patients will be evaluated every three months for two years and every six months there-after.

STUDY OF MN PROTEIN EXPRESSION AS A POTENTIAL DIAGNOSTIC BIOMARKER OF CERVICAL DYSPLASIA AND/OR NEOPLASIA IN PATIENTS WITH ATYPICAL GLANDULAR CELLS OF UNDETERMINED SIGNIFICANCE

This diagnostic trial is designed to evaluate the effectiveness of the presence of a specific protein as a potential biomarker of cervical dysplasia and/or cancer. The presence of specific proteins may allow a doctor to determine whether or not a patient has cervical dysplasia and/or cancer.

Patients will undergo a Pap smear and a colposcopic exam. Patients may have tissue samples removed from the cervix and/or endometrium. Specimens will be examined to determine if a particular protein is present. Some patients may undergo a hysterectomy. Patients who do not undergo hysterectomy will be evaluated every six months for two years.

STUDY OF PRIMARY SCREENING STRATEGIES FOR THE DETECTION OF CERVICAL NEOPLASIA

This screening trial is designed to compare different types of screening tests used to detect cervical neoplasia. Screening tests may help doctors detect abnormal cells in the cervix early and plan effective treatment.

Participants will undergo several screening procedures including Pap smear and colposcopy. They may undergo a biopsy. Some patients may also undergo procedures to remove abnormal cervical cells.

STUDY OF VAGINAL LENGTH, ELASTICITY, LUBRICATION, AND SEXUAL FUNCTION IN PATIENTS WITH STAGE IB2 CERVICAL CANCER

This clinical trial is designed to determine the type of vaginal changes that occur in patients receiving treatment for cervical cancer and the effect these changes have on sexual function.

Patients will undergo a pelvic exam to determine the size of the vagina, and will then complete questionnaires over a two-year period about vaginal dryness and sexual activity, response, and satisfaction. Pelvic exams will be repeated periodically

for two years. Patients will be evaluated every three months for two years, every six months for three years, and once a year thereafter.

ENDOMETRIAL CANCER

NCI HIGH PRIORITY CLINICAL TRIAL—PHASE III RANDOMIZED STUDY OF ESTROGEN REPLACEMENT THERAPY VERSUS PLACEBO IN WOMEN WITH STAGE I OR II ENDOMETRIAL ADENOCARCINOMA

This randomized, double-blinded Phase III trial is designed to determine the effectiveness of estrogen replacement therapy in treating women who have stage I or stage II endometrial cancer. Estrogen replacement therapy may improve quality of life in postmenopausal women with endometrial cancer. It is not yet known whether estrogen replacement therapy will affect cancer recurrence.

Patients will be randomly assigned to one of two groups. Patients in group one will receive estrogen by mouth once a day for three years. Patients in group two will receive a placebo by mouth once a day for three years. All patients will be evaluated every six months for three years and then once a year for two years.

PHASE I STUDY OF DOXORUBICIN AND CISPLATIN FOLLOWED BY RADIOTHERAPY IN PATIENTS WITH STAGE III OR IV ENDOMETRIAL CANCER

This Phase I trial is designed to study the effectiveness of combination chemotherapy plus radiation therapy in treating women who have stage III or stage IV endometrial cancer.

Patients will receive infusions of doxorubicin and cisplatin every three weeks for three courses. Patients will then receive radiation therapy to the abdomen five days a week for four to six weeks. Patients will receive follow-up evaluations every three months for two years, every six months for three years, and once a year thereafter.

PHASE I STUDY OF INTERLEUKIN-12, PACLITAXEL, AND TRASTUZUMAB (HERCEPTIN) IN PATIENTS WITH HER2/NEU-OVEREXPRESSING MALIGNANCIES

This Phase I trial is designed to study the effectiveness of interleukin-12, paclitaxel, and trastuzumab in treating patients who have solid tumors. Chemotherapy use different ways to stop tumor cells from dividing so they stop growing or die. Interleukin-12 may kill tumor cells by stopping blood flow to the tumor and by stimulating a person's white blood cells to kill cancer cells. Monoclonal antibodies such as trastuzumab can locate tumor cells and either kill them or deliver tumor-killing substances to them without harming normal cells. Combining interleukin-12, chemotherapy, and monoclonal antibody therapy may kill more tumor cells.

Patients will receive an infusion of trastuzumab once a week for three weeks and an infusion of paclitaxel on day 1 of week 1. Beginning with course two, patients will receive trastuzumab and paclitaxel as in course one and infusions of interleukin-12 twice a week for up to a year. Patients will be evaluated every three months for a year and every six months thereafter.

PHASE I STUDY OF PACLITAXEL AND CISPLATIN WITH RADIOTHERAPY IN PATIENTS WITH STAGE III OR IV ENDOMETRIAL CANCER

This Phase I trial is designed to study the effectiveness of combination chemotherapy plus radiation therapy in treating women who have stage III or stage IV endometrial cancer.

Patients will receive an infusion of paclitaxel and cisplatin once a week for six weeks. They will also receive radiation therapy five days a week for six weeks. Patients will receive follow-up evaluations every three months for two years, every six months for three years, and then once a year thereafter.

PHASE I/II STUDY OF DOXORUBICIN HCL LIPOSOME AND CARBOPLATIN IN PATIENTS WITH GYNECOLOGICAL TUMORS

This Phase I/II trial is designed to study the effectiveness of combining liposomal doxorubicin with carboplatin in treating patients who have gynecologic cancer.

Patients will receive an infusion of liposomal doxorubicin followed by an infusion of carboplatin once every four weeks for six courses. Patients will be evaluated at four to six weeks and every three months thereafter.

PHASE II RANDOMIZED STUDY OF MEDROXYPROGESTERONE VERSUS ETHINYL ESTRADIOL AND NORGESTREL FOR THE PREVENTION OF ENDOMETRIAL CARCINOGENESIS IN WOMEN WITH A KNOWN HEREDITARY NON-POLYPOSIS COLON CANCER–ASSOCIATED GENE MUTATION

This randomized Phase II trial is designed to compare different hormone therapy regimens in preventing endometrial cancer in women who have a genetic risk for endometrial cancer. Hormone therapy may prevent the development of endometrial cancer, but it is not yet known which hormone therapy regimen is more effective in preventing endometrial cancer.

All participants will undergo a transvaginal ultrasound and endometrial biopsy. Participants will then be randomly assigned to one of two groups. Participants in group one will receive an injection of medroxyprogesterone followed three months later by a second transvaginal ultrasound and endometrial biopsy. Participants in group two will receive birth control pills by mouth once a day for three weeks followed by a placebo by mouth once a day for one week. Treatment may be repeated every four weeks for up to four courses. Approximately one week after starting the fourth hormone treatment, participants will undergo a second transvaginal ultrasound and endometrial biopsy as in group one. All participants will be evaluated at six weeks. Participants may undergo additional endometrial screening at six months.

PHASE II STUDY OF DOCETAXEL AND CARBOPLATIN IN PATIENTS WITH SUBOPTIMALLY DEBULKED STAGE III OR STAGE IV OVARIAN CARCINOMA, FALLOPIAN TUBE CARCINOMA, PAPILLARY SEROUS CANCER OF THE UTERUS, OR PRIMARY PERITONEAL CARCINOMA

This Phase II trial is designed to study the effectiveness of combining docetaxel and carboplatin in treating patients who have stage III or stage IV ovarian cancer, fallopian tube cancer, or primary peritoneal cancer.

Patients will receive infusions of docetaxel and carboplatin every three weeks. Treatment may be repeated for up to six courses. Quality of life will be assessed before treatment and then after every three courses of chemotherapy.

PHASE II STUDY OF ERLOTINIB IN PATIENTS WITH LOCALLY ADVANCED AND/OR METASTATIC CARCINOMA OF THE ENDOMETRIUM

This Phase II trial is designed to determine the effectiveness of erlotinib in treating patients who have locally advanced and/or metastatic endometrial cancer. Biological therapies such as erlotinib may interfere with the growth of tumor cells and slow the growth of the tumor.

Patients will receive erlotinib by mouth once a day for as long as benefit is shown, and will be evaluated at one month and periodically thereafter.

PHASE II STUDY OF FLAVOPIRIDOL IN PATIENTS WITH RECURRENT OR PERSISTENT ENDOMETRIAL CARCINOMA

This Phase II trial is designed to study the effectiveness of flavopiridol in treating patients who have recurrent or persistent endometrial cancer.

Patients will receive a one-hour infusion of flavopiridol on days 1 through 3. Treatment may be repeated every three weeks for as long as benefit is shown. Patients will be evaluated every three months for two years, every six months for three years, and once a year thereafter.

PHASE II STUDY OF GEFITINIB IN PATIENTS WITH PERSISTENT OR RECURRENT ENDOMETRIAL CARCINOMA

This Phase II trial is designed to study the effectiveness of gefitinib in treating patients who have persistent or recurrent endometrial cancer. Biological therapies such as gefitinib may interfere with the growth of tumor cells and slow the growth of endometrial cancer.

Patients will receive gefitinib by mouth once a day for as long as benefit is shown, and will then be evaluated every three months for two years, every six months for three years, and once a year thereafter.

PHASE II STUDY OF ICI 182780 IN PATIENTS WITH RECURRENT OR METASTATIC ENDOMETRIAL CANCER

This Phase II trial is designed to study the effectiveness of ICI 182780 in treating patients who

have recurrent, persistent, or metastatic endometrial cancer. Estrogen can stimulate the growth of cancer cells. Hormone therapy using ICI 182780 may fight cancer by blocking the uptake of estrogen by the tumor cells.

Patients will receive injections of ICI 182780 every four weeks. Treatment may continue for at least two courses. Patients will receive follow-up evaluations every three months for two years, every six months for three years, and then once a year thereafter.

PHASE II STUDY OF TRASTUZUMAB (HERCEPTIN) IN PATIENTS WITH RECURRENT OR ADVANCED ENDOMETRIAL ADENOCARCINOMA

This Phase II trial is designed to study the effectiveness of trastuzumab in treating patients who have stage III, stage IV, or recurrent endometrial cancer. Monoclonal antibodies such as trastuzumab can locate tumor cells and either kill them or deliver tumor-killing substances to them without harming normal cells.

Patients will receive an infusion of trastuzumab once a week for as long as benefit is shown. Patients will be evaluated every two months.

PHASE II STUDY OF WHOLE BODY HYPERTHERMIA COMBINED WITH DOXORUBICIN HCL LIPOSOME AND FLUOROURACIL IN PATIENTS WITH METASTATIC BREAST, OVARIAN, ENDOMETRIAL, OR CERVICAL CANCER

This Phase II trial is designed to study the effectiveness of fluorouracil and liposomal doxorubicin combined with systemic hyperthermia in treating patients with metastatic breast, ovarian, endometrial, or cervical cancer. Hyperthermia therapy kills tumor cells by heating them to several degrees above body temperature. Drugs used in chemotherapy use different ways to stop tumor cells from dividing so they stop growing or die. Combining chemotherapy with hyperthermia may kill more tumor cells.

Patients will receive a 24-hour continuous infusion of fluorouracil on days 1 through 5 followed by an infusion of liposomal doxorubicin on day 6. One day later, patients will receive up to four six-hour hyperthermia treatments. Treatment may be repeated every four to five weeks for four courses. Some patients may receive further chemotherapy without hyperthermia. Patients will be evaluated at four weeks and every six months for a year.

PHASE III RANDOMIZED ADJUVANT STUDY OF TUMOR VOLUME-DIRECTED PELVIC RADIOTHERAPY WITH OR WITHOUT PARAAORTIC RADIOTHERAPY FOLLOWED BY CISPLATIN AND DOXORUBICIN WITH OR WITHOUT PACLITAXEL IN PATIENTS WITH STAGE III OR IV ENDOMETRIAL CARCINOMA

This randomized Phase III trial is designed to compare the effectiveness of two combination chemotherapy regimens plus radiation therapy in treating patients who have stage III or stage IV endometrial cancer. It is not yet known which combination chemotherapy regimen plus radiation therapy is more effective for endometrial cancer.

Patients will undergo radiation therapy to the pelvis, with or without radiation therapy to the lymph nodes, once a day, five days a week for up to 16 weeks. Patients will be randomly assigned to one of two groups within eight weeks after completion of radiation therapy. Patients in group one will receive infusions of doxorubicin and cisplatin on day 1 and injections of filgrastim or pegfilgrastim on days 2–11. Patients in group two will receive the same doxorubicin and cisplatin plus an infusion of paclitaxel on day 2 and injections of filgrastim or pegfilgrastim on days 3 through 12. Treatment in both groups may be repeated every three weeks for up to six courses. Patients will be evaluated every three months for two years, every six months for three years, and once a year thereafter.

PHASE III RANDOMIZED STUDY OF ADJUVANT RADIATION WITH OR WITHOUT CHEMOTHERAPY IN PATIENTS WITH HIGH RISK ENDOMETRIAL CARCINOMA

This randomized Phase III trial is designed to compare the effectiveness of radiation therapy with or without chemotherapy in treating patients who have endometrial cancer. All patients will undergo surgery to remove the uterus, fallopian tubes, ovaries, and affected lymph nodes. Patients will be randomly assigned to one of two groups. Patients in group one will receive radiation therapy for five

to seven weeks. Patients in group two will receive radiation for five to seven weeks. Chemotherapy, consisting of an infusion of cisplatin and an infusion of doxorubicin or epirubicin every three weeks for four courses, will be given before or after radiation therapy. Patients will receive follow-up evaluations at three and six months and then every six months for five years.

PHASE III RANDOMIZED STUDY OF ADJUVANT RADIOTHERAPY WITH OR WITHOUT CISPLATIN AND PACLITAXEL AFTER TOTAL ABDOMINAL HYSTERECTOMY AND BILATERAL SALPINGO-OOPHORECTOMY IN PATIENTS WITH STAGE I OR II ENDOMETRIAL CANCER

This randomized Phase III trial is designed to compare the effectiveness of radiation therapy with or without combination chemotherapy following surgery in treating patients who have stage I or stage II endometrial cancer.

Patients will be randomly assigned to one of two groups. Patients in group one will receive radiation therapy once a day five days a week for five and a half weeks. Patients in group two will receive radiation therapy as in group one plus infusions of cisplatin on days 1 and 28. In addition, these patients will receive an infusion of paclitaxel followed by infusions of cisplatin in weeks 8, 12, 16, and 20. Patients will receive follow-up evaluations every three months for a year, every six months for three years, and once a year thereafter.

PHASE III RANDOMIZED STUDY OF DOXORUBICIN AND CISPLATIN WITH OR WITHOUT PACLITAXEL IN PATIENTS WITH LOCALLY ADVANCED, METASTATIC, AND/OR RELAPSED ENDOMETRIAL CANCER

This randomized Phase III trial is designed to compare the effectiveness of doxorubicin and cisplatin combined with paclitaxel to that of doxorubicin and cisplatin alone in treating patients who have locally advanced, metastatic, and/or relapsed endometrial cancer.

Patients will be randomly assigned to one of two groups. Patients in group one will receive a 30-minute infusion of doxorubicin, a three-hour infusion of paclitaxel, and a one-hour infusion of cisplatin on day 1. Patients in group two will receive doxorubicin and cisplatin alone as in group one. Treatment in both groups may be repeated every three weeks for up to six courses. Quality of life will be assessed periodically. Patients will be evaluated every three months for two years, every six months for three years, and once a year thereafter.

PHASE III RANDOMIZED STUDY OF LYMPHADENECTOMY AND ADJUVANT EXTERNAL BEAM RADIOTHERAPY IN PATIENTS WITH ENDOMETRIAL CANCER

This randomized Phase III trial is designed to compare the effectiveness of conventional surgery with or without lymphadenectomy and/or radiation therapy in treating patients who have stage I endometrial cancer. It is not yet known whether conventional surgery is more effective with or without lymphadenectomy and/or radiation therapy in treating this level of endometrial cancer.

Patients will be randomly assigned to one of two groups and will receive either conventional surgery alone or conventional surgery plus lymphadenectomy and/or radiation therapy. Quality of life will be assessed periodically, and patients will be evaluated every three months for a year, every six months for two years, and once a year thereafter.

PHASE III RANDOMIZED STUDY OF MEDROXYPROGESTERONE ACETATE VERSUS OBSERVATION FOR PREVENTION OF ENDOMETRIAL PATHOLOGY IN POSTMENOPAUSAL WOMEN WITH BREAST CANCER TREATED WITH ADJUVANT TAMOXIFEN

This randomized Phase III trial is designed to study the effectiveness of medroxyprogesterone in preventing endometrial disorders in postmenopausal women who have ductal carcinoma in situ, lobular carcinoma in situ, Paget's disease of the nipple, stage I breast cancer, or stage II breast cancer and who are taking tamoxifen. It is not yet known whether medroxyprogesterone is effective in preventing endometrial disorders in patients with breast cancer who are taking tamoxifen.

Patients will be randomly assigned to one of two groups. Patients in group one will receive tamoxifen by mouth once a day for five years and will undergo observation. Patients in group two will

receive tamoxifen by mouth once a day for five years; they will also receive medroxyprogesterone by mouth once a day for two weeks. Treatment may be repeated every three months for five years. Patients will be evaluated every six months for two years and once a year thereafter.

PHASE III RANDOMIZED STUDY OF OCTREOTIDE FOR PREVENTION OF ACUTE DIARRHEA IN PATIENTS RECEIVING RADIOTHERAPY TO THE PELVIS

This randomized Phase III trial is designed to determine the effectiveness of octreotide in preventing diarrhea in patients who are undergoing radiation therapy to the pelvis.

No more than four days after beginning radiation therapy, patients will be randomly assigned to one of two groups. Patients in group one will receive an injection of short-acting octreotide on day 1 and an injection of long-acting octreotide on days 2 and 29. Patients in group two will receive an injection of a placebo as in group one. Treatment in both groups may continue for as long as benefit is shown. Patients will complete questionnaires periodically, and they will be evaluated once a week for four weeks, at one year, and at two years.

PHASE III RANDOMIZED STUDY OF PELVIC RADIOTHERAPY VERSUS OBSERVATION AFTER LAPAROSCOPICALLY-ASSISTED VAGINAL HYSTERECTOMY OR TOTAL ABDOMINAL HYSTERECTOMY IN PATIENTS WITH INTERMEDIATE-RISK, STAGE I ENDOMETRIAL CANCER

This is a randomized Phase III trial designed to compare the effectiveness of radiation therapy with that of no further therapy following surgery in treating patients who have stage I endometrial cancer. It is not yet known whether receiving radiation therapy after surgery is more effective than receiving no further therapy after surgery for endometrial cancer.

Following surgery, patients will be randomly assigned to one of two groups. Patients in group one will receive no further therapy. Patients in group two will receive radiation therapy to the pelvis five days a week for five weeks. Patients will receive follow-up evaluations every three months for two years, every four months for a year, every six months for two years, and once a year thereafter.

PHASE III RANDOMIZED STUDY OF VAGINAL HYSTERECTOMY AND BILATERAL SALPINGO-OOPHORECTOMY (BSO) VIA LAPAROSCOPY VERSUS TOTAL ABDOMINAL HYSTERECTOMY AND BSO VIA CONVENTIONAL LAPAROTOMY PLUS PELVIC AND PARA-AORTIC LYMPH NODE SAMPLING IN PATIENTS WITH STAGE I OR IIA, GRADE I–III ENDOMETRIAL CANCER OR UTERINE CANCER

This randomized Phase III trial is designed to compare the effectiveness of laparoscopic surgery with standard surgery in treating patients with endometrial cancer or cancer of the uterus. Laparoscopic surgery is a less invasive type of surgery for cancer of the uterus and may have fewer side effects and improve recovery. It is not known whether laparoscopic surgery is more effective than standard surgery in treating endometrial cancer.

Patients will be randomly assigned to receive either laparoscopic surgery or standard surgery. Quality of life will be assessed periodically. Patients will be evaluated at six weeks, every three months for two years, and every six months for three years following surgery.

PROSPECTIVE STUDY OF IMMEDIATE HYSTERECTOMY AND PHASE II RANDOMIZED STUDY OF MEDROXYPROGESTERONE ACETATE (PROVERA) VERSUS MEDROXYPROGESTERONE ACETATE SUSPENSION (DEPO-PROVERA) PRIOR TO HYSTERECTOMY IN PATIENTS WITH ATYPICAL ENDOMETRIAL HYPERPLASIA

This Phase II trial is designed to compare the effectiveness of surgery alone with that of medroxyprogesterone followed by surgery in preventing endometrial cancer in patients who have endometrial hyperplasia. The use of surgery with or without medroxyprogesterone may be an effective way to prevent the development of endometrial cancer in patients who have endometrial hyperplasia.

Some patients will immediately undergo a hysterectomy. Other patients will be randomly assigned to receive either medroxyprogesterone by mouth once a day for three months followed by a hysterectomy or an injection of medroxyprogesterone once a month for three months followed by a hysterectomy. Patients will be evaluated every three months for two years, every six months for three years, and once a year thereafter.

FALLOPIAN TUBE CANCER

PHASE I STUDY OF OXALIPLATIN AND TOPOTECAN IN PATIENTS WITH PREVIOUSLY TREATED OVARIAN EPITHELIAL CANCER, PRIMARY PERITONEAL CANCER, OR FALLOPIAN TUBE CANCER

This Phase I trial is designed to study the effectiveness of combining oxaliplatin and topotecan in treating patients who have previously treated ovarian epithelial, primary peritoneal, or fallopian tube cancer.

Patients will receive a 15-day continuous infusion of topotecan plus an infusion of oxaliplatin on days 1 and 15. Treatment may be repeated every four weeks for up to six courses. Patients will be evaluated through day 30.

PHASE I STUDY OF PACLITAXEL, CARBOPLATIN, AND DOXORUBICIN HCL LIPOSOME IN PATIENTS WITH PREVIOUSLY UNTREATED OVARIAN EPITHELIAL, PERITONEAL, OR FALLOPIAN TUBE CANCER

This Phase I trial is designed to study the effectiveness of combination chemotherapy consisting of liposomal doxorubicin, paclitaxel, and carboplatin in treating patients who have untreated ovarian, peritoneal, or fallopian tube cancer.

Patients will receive an infusion of liposomal doxorubicin in week 1 and an infusion of carboplatin in weeks 1 and 4. They will also receive an infusion of paclitaxel once a week in weeks 1 through 6. Treatment may be repeated every six weeks for up to four courses. Patients will receive follow-up evaluations every three months for two years, every six months for three years, and once a year thereafter.

PHASE I/II STUDY OF DOXORUBICIN HCL LIPOSOME AND CARBOPLATIN IN PATIENTS WITH GYNECOLOGICAL TUMORS

This Phase I/II trial is designed to study the effectiveness of combining liposomal doxorubicin with carboplatin in treating patients who have gynecologic cancer.

Patients will receive an infusion of liposomal doxorubicin followed by an infusion of carboplatin once every four weeks for six courses. Patients will be evaluated at four to six weeks and every three months thereafter.

PHASE II PILOT STUDY OF GEFITINIB IN PATIENTS WITH OVARIAN EPITHELIAL CANCER OR CERVICAL CANCER

This Phase II trial is designed to study the effectiveness of gefitinib in treating patients who have ovarian epithelial cancer or cervical cancer. Biological therapies such as gefitinib may interfere with the growth of the tumor cells and slow the growth of ovarian epithelial cancer or cervical cancer. Comparing results of diagnostic procedures performed before, during, and after treatment with gefitinib may help doctors predict a patient's response to treatment and help plan the most effective treatment.

Patients will receive gefitinib by mouth once a day for as long as benefit is shown. Patients will undergo biopsies of the sentinel lymph node and areas of normal skin at the start of the study and after four weeks of treatment. Patients will be evaluated once a month.

PHASE II STUDY OF BRYOSTATIN 1 AND CISPLATIN IN PATIENTS WITH ADVANCED RECURRENT OR RESIDUAL OVARIAN EPITHELIAL, FALLOPIAN TUBE, OR PRIMARY PAPILLARY PERITONEAL CANCER

This Phase II trial is designed to study the effectiveness of combining bryostatin 1 and cisplatin in treating patients who have advanced recurrent or residual ovarian epithelial, fallopian tube, or primary peritoneal cancer. Patients will receive a three-day continuous infusion of bryostatin 1 followed by an infusion of cisplatin on day 4. Treatment may continue every three weeks for at least two courses. Patients will receive follow-up evaluations.

PHASE II STUDY OF CARBOXYAMIDOTRIAZOLE IN PATIENTS WITH REFRACTORY OR RECURRENT OVARIAN EPITHELIAL, FALLOPIAN TUBE, OR PRIMARY PERITONEAL CANCER

This Phase II trial is designed to study the effectiveness of carboxyamidotriazole in treating patients with refractory or recurrent ovarian epithelial, fallopian tube, or primary peritoneal cancer. Patients will receive carboxyamidotriazole by mouth once a day. Treatment may continue for as long as benefit is shown.

PHASE II STUDY OF CYCLOPHOSPHAMIDE, PACLITAXEL, AND CISPLATIN WITH FILGRASTIM (G-CSF) IN PATIENTS WITH NEWLY DIAGNOSED STAGE III OR IV OVARIAN EPITHELIAL CANCER

This Phase II trial is designed to study the effectiveness of combination chemotherapy consisting of cisplatin, cyclophosphamide, and paclitaxel plus filgrastim in treating patients with newly-diagnosed and resected stage III ovarian cancer or stage IV ovarian epithelial cancer.

Patients will receive an infusion of cyclophosphamide and a 24-hour infusion of paclitaxel on day 1 and an infusion of cisplatin on day 2. They will then receive injections of filgrastim once a day for nine days. Treatment will be repeated every three weeks for at least six courses. Cisplatin will not be repeated after the sixth course. Some patients may undergo laparoscopy, second-look laparotomy, or surgery to reduce the size of the tumor. Patients will receive follow-up evaluations every three months for three years, every six months for one year, and once a year thereafter.

PHASE II STUDY OF DOCETAXEL AND CARBOPLATIN IN PATIENTS WITH SUBOPTIMALLY DEBULKED STAGE III OR STAGE IV OVARIAN CARCINOMA, FALLOPIAN TUBE CARCINOMA, PAPILLARY SEROUS CANCER OF THE UTERUS, OR PRIMARY PERITONEAL CARCINOMA

This Phase II trial is designed to study the effectiveness of combining docetaxel and carboplatin in treating patients who have stage III or stage IV ovarian cancer, fallopian tube cancer, or primary peritoneal cancer.

Patients will receive infusions of docetaxel and carboplatin every three weeks. Treatment may be repeated for up to six courses. Quality of life will be assessed before treatment and then after every three courses of chemotherapy.

PHASE II STUDY OF IMATINIB MESYLATE IN PATIENTS WITH REFRACTORY OR RELAPSED OVARIAN EPITHELIAL, FALLOPIAN TUBE, OR PRIMARY PERITONEAL CANCER OR OVARIAN LOW MALIGNANT POTENTIAL TUMOR

This Phase II trial is designed to determine the effectiveness of imatinib mesylate in treating patients who have refractory or relapsed ovarian epithelial, fallopian tube, or primary peritoneal cancer. Imatinib mesylate may stop the growth of cancer cells by blocking the enzymes necessary for cancer cell growth.

Patients will receive imatinib mesylate by mouth once a day. Treatment may continue for as long as benefit is shown.

PHASE II STUDY OF IRINOTECAN IN PATIENTS WITH PLATINUM AND TAXANE REFRACTORY OVARIAN EPITHELIAL, PRIMARY PERITONEAL, OR FALLOPIAN TUBE CANCER

This Phase II trial is designed to study the effectiveness of irinotecan in treating patients who have refractory ovarian epithelial, primary peritoneal, or fallopian tube cancer. Patients will receive a 1.5-hour infusion of irinotecan once a week for two weeks. Treatment may be repeated every three weeks for as long as benefit is shown. Patients will be evaluated every six months for three years.

PHASE II STUDY OF NEOADJUVANT PACLITAXEL AND CARBOPLATIN FOLLOWED BY SURGERY AND ADJUVANT PACLITAXEL AND CARBOPLATIN IN PATIENTS WITH STAGE III OR IV OVARIAN EPITHELIAL CANCER, PRIMARY PERITONEAL CANCER, OR FALLOPIAN TUBE CANCER

This Phase II trial is designed to study the effectiveness of combination chemotherapy and surgery in treating patients who have stage III or stage IV ovarian epithelial cancer, primary peritoneal cancer, or fallopian tube cancer.

Patients will receive infusions of paclitaxel and carboplatin every three weeks for three courses. Within five weeks of the last course, some patients will undergo surgery to remove the tumor. Within five weeks of surgery, some patients will receive an infusion of paclitaxel followed by an intraperitoneal infusion of carboplatin on day 1, and an intraperitoneal infusion of paclitaxel on day 8. Treatment may be repeated every four weeks for up to six courses. Patients will receive follow-up evaluations every three months for a year, every six months for two years, and once a year for up to five years.

PHASE II STUDY OF PACLITAXEL, CISPLATIN, AND DOXORUBICIN HCL LIPOSOME IN PATIENTS WITH OPTIMALLY DEBULKED STAGE III OVARIAN EPITHELIAL, FALLOPIAN TUBE, OR PRIMARY PERITONEAL CANCER

This Phase II trial is designed to study the effectiveness of combining paclitaxel, cisplatin, and liposomal doxorubicin in treating women who have undergone surgery for stage III ovarian cancer, fallopian tube cancer, or primary peritoneal cancer.

Patients will receive an infusion of paclitaxel on day 1, an intraperitoneal infusion of cisplatin on day 2, and an intraperitoneal infusion of paclitaxel plus an infusion of liposomal doxorubicin on day 8. Treatment may be repeated every four weeks for up to six courses. Patients will receive follow-up evaluations every six months for two years and once a year thereafter.

PHASE II STUDY OF THALIDOMIDE IN PATIENTS WITH OVARIAN, FALLOPIAN TUBE, OR PRIMARY PERITONEAL CANCER WHO EXHIBIT AN ASYMPTOMATIC RISE IN CA 125 AFTER PRIOR CHEMOTHERAPY

This Phase II trial is designed to study the effectiveness of thalidomide in treating patients who have ovarian, fallopian tube, or primary peritoneal cancer. Thalidomide may stop the growth of cancer by stopping blood flow to the tumor.

Patients will receive thalidomide by mouth once a day for seven days. Treatment may be repeated every four weeks for as long as benefit is shown.

PHASE II/III RANDOMIZED STUDY OF CARBOPLATIN AND IFOSFAMIDE WITH OR WITHOUT WHOLE BODY HYPERTHERMIA IN PATIENTS WITH RECURRENT OVARIAN EPITHELIAL, FALLOPIAN TUBE, OR EXTRAOVARIAN PERITONEAL CANCER

This randomized Phase II/III trial is designed to compare the effectiveness of chemotherapy with or without whole-body hyperthermia in treating patients who have recurrent ovarian epithelial, fallopian tube, or peritoneal cancer.

Patients will be randomly assigned to one of two groups. Patients in group one will receive infusions of ifosfamide and carboplatin. They will also undergo whole-body hyperthermia for at least one hour. Patients in group two will receive ifosfamide and carboplatin as in group one. All treatment may be repeated every four weeks for up to six courses. Quality of life will be assessed periodically. Patients will be evaluated at one month and every three months for two years.

PHASE III RANDOMIZED ADJUVANT STUDY OF CARBOPLATIN AND PACLITAXEL WITH OR WITHOUT GEMCITABINE IN PATIENTS WITH STAGE I–IV OVARIAN EPITHELIAL OR FALLOPIAN TUBE CANCER

This randomized Phase III trial is designed to compare the effectiveness of carboplatin and paclitaxel combined with gemcitabine to that of paclitaxel and carboplatin alone in treating patients who have undergone surgery for ovarian epithelial or fallopian tube cancer. Patients will be randomly assigned to one of two groups. Patients in group one will receive a 30- to 60-minute infusion of carboplatin and a three-hour infusion of paclitaxel on day 1. They will also receive a 30- to 60-minute infusion of gemcitabine on days 1 and 8. Patients in group two will receive carboplatin and paclitaxel alone as in group one. Treatment in both groups may be repeated every three weeks for up to 10 courses. Some patients in both groups may undergo a second surgery. Quality of life will be assessed periodically. Patients will be evaluated every three months for two years, every six months for up to five years, and once a year thereafter.

PHASE III RANDOMIZED STUDY OF CISPLATIN AND TOPOTECAN FOLLOWED BY PACLITAXEL AND CARBOPLATIN VERSUS PACLITAXEL AND CARBOPLATIN ALONE IN PATIENTS WITH NEWLY DIAGNOSED STAGE IIB–IV OVARIAN EPITHELIAL, PRIMARY PERITONEAL, OR FALLOPIAN TUBE CANCER

This randomized Phase III trial is designed to compare the effectiveness of different combination chemotherapy regimens in treating patients who have stage IIB, stage III, or stage IV ovarian epithelial cancer, primary peritoneal cancer, or fallopian tube cancer.

Patients will be randomly assigned to one of two groups. Patients in group one will receive an infusion of cisplatin on day 1 and infusions of topotecan on days 1 through 5, repeated every three weeks for four courses. They will then receive an infusion of carboplatin and an infusion of paclitaxel, repeated every three weeks for four courses. Patients in group two will receive infusions of paclitaxel and carboplatin once every three weeks for up to eight courses. Quality of life will be assessed periodically. Patients will be evaluated every three months for three years, every six months for two years, and once a year thereafter.

PHASE III RANDOMIZED STUDY OF NEOADJUVANT CHEMOTHERAPY FOLLOWED BY INTERVAL DEBULKING SURGERY VERSUS UP-FRONT CYTOREDUCTIVE SURGERY FOLLOWED BY CHEMOTHERAPY WITH OR WITHOUT INTERVAL DEBULKING SURGERY IN PATIENTS WITH STAGE IIIC OR IV OVARIAN EPITHELIAL, PERITONEAL, OR FALLOPIAN TUBE CANCER

This randomized Phase III trial is designed to compare the effectiveness of chemotherapy before surgery with that of chemotherapy after surgery, with or without additional surgery, in treating patients who have stage IIIC or stage IV ovarian cancer, peritoneal cancer, or fallopian tube cancer.

Patients will be randomly assigned to one of two groups. Patients in group one will undergo surgery followed by an infusion of cisplatin or carboplatin every three weeks for three courses. Some of these patients will undergo additional surgery followed by three more courses of chemotherapy. Patients in group two will receive chemotherapy as in group one followed by surgery and three additional courses of chemotherapy. Patients in both groups may undergo second-look surgery. Quality of life will be assessed periodically. All patients will be evaluated every three months for two years, every six months for three years, and once a year thereafter.

PHASE III RANDOMIZED STUDY OF OCTREOTIDE FOR PREVENTION OF ACUTE DIARRHEA IN PATIENTS RECEIVING RADIOTHERAPY TO THE PELVIS

This randomized Phase III trial is designed to determine the effectiveness of octreotide in preventing diarrhea in patients who are undergoing radiation therapy to the pelvis. No more than four days after beginning radiation therapy, patients will be randomly assigned to one of two groups. Patients in group one will receive an injection of short-acting octreotide on day 1 and an injection of long-acting octreotide on days 2 and 29. Patients in group two will receive an injection of a placebo as in group one. Treatment in both groups may continue for as long as benefit is shown. Patients will complete questionnaires periodically. They will be evaluated once a week for four weeks, at one year, and at two years.

PHASE III RANDOMIZED STUDY OF PACLITAXEL AND CARBOPLATIN WITH OR WITHOUT EPIRUBICIN AS INITIAL TREATMENT IN PATIENTS WITH STAGE IIB, III, OR IV INVASIVE OVARIAN EPITHELIAL, FALLOPIAN TUBE, OR PERITONEAL CANCER

This randomized Phase III trial is designed to compare the effectiveness of paclitaxel and carboplatin with or without epirubicin in treating patients who have stage IIB, stage III, or stage IV invasive ovarian epithelial, fallopian tube, or peritoneal cancer.

Patients will undergo surgery either before or after three courses of chemotherapy. Patients will be randomly assigned to one of two chemotherapy groups. Patients in group one will receive infusions of epirubicin, paclitaxel, and carboplatin on day 1. Treatment may be repeated every three weeks for six to nine courses. Patients in group two will receive treatment with paclitaxel and carboplatin alone as in group one. Quality of life will be assessed periodically. Patients will receive follow-up evaluations every three months for two years, every six months for three years, and once a year thereafter.

PHASE III RANDOMIZED STUDY OF TAMOXIFEN VERSUS THALIDOMIDE IN PATIENTS WITH ONLY A BIOCHEMICAL RECURRENCE OF OVARIAN EPITHELIAL, FALLOPIAN TUBE, OR PRIMARY PERITONEAL CANCER AFTER FIRST-LINE CHEMOTHERAPY

This randomized Phase III trial is designed to compare the effectiveness of tamoxifen with that of thalidomide in treating women who have ovarian epithelial cancer, fallopian tube cancer, or primary peritoneal cancer. Estrogen can stimulate the growth of some types of cancer cells. Hormone therapy using tamoxifen may fight cancer by blocking the uptake of estrogen. Thalidomide may stop the growth of cancer by stopping blood flow to the tumor.

Patients will be randomly assigned to one of two groups. Patients in group one will receive thalidomide by mouth once a day. Patients in group two will receive tamoxifen by mouth twice a day. Treatment may continue for as long as benefit is shown. Patients will be evaluated every three months for two years, every six months for three years, and once a year thereafter.

PILOT DIAGNOSTIC STUDY OF PROTEOMIC EVALUATION IN PATIENTS WITH STAGE III OR IV PRIMARY PERITONEAL, FALLOPIAN TUBE, OR OVARIAN EPITHELIAL CANCER, OR STAGE IIC OVARIAN CLEAR CELL CYSTADENOCARCINOMA IN FIRST CLINICAL REMISSION TO DEVELOP A PROTEIN PROFILE ASSOCIATED WITH RELAPSE

This diagnostic trial is designed to study the effectiveness of protein evaluation in predicting disease relapse in patients who have stage III or stage IV primary peritoneal or fallopian tube cancer, or stage II, stage III, or stage IV ovarian epithelial cancer that is in remission, or stage IIC ovarian clear cell cystadenocarcinoma.

Patients will be evaluated at one month and every three months until disease relapse. Protein samples will be collected and analyzed.

OVARIAN CANCER

NATIONAL OVARIAN CANCER EARLY DETECTION PROGRAM: SCREENING AND GENETIC STUDY

This clinical trial is designed to determine effective methods of identifying women who are at increased risk for developing ovarian cancer. Screening and genetic testing may help doctors detect cancer cells early and plan more effective treatment for ovarian cancer.

Participants will complete questionnaires and a medical history and will meet with a genetic counselor. Blood samples will be collected and analyzed, and participants will undergo laparoscopy to examine the ovaries and collect ovarian cells for testing. Participants will be evaluated every six months.

PHASE I STUDY OF ALLOGENEIC PERIPHERAL BLOOD MONONUCLEAR CELL-STIMULATED PERIPHERAL BLOOD LYMPHOCYTES TRANSDUCED WITH A GENE ENCODING CHIMERIC T-CELL RECEPTOR REACTIVE WITH FOLATE-BINDING PROTEIN IN PATIENTS WITH ADVANCED OVARIAN EPITHELIAL CANCER

This Phase I trial is designed to study the effectiveness of interleukin-2 plus gene-modified white blood cells in treating patients who have advanced ovarian epithelial cancer. Interleukin-2 may stimulate a person's white blood cells to kill ovarian cancer cells. Interleukin-2, combined with white blood cells that are gene-modified to recognize and kill ovarian cancer cells, may be an effective treatment for recurrent or residual ovarian cancer.

White blood cells will be collected from patients' blood and treated in the laboratory with either a monoclonal antibody or donor white blood cells and an antiovarian cancer gene. Patients will receive an infusion of the gene-modified cells followed by either an infusion of interleukin-2 every 12 hours for up to eight doses or an injection of donor white blood cells on days 1 and 8. Treatment may be repeated two to three weeks later. Patients will be evaluated at four and eight weeks and periodically thereafter.

PHASE I STUDY OF ANTI-CYTOTOXIC T-LYMPHOCYTE-ASSOCIATED ANTIGEN-4 MONOCLONAL ANTIBODY IN PATIENTS WITH OVARIAN EPITHELIAL CANCER, MELANOMA, ACUTE MYELOID LEUKEMIA, MYELODYSPLASTIC SYNDROMES, OR NON–SMALL CELL LUNG CANCER PREVIOUSLY TREATED WITH SARGRAMOSTIM (GM-CSF)-BASED AUTOLOGOUS TUMOR VACCINE

This Phase I trial is designed to study the effectiveness of monoclonal antibody therapy in treating patients who have ovarian epithelial cancer, melanoma, acute myeloid leukemia, myelodysplastic syndrome, or non–small cell lung cancer. Monoclonal antibodies can locate tumor cells and either kill them or deliver tumor-killing substances to them without harming normal cells.

Patients will receive a 90-minute infusion of monoclonal antibody every three months for as long as benefit is shown. Patients will be evaluated once a month.

PHASE I STUDY OF BMS-247550 IN PATIENTS WITH ADVANCED OR RECURRENT SOLID TUMORS, OVARIAN CANCER, OR BREAST CANCER

This Phase I trial is designed to study the effectiveness of BMS-247550 in treating patients who have metastatic, recurrent, or locally advanced ovarian cancer, breast cancer, or metastatic or unresectable solid tumors.

Patients will receive an infusion of BMS-247550 once every three weeks. Treatment will continue for as long as benefit is shown. Patients will be evaluated at two months.

PHASE I STUDY OF LMB-9 IMMUNOTOXIN IN PATIENTS WITH ADVANCED COLON, BREAST, NON–SMALL CELL LUNG, BLADDER, PANCREAS, OR OVARIAN CANCER

This Phase I trial is designed to study the effectiveness of LMB-9 immunotoxin in treating patients who have advanced colon, breast, non–small cell lung, bladder, pancreatic, or ovarian cancer. The LMB-9 immunotoxin can locate tumor cells and kill them without harming normal cells.

Patients will receive a 10-day continuous infusion of LMB-9 immunotoxin. Treatment may be repeated every 30 days for as long as benefit is shown. Patients will be evaluated at three weeks and then every two months thereafter.

PHASE I STUDY OF OXALIPLATIN AND TOPOTECAN IN PATIENTS WITH PREVIOUSLY TREATED OVARIAN EPITHELIAL CANCER, PRIMARY PERITONEAL CANCER, OR FALLOPIAN TUBE CANCER

This Phase I trial is designed to study the effectiveness of combining oxaliplatin and topotecan in treating patients who have previously treated ovarian epithelial, primary peritoneal, or fallopian tube cancer.

Patients will receive a 15-day continuous infusion of topotecan plus an infusion of oxaliplatin on days 1 and 15. Treatment may be repeated every four weeks for up to six courses. Patients will be evaluated through day 30.

PHASE I STUDY OF PACLITAXEL, CARBOPLATIN, AND DOXORUBICIN HCL LIPOSOME IN PATIENTS WITH PREVIOUSLY UNTREATED OVARIAN EPITHELIAL, PERITONEAL, OR FALLOPIAN TUBE CANCER

This Phase I trial is designed to study the effectiveness of combination chemotherapy consisting of liposomal doxorubicin, paclitaxel, and carboplatin in treating patients who have untreated ovarian, peritoneal, or fallopian tube cancer.

Patients will receive an infusion of liposomal doxorubicin in week 1 and an infusion of carboplatin in weeks 1 and 4. They will also receive an infusion of paclitaxel once a week in weeks 1 through 6. Treatment may be repeated every six weeks for up to four courses. Patients will receive follow-up evaluations every three months for two years, every six months for three years, and once a year thereafter.

PHASE I STUDY OF PACLITAXEL, CISPLATIN, AND TOPOTECAN WITH OR WITHOUT FILGRASTIM (G-CSF) IN PATIENTS WITH NEWLY DIAGNOSED ADVANCED OVARIAN CANCER

This Phase I trial is designed to study the effectiveness of paclitaxel, cisplatin, and topotecan with or without filgrastim in treating patients who have newly diagnosed stage III or stage IV epithelial ovarian cancer. Colony-stimulating factors such as filgrastim may increase the number of immune cells found in bone marrow or peripheral blood and may help a person's immune system recover from the side effects of chemotherapy.

Patients will receive infusions of paclitaxel and cisplatin on day 1, followed by infusions of topotecan on days 1 through 3. Patients will then receive injections of filgrastim beginning on day 4 and continuing until blood counts return to normal. Treatment may be repeated every three weeks. Patients will receive follow-up evaluations.

PHASE I STUDY OF PS-341 AND CARBOPLATIN IN PATIENTS WITH RECURRENT OR PROGRESSIVE OVARIAN EPITHELIAL OR PRIMARY PERITONEAL CANCER

This Phase I trial is designed to study the effectiveness of combining PS-341 and carboplatin in treating patients who have recurrent or progressive ovarian epithelial or primary peritoneal cancer. PS-341 may stop the growth of tumor cells by blocking the enzymes necessary for tumor cell growth. Combining PS-341 with chemotherapy may kill more tumor cells.

Patients will receive an infusion of carboplatin once a week for two weeks followed by a one-week rest. Patients will then receive infusions of PS-341 twice a week and infusions of carboplatin once a week for two weeks. Combined treatment may be repeated every three weeks for up to six courses.

PHASE I STUDY OF YTTRIUM Y 90 MONOCLONAL ANTIBODY MN-14 IN PATIENTS WITH CHEMOTHERAPY-RESISTANT OR REFRACTORY ADVANCED OVARIAN EPITHELIAL CANCER

This Phase I trial is designed to study the effectiveness of radiolabeled monoclonal antibody therapy in treating patients who have metastatic or recurrent ovarian epithelial cancer. Radiolabeled monoclonal antibodies can locate tumor cells and either kill them or deliver tumor-killing substances to them without harming normal cells.

Patients will receive an infusion of radiolabeled monoclonal antibody followed by imaging procedures. One week later, patients will receive an infusion of radiolabeled monoclonal antibody. Patients will be evaluated every three months for two years and every six months for three years.

PHASE I/II STUDY OF DOXORUBICIN HCL LIPOSOME AND CARBOPLATIN IN PATIENTS WITH GYNECOLOGICAL TUMORS

This Phase I/II trial is designed to study the effectiveness of combining liposomal doxorubicin with carboplatin in treating patients who have gynecologic cancer.

Patients will receive an infusion of liposomal doxorubicin followed by an infusion of carboplatin once every four weeks for six courses. Patients will be evaluated at four to six weeks and every three months thereafter.

PHASE I/II STUDY OF ORAL TOPOTECAN, CARBOPLATIN, AND PACLITAXEL IN PATIENTS WITH STAGE IIB, IIC, III, OR IV OVARIAN EPITHELIAL CANCER

This Phase I/II trial is designed to study the effectiveness of topotecan combined with carboplatin and paclitaxel in treating patients who have stage II, stage III, or stage IV ovarian epithelial cancer.

Patients will receive topotecan by mouth for five days plus infusions of paclitaxel and carboplatin on day 5. Treatment will be repeated every three weeks for up to six courses. Patients will receive follow-up evaluations every three months for two years and then every six months for three years.

PHASE II PILOT STUDY OF CONSOLIDATION THERAPY WITH INTRAPERITONEAL FLOXURIDINE AND CISPLATIN AND/OR CARBOPLATIN IN PATIENTS WITH STAGE III OVARIAN EPITHELIAL OR GASTROINTESTINAL CANCER

This Phase II trial is designed to study the effectiveness of intraperitoneal combination chemotherapy in treating patients who have stage III ovarian epithelial cancer or gastrointestinal cancer.

Patients will receive intraperitoneal infusions of floxuridine on days 1 through 3 and cisplatin and/or carboplatin on day 3. Treatment may be repeated every three weeks for up to six courses. Patients will be evaluated at four and six weeks and then every six months for two years.

PHASE II PILOT STUDY OF GEFITINIB IN PATIENTS WITH OVARIAN EPITHELIAL CANCER OR CERVICAL CANCER

This Phase II trial is designed to study the effectiveness of gefitinib in treating patients who have ovarian epithelial cancer or cervical cancer. Biological therapies such as gefitinib may interfere with the growth of the tumor cells and slow the growth of ovarian epithelial cancer or cervical cancer. Comparing results of diagnostic procedures performed before, during, and after treatment with gefitinib may help doctors predict a patient's response to treatment and help plan the most effective treatment.

Patients will receive gefitinib by mouth once a day for as long as benefit is shown. Patients will undergo biopsies of the sentinel lymph node and areas of normal skin at the start of the study and after four weeks of treatment. Patients will be evaluated once a month.

PHASE II PILOT STUDY OF P53 VACCINE IN PATIENTS WITH ADENOCARCINOMA OF THE OVARY WHO HAVE NO EVIDENCE OF DISEASE OR MARKER DISEASE ONLY

This Phase II trial is designed to study the effectiveness of vaccine therapy in treating patients who have stage III, stage IV, or recurrent ovarian cancer.

Patients will be assigned to one of two groups. Patients in group one will receive an injection of the vaccine plus an injection of sargramostim. Patients in group two will have peripheral stem cells collected and treated in the laboratory with sargramostim, interleukin-4 and the vaccine. Eight days later the treated stem cells will be reinfused. Treatment for both groups may be repeated every three weeks for four doses. During the third course of treatment, patients will receive an injection of interleukin-2 once a day for two weeks. Treatment may continue for up to two years. Patients will be evaluated at one month.

PHASE II RANDOMIZED STUDY OF CARBOPLATIN WITH OR WITHOUT THALIDOMIDE IN PATIENTS WITH STAGE IC–IV OVARIAN EPITHELIAL CANCER

This randomized Phase II trial is designed to compare the effectiveness of carboplatin with or without thalidomide in treating patients who have ovarian epithelial cancer.

Patients will be randomly assigned to one of two groups. Patients in group one will receive an infusion of carboplatin every four weeks for up to six courses. Patients in group two will receive carboplatin as in group one plus thalidomide by mouth once a day for up to 24 weeks.

PHASE II RANDOMIZED STUDY OF TOREMIFENE IN PATIENTS WITH CHEMOTHERAPY-RESISTANT PAPILLARY CARCINOMA OF THE OVARY

This randomized Phase II trial is designed to study the effectiveness of toremifene in treating patients who have recurrent or refractory ovarian cancer.

Patients will receive one of two doses of toremifene by mouth once a day for four weeks. Treatment may continue for as long as benefit is shown. Quality of life will be assessed before therapy and then every four weeks during therapy. Patients will receive follow-up evaluations once every three months.

PHASE II STUDY OF ANTINEOPLASTONS A10 AND AS2-1 IN PATIENTS WITH STAGE III OR IV OVARIAN CANCER

This Phase II trial is designed to study the effectiveness of antineoplaston therapy in treating patients with stage III or stage IV ovarian cancer.

Patients will receive infusions of antineoplastons six times a day. Treatment may be repeated for as long as benefit is shown. Patients will be evaluated every two months for a year and then every three months for a year.

PHASE II STUDY OF BEVACIZUMAB IN PATIENTS WITH PERSISTENT OR RECURRENT OVARIAN EPITHELIAL OR PRIMARY PERITONEAL CANCER

This Phase II trial is designed to study the effectiveness of bevacizumab in treating patients who have persistent or recurrent ovarian epithelial cancer or primary peritoneal cancer.

Patients will receive an infusion of bevacizumab once every three weeks for as long as benefit is shown. Patients will be evaluated every three months for two years, every six months for three years, and once a year thereafter.

PHASE II STUDY OF BMS-247550 IN PATIENTS WITH RECURRENT OR PERSISTENT PLATINUM- AND PACLITAXEL-REFRACTORY OVARIAN EPITHELIAL OR PRIMARY PERITONEAL CANCER

This Phase II trial is designed to study the effectiveness of BMS-247550 in treating patients who have recurrent or persistent ovarian epithelial or primary peritoneal cancer that has not responded to previous chemotherapy.

Patients will receive an infusion of BMS-247550 once every three weeks for as long as benefit is shown. Patients will be evaluated every three months for two years and every six months for three years.

PHASE II STUDY OF BMS-247550 IN PATIENTS WITH RELAPSED AND/OR REFRACTORY STAGE III OR IV OVARIAN EPITHELIAL OR PRIMARY PERITONEAL CANCER

This Phase II trial is designed to study the effectiveness of BMS-247550 in treating patients who have relapsed and/or refractory stage III or stage IV ovarian epithelial cancer or primary peritoneal cancer.

Patients will receive a one-hour infusion of BMS-247550 once a week for three weeks. Treatment may be repeated every four weeks for as long as benefit is shown.

PHASE II STUDY OF BRYOSTATIN 1 AND CISPLATIN IN PATIENTS WITH ADVANCED RECURRENT OR RESIDUAL OVARIAN EPITHELIAL, FALLOPIAN TUBE, OR PRIMARY PAPILLARY PERITONEAL CANCER

This Phase II trial is designed to study the effectiveness of combining bryostatin 1 and cisplatin in treating patients who have advanced recurrent or residual ovarian epithelial, fallopian tube, or primary peritoneal cancer.

Patients will receive a three-day continuous infusion of bryostatin 1 followed by an infusion of cisplatin on day 4. Treatment may continue every three weeks for at least two courses. Patients will receive follow-up evaluations.

PHASE II STUDY OF CARBOXYAMIDOTRIAZOLE IN PATIENTS WITH REFRACTORY OR RECURRENT OVARIAN EPITHELIAL, FALLOPIAN TUBE, OR PRIMARY PERITONEAL CANCER

This Phase II trial is designed to study the effectiveness of carboxyamidotriazole in treating patients with refractory or recurrent ovarian epithelial, fallopian tube, or primary peritoneal cancer.

Patients will receive carboxyamidotriazole by mouth once a day. Treatment may continue for as long as benefit is shown.

PHASE II STUDY OF CISPLATIN AND PROLONGED TOPOTECAN FOLLOWED BY PACLITAXEL AND CARBOPLATIN IN PATIENTS WITH ADVANCED OVARIAN EPITHELIAL CARCINOMA

This Phase II trial is designed to study the effectiveness of combination chemotherapy in treating patients who have advanced ovarian epithelial cancer.

Patients will receive an infusion of cisplatin on day 1 of each course. Topotecan will be given by continuous infusion for two weeks for course 1 and by mouth twice a day for two weeks for all other courses. Treatment may be repeated every four weeks for four courses. Patients will then receive infusions of paclitaxel and carboplatin every three weeks for four courses.

PHASE II STUDY OF CT-2103 AS THIRD-LINE TREATMENT IN PATIENTS WITH RECURRENT OR PERSISTENT OVARIAN EPITHELIAL OR PRIMARY PERITONEAL CANCER

This Phase II trial is designed to study the effectiveness of CT-2103 in treating patients who have recurrent or persistent ovarian epithelial cancer or primary peritoneal cancer.

Patients will receive an infusion of CT-2103 every three weeks for up to six courses. Patients will be evaluated every three months for two years, every six months for three years, and once a year thereafter.

PHASE II STUDY OF CYCLOPHOSPHAMIDE, PACLITAXEL, AND CISPLATIN WITH FILGRASTIM (G-CSF) IN PATIENTS WITH NEWLY DIAGNOSED STAGE III OR IV OVARIAN EPITHELIAL CANCER

This Phase II trial is designed to study the effectiveness of combination chemotherapy consisting of cisplatin, cyclophosphamide, and paclitaxel plus filgrastim in treating patients with newly diagnosed and resected stage III ovarian cancer or stage IV ovarian epithelial cancer.

Patients will receive an infusion of cyclophosphamide and a 24-hour infusion of paclitaxel on day 1 and an infusion of cisplatin on day 2. They will then receive injections of filgrastim once a day for nine days. Treatment will be repeated every three weeks for at least six courses. Cisplatin will not be repeated after the sixth course. Some patients may undergo laparoscopy, second-look laparotomy, or surgery to reduce the size of the tumor. Patients will receive follow-up evaluations every three months for three years, every six months for one year, and once a year thereafter.

PHASE II STUDY OF DOCETAXEL AND CARBOPLATIN IN PATIENTS WITH SUBOPTIMALLY DEBULKED STAGE III OR STAGE IV OVARIAN CARCINOMA, FALLOPIAN TUBE CARCINOMA, PAPILLARY SEROUS CANCER OF THE UTERUS, OR PRIMARY PERITONEAL CARCINOMA

This Phase II trial is designed to study the effectiveness of combining docetaxel and carboplatin in treating patients who have stage III or stage IV ovarian cancer, fallopian tube cancer, or primary peritoneal cancer.

Patients will receive infusions of docetaxel and carboplatin every three weeks. Treatment may be repeated for up to six courses. Quality of life will be assessed before treatment and then after every three courses of chemotherapy.

PHASE II STUDY OF DOCETAXEL IN WOMEN WITH PLATINUM RESISTANT, REFRACTORY OVARIAN EPITHELIAL OR PRIMARY PERITONEAL SEROUS CANCER

This Phase II trial is designed to study the effectiveness of docetaxel in treating women who have ovarian epithelial cancer or primary peritoneal cancer that has not responded to previous treatment.

Patients will receive an infusion of docetaxel once a week for three weeks. Treatment may be repeated every four weeks for as long as benefit is shown.

PHASE II STUDY OF FENRETINIDE IN PATIENTS WITH RECURRENT OR METASTATIC OVARIAN EPITHELIAL OR PRIMARY PERITONEAL CANCER

This Phase II trial is designed to study the effectiveness of fenretinide in treating patients who have recurrent or metastatic ovarian epithelial or primary peritoneal cancer.

Patients will receive fenretinide by mouth twice a day for one week. Treatment may be repeated every three weeks for as long as benefit is shown.

PHASE II STUDY OF GEMCITABINE AND CISPLATIN IN PATIENTS WITH RECURRENT OR REFRACTORY PLATINUM RESISTANT OVARIAN EPITHELIAL CANCER OR PRIMARY PERITONEAL CARCINOMA

This Phase II trial is designed to study the effectiveness of gemcitabine plus cisplatin in treating patients who have primary ovarian epithelial cancer or primary peritoneal cancer that is recurrent or has not responded to platinum-based chemotherapy.

Patients will receive a one-hour infusion of cisplatin and gemcitabine once a week for two weeks. Treatment may be repeated every four weeks for as long as benefit is shown. Patients will be evaluated every three months for two years, every six months for three years, and once a year thereafter.

PHASE II STUDY OF HIGH-DOSE CYCLOPHOSPHAMIDE, CARBOPLATIN, AND MITOXANTRONE FOLLOWED BY AUTOLOGOUS BONE MARROW TRANSPLANTATION IN PATIENTS WITH REFRACTORY OR RELAPSED OVARIAN EPITHELIAL CANCER

This Phase II trial is designed to study the effectiveness of combination chemotherapy with cyclophosphamide, carboplatin, mitoxantrone and autologous bone marrow transplantation in treating patients with refractory or recurrent ovarian cancer.

Prior to chemotherapy, bone marrow will be harvested from the patient and preserved. Patients will receive infusions of cyclophosphamide and mitoxantrone on days 1, 3, and 5, and a five-day continuous infusion of carboplatin beginning on day 1. Marrow will be reinfused no sooner than 60 hours following completion of carboplatin infusion.

PHASE II STUDY OF IMATINIB MESYLATE IN PATIENTS WITH PERSISTENT OR RECURRENT OVARIAN EPITHELIAL OR PRIMARY PERITONEAL CARCINOMA

This Phase II trial is designed to study the effectiveness of imatinib mesylate in treating patients who have persistent or recurrent ovarian epithelial or primary peritoneal cancer.

Patients will receive imatinib mesylate by mouth twice a day for as long as benefit is shown. Patients will be evaluated every three months for two years, every six months for three years, and once a year thereafter.

PHASE II STUDY OF IMATINIB MESYLATE IN PATIENTS WITH PLATINUM- AND TAXANE-REFRACTORY STAGE III OR IV OVARIAN EPITHELIAL OR PRIMARY PERITONEAL CANCER

This Phase II trial is designed to study the effectiveness of imatinib mesylate in treating patients

who have stage III or stage IV ovarian epithelial or primary peritoneal cancer that has not responded to previous treatment. Imatinib mesylate may stop the growth of tumor cells by blocking the enzymes necessary for cancer cell growth.

Patients will receive imatinib mesylate by mouth twice a day for as long as benefit is shown. Patients will be evaluated every three months for a year, every six months for two years, and once a year thereafter.

PHASE II STUDY OF IMATINIB MESYLATE IN PATIENTS WITH REFRACTORY OR RELAPSED OVARIAN EPITHELIAL, FALLOPIAN TUBE, OR PRIMARY PERITONEAL CANCER OR OVARIAN LOW MALIGNANT POTENTIAL TUMOR

This Phase II trial is designed to determine the effectiveness of imatinib mesylate in treating patients who have refractory or relapsed ovarian epithelial, fallopian tube, or primary peritoneal cancer.

Patients will receive imatinib mesylate by mouth once a day. Treatment may continue for as long as benefit is shown.

PHASE II STUDY OF INTRAPERITONEAL INTERLEUKIN-12 IN PATIENTS WITH PERITONEAL CARCINOMATOSIS ASSOCIATED WITH OVARIAN EPITHELIAL CANCER OR PRIMARY PERITONEAL CARCINOMA

This Phase II trial is designed to study the effectiveness of intraperitoneal interleukin-12 in treating patients who have ovarian epithelial cancer or primary peritoneal cancer.

Patients will receive intraperitoneal infusions of interleukin-12 once a week. Treatment may be repeated every four weeks for up to six courses. Quality of life will be assessed periodically. Patients will be evaluated every two months for a year and then every three months for a year.

PHASE II STUDY OF IRINOTECAN IN PATIENTS WITH PLATINUM AND TAXANE REFRACTORY OVARIAN EPITHELIAL, PRIMARY PERITONEAL, OR FALLOPIAN TUBE CANCER

This Phase II trial is designed to study the effectiveness of irinotecan in treating patients who have refractory ovarian epithelial, primary peritoneal, or fallopian tube cancer.

Patients will receive a 1.5-hour infusion of irinotecan once a week for two weeks. Treatment may be repeated every three weeks for as long as benefit is shown. Patients will be evaluated every six months for three years.

PHASE II STUDY OF IROFULVEN IN PATIENTS WITH RECURRENT OR PERSISTENT PLATINUM-SENSITIVE OVARIAN EPITHELIAL OR PRIMARY PERITONEAL CANCER

This Phase II trial is designed to study the effectiveness of irofulven in treating patients who have recurrent or persistent ovarian epithelial cancer or primary peritoneal cancer.

Patients will receive an infusion of irofulven once a week for two weeks. Treatment may be repeated every three weeks for as long as benefit is shown. Patients will be evaluated at one month, every three months for two years, and every six months for three years.

PHASE II STUDY OF KARENITECIN AS THIRD-LINE TREATMENT IN PATIENTS WITH PERSISTENT OR RECURRENT PLATINUM-RESISTANT OVARIAN EPITHELIAL OR PRIMARY PERITONEAL CANCER

This Phase II trial is designed to study the effectiveness of karenitecin in treating patients who have persistent or recurrent ovarian epithelial cancer or primary peritoneal cancer.

Patients will receive a one-hour infusion of karenitecin for five days. Treatment may be repeated every three weeks for as long as benefit is shown. Patients will be evaluated every three months for two years, every six months for three years, and once a year thereafter.

PHASE II STUDY OF NEOADJUVANT PACLITAXEL AND CARBOPLATIN FOLLOWED BY SURGERY AND ADJUVANT PACLITAXEL AND CARBOPLATIN IN PATIENTS WITH STAGE III OR IV OVARIAN EPITHELIAL CANCER, PRIMARY PERITONEAL CANCER, OR FALLOPIAN TUBE CANCER

This Phase II trial is designed to study the effectiveness of combination chemotherapy and surgery in treating patients who have stage III or stage IV ovarian epithelial cancer, primary peritoneal cancer, or fallopian tube cancer.

Patients will receive infusions of paclitaxel and carboplatin every three weeks for three courses. Within five weeks of the last course, some patients will undergo surgery to remove the tumor. Within five weeks of surgery, some patients will receive an infusion of paclitaxel followed by an intraperitoneal infusion of carboplatin on day 1, and an intraperitoneal infusion of paclitaxel on day 8. Treatment may be repeated every four weeks for up to six courses. Patients will receive follow-up evaluations every three months for a year, every six months for two years, and once a year for up to five years.

PHASE II STUDY OF NITROCAMPTOTHECIN IN PATIENTS WITH ADVANCED OVARIAN CANCER

This Phase II trial is designed to study the effectiveness of nitrocamptothecin in treating patients who have advanced ovarian cancer.

Patients will receive nitrocamptothecin by mouth once a day five days a week for three weeks. Treatment may be repeated every three weeks for as long as benefit is shown. Patients will be evaluated every six weeks.

PHASE II STUDY OF NITROCAMPTOTHECIN IN PATIENTS WITH RECURRENT OR METASTATIC OVARIAN EPITHELIAL OR PRIMARY PERITONEAL CANCER

This Phase II trial is designed to study the effectiveness of nitrocamptothecin in treating patients who have recurrent or metastatic ovarian epithelial or primary peritoneal cancer.

Patients will receive nitrocamptothecin by mouth on days 1 through 5. Treatment may be repeated every week for as long as benefit is shown. Patients will be evaluated at two weeks, every three months for two years, and then every six months for three years.

PHASE II STUDY OF PACLITAXEL, CISPLATIN, AND DOXORUBICIN HCL LIPOSOME IN PATIENTS WITH OPTIMALLY DEBULKED STAGE III OVARIAN EPITHELIAL, FALLOPIAN TUBE, OR PRIMARY PERITONEAL CANCER

This Phase II trial is designed to study the effectiveness of combining paclitaxel, cisplatin, and liposomal doxorubicin in treating women who have undergone surgery for stage III ovarian cancer, fallopian tube cancer, or primary peritoneal cancer.

Patients will receive an infusion of paclitaxel on day 1, an intraperitoneal infusion of cisplatin on day 2, and an intraperitoneal infusion of paclitaxel plus an infusion of liposomal doxorubicin on day 8. Treatment may be repeated every four weeks for up to six courses. Patients will receive follow-up evaluations every six months for two years and once a year thereafter.

PHASE II STUDY OF THALIDOMIDE IN PATIENTS WITH OVARIAN, FALLOPIAN TUBE, OR PRIMARY PERITONEAL CANCER WHO EXHIBIT AN ASYMPTOMATIC RISE IN CA 125 AFTER PRIOR CHEMOTHERAPY

This Phase II trial is designed to study the effectiveness of thalidomide in treating patients who have ovarian, fallopian tube, or primary peritoneal cancer.

Patients will receive thalidomide by mouth once a day for seven days. Treatment may be repeated every four weeks for as long as benefit is shown.

PHASE II STUDY OF THALIDOMIDE IN PATIENTS WITH PLATINUM-REFRACTORY OR RESISTANT OVARIAN EPITHELIAL CARCINOMA

This Phase II trial is designed to study the effectiveness of thalidomide in treating women who have epithelial ovarian cancer that has not responded to previous therapy.

Patients will receive thalidomide by mouth once a day for as long as benefit is shown. Quality of life will be assessed periodically.

PHASE II STUDY OF WHOLE BODY HYPERTHERMIA COMBINED WITH DOXORUBICIN HCL LIPOSOME AND FLUOROURACIL IN PATIENTS WITH METASTATIC BREAST, OVARIAN, ENDOMETRIAL, OR CERVICAL CANCER

This Phase II trial is designed to study the effectiveness of fluorouracil and liposomal doxorubicin combined with systemic hyperthermia in treating patients with metastatic breast, ovarian, endometrial, or cervical cancer. Hyperthermia therapy kills tumor cells by heating them to several degrees above body temperature. Combining chemotherapy with hyperthermia may kill more tumor cells.

Patients will receive a 24-hour continuous infusion of fluorouracil on days 1 through 5 followed by an infusion of liposomal doxorubicin on day 6. One day later, patients will receive up to four six-hour hyperthermia treatments. Treatment may be repeated every four to five weeks for four courses. Some patients may receive further chemotherapy without hyperthermia. Patients will be evaluated at four weeks and every six months for a year.

PHASE II/III RANDOMIZED STUDY OF CARBOPLATIN AND IFOSFAMIDE WITH OR WITHOUT WHOLE-BODY HYPERTHERMIA IN PATIENTS WITH RECURRENT OVARIAN EPITHELIAL, FALLOPIAN TUBE, OR EXTRAOVARIAN PERITONEAL CANCER

This randomized Phase II/III trial is designed to compare the effectiveness of chemotherapy with or without whole-body hyperthermia in treating patients who have recurrent ovarian epithelial, fallopian tube, or peritoneal cancer.

Patients will be randomly assigned to one of two groups. Patients in group one will receive infusions of ifosfamide and carboplatin. They will also undergo whole-body hyperthermia for at least one hour. Patients in group two will receive ifosfamide and carboplatin as in group one. All treatment may be repeated every four weeks for up to six courses. Quality of life will be assessed periodically. Patients will be evaluated at one month and every three months for two years.

PHASE III RANDOMIZED ADJUVANT STUDY OF CARBOPLATIN AND PACLITAXEL WITH OR WITHOUT GEMCITABINE IN PATIENTS WITH STAGE I–IV OVARIAN EPITHELIAL OR FALLOPIAN TUBE CANCER

This randomized Phase III trial is designed to compare the effectiveness of carboplatin and paclitaxel combined with gemcitabine to that of paclitaxel and carboplatin alone in treating patients who have undergone surgery for ovarian epithelial or fallopian tube cancer.

Patients will be randomly assigned to one of two groups. Patients in group one will receive a 30- to 60-minute infusion of carboplatin and a three-hour infusion of paclitaxel on day 1. They will also receive a 30- to 60-minute infusion of gemcitabine on days 1 and 8. Patients in group two will receive carboplatin and paclitaxel alone as in group one.

Treatment in both groups may be repeated every three weeks for up to 10 courses. Some patients in both groups may undergo a second surgery. Quality of life will be assessed periodically. Patients will be evaluated every three months for two years, every six months for up to five years, and once a year thereafter.

PHASE III RANDOMIZED STUDY OF CARBOPLATIN AND PACLITAXEL WITH OR WITHOUT LOW-DOSE PACLITAXEL IN PATIENTS WITH EARLY STAGE OVARIAN CARCINOMA

This randomized Phase III trial is designed to study the effectiveness of combined carboplatin and paclitaxel with or without continued low-dose paclitaxel in treating patients with early-stage ovarian cancer.

Patients will be randomly assigned to one of two groups. All patients will receive a three-hour infusion of paclitaxel followed by an infusion of carboplatin every three weeks for three courses. Four weeks after the third course, patients in group one will receive a one-hour infusion of low-dose paclitaxel once a week for 24 weeks. Patients in group two will receive no further treatment but will undergo observation. All patients will be evaluated every three months for two years, every six months for three years, and once a year thereafter.

PHASE III RANDOMIZED STUDY OF CARBOPLATIN WITH OR WITHOUT PEGYLATED DOXORUBICIN HCL LIPOSOME IN PATIENTS WITH PLATINUM-SENSITIVE RECURRENT OVARIAN EPITHELIAL OR PRIMARY PERITONEAL CANCER

This randomized Phase III trial is designed to determine the effectiveness of carboplatin with or without liposomal doxorubicin in treating patients who have recurrent ovarian epithelial or primary peritoneal cancer.

Patients will be randomly assigned to one of two groups. Patients in group one will receive an infusion of carboplatin and a one-hour infusion of liposomal doxorubicin. Patients in group two will receive an infusion of carboplatin alone as in group one. Treatment in both groups may be repeated every four weeks for as long as benefit is shown. Patients will be evaluated at four weeks, every six

months for three years, and once a year for seven years.

PHASE III RANDOMIZED STUDY OF CISPLATIN AND TOPOTECAN FOLLOWED BY PACLITAXEL AND CARBOPLATIN VERSUS PACLITAXEL AND CARBOPLATIN ALONE IN PATIENTS WITH NEWLY DIAGNOSED STAGE IIB–IV OVARIAN EPITHELIAL, PRIMARY PERITONEAL, OR FALLOPIAN TUBE CANCER

This randomized Phase III trial is designed to compare the effectiveness of different combination chemotherapy regimens in treating patients who have stage IIB, stage III, or stage IV ovarian epithelial cancer, primary peritoneal cancer, or fallopian tube cancer.

Patients will be randomly assigned to one of two groups. Patients in group one will receive an infusion of cisplatin on day 1 and infusions of topotecan on days 1 through 5, repeated every three weeks for four courses. They will then receive an infusion of carboplatin and an infusion of paclitaxel, repeated every three weeks for four courses. Patients in group two will receive infusions of paclitaxel and carboplatin once every three weeks for up to eight courses. Quality of life will be assessed periodically. Patients will be evaluated every three months for three years, every six months for two years, and once a year thereafter.

PHASE III RANDOMIZED STUDY OF HIGH DOSE SEQUENTIAL CHEMOTHERAPY VERSUS STANDARD CHEMOTHERAPY IN PATIENTS WITH OPTIMALLY DEBULKED STAGE III OR IV OVARIAN EPITHELIAL CANCER

This randomized Phase III trial is designed to compare the effectiveness of high-dose chemotherapy with that of standard chemotherapy in treating patients who have stage III or stage IV ovarian epithelial cancer that has been removed during surgery.

Patients will be randomly assigned to one of two groups. Patients in group one will receive five courses of high-dose combination chemotherapy plus peripheral stem cell transplantation. Treatment may be repeated every three to four weeks. Patients in group two will receive standard combination chemotherapy every four weeks for six courses. Quality of life will be assessed before treatment and periodically after treatment. Patients will receive follow-up evaluations every three months for two years, every six months for a year, and once a year thereafter.

PHASE III RANDOMIZED STUDY OF NEOADJUVANT CHEMOTHERAPY FOLLOWED BY INTERVAL DEBULKING SURGERY VERSUS UP-FRONT CYTOREDUCTIVE SURGERY FOLLOWED BY CHEMOTHERAPY WITH OR WITHOUT INTERVAL DEBULKING SURGERY IN PATIENTS WITH STAGE IIIC OR IV OVARIAN EPITHELIAL, PERITONEAL, OR FALLOPIAN TUBE CANCER

This randomized Phase III trial is designed to compare the effectiveness of chemotherapy before surgery with that of chemotherapy after surgery, with or without additional surgery, in treating patients who have stage III or stage IV ovarian cancer, peritoneal cancer, or fallopian tube cancer.

Patients will be randomly assigned to one of two groups. Patients in group one will undergo surgery followed by an infusion of cisplatin or carboplatin every three weeks for three courses. Some of these patients will undergo additional surgery followed by three more courses of chemotherapy. Patients in group two will receive chemotherapy as in group one followed by surgery and three additional courses of chemotherapy. Patients in both groups may undergo second-look surgery. Quality of life will be assessed periodically. All patients will be evaluated every three months for two years, every six months for three years, and once a year thereafter.

PHASE III RANDOMIZED STUDY OF OCTREOTIDE FOR PREVENTION OF ACUTE DIARRHEA IN PATIENTS RECEIVING RADIOTHERAPY TO THE PELVIS

This randomized Phase III trial is designed to determine the effectiveness of octreotide in preventing diarrhea in patients who are undergoing radiation therapy to the pelvis. No more than four days after beginning radiation therapy, patients will be randomly assigned to one of two groups.

Patients in group one will receive an injection of short-acting octreotide on day 1 and an injection of long-acting octreotide on days 2 and 29. Patients in group two will receive an injection of a placebo as

in group one. Treatment in both groups may continue for as long as benefit is shown. Patients will complete questionnaires periodically. They will be evaluated once a week for four weeks, at a year, and at two years.

PHASE III RANDOMIZED STUDY OF PACLITAXEL AND CARBOPLATIN WITH OR WITHOUT EPIRUBICIN AS INITIAL TREATMENT IN PATIENTS WITH STAGE IIB, III, OR IV INVASIVE OVARIAN EPITHELIAL, FALLOPIAN TUBE, OR PERITONEAL CANCER

This randomized Phase III trial is designed to compare the effectiveness of paclitaxel and carboplatin with or without epirubicin in treating patients who have stage IIB, stage III, or stage IV invasive ovarian epithelial, fallopian tube, or peritoneal cancer.

Patients will undergo surgery either before or after three courses of chemotherapy. Patients will be randomly assigned to one of two chemotherapy groups. Patients in group one will receive infusions of epirubicin, paclitaxel, and carboplatin on day 1. Treatment may be repeated every three weeks for six to nine courses. Patients in group two will receive treatment with paclitaxel and carboplatin alone as in group one. Quality of life will be assessed periodically. Patients will receive follow-up evaluations every three months for two years, every six months for three years, and once a year thereafter.

PHASE III RANDOMIZED STUDY OF PACLITAXEL AND CARBOPLATIN WITH OR WITHOUT GEMCITABINE, DOXORUBICIN HCL LIPOSOME, OR TOPOTECAN IN PATIENTS WITH STAGE III OR IV OVARIAN EPITHELIAL OR SEROUS PRIMARY PERITONEAL CARCINOMA

This randomized Phase III trial is designed to compare the effectiveness of various combination chemotherapy regimens in treating patients who have stage III or stage IV ovarian cancer or primary peritoneal cancer.

Patients will be randomly assigned to one of five groups. Each group of patients will receive infusions of different combination chemotherapy regimens one to three times a week. Treatment may be repeated every three weeks for up to eight courses. Some patients may undergo surgery. All patients will receive follow-up evaluations every three months for two years and every six months thereafter.

PHASE III RANDOMIZED STUDY OF PACLITAXEL WITH EITHER CARBOPLATIN OR CISPLATIN VERSUS CONVENTIONAL PLATINUM-BASED CHEMOTHERAPY IN PATIENTS WITH RELAPSED OVARIAN EPITHELIAL OR PERITONEAL CANCER

This randomized Phase III trial is designed to compare the effectiveness of platinum-based chemotherapy with or without paclitaxel in treating patients with relapsed ovarian epithelial cancer.

Patients will be randomly assigned to one of two groups. Patients in group one will receive platinum-based chemotherapy consisting of either cisplatin or carboplatin alone or cisplatin combined with other drugs. Patients in group two will receive a three-hour infusion of paclitaxel followed by either carboplatin or cisplatin. Treatment for both groups may be repeated every three weeks for up to six courses. Patients will receive follow-up evaluations at six months, then every three months for two years, every six months for three years, and once a year thereafter.

PHASE III RANDOMIZED STUDY OF TAMOXIFEN VERSUS THALIDOMIDE IN PATIENTS WITH ONLY A BIOCHEMICAL RECURRENCE OF OVARIAN EPITHELIAL, FALLOPIAN TUBE, OR PRIMARY PERITONEAL CANCER AFTER FIRST-LINE CHEMOTHERAPY

This randomized Phase III trial is designed to compare the effectiveness of tamoxifen with that of thalidomide in treating women who have ovarian epithelial cancer, fallopian tube cancer, or primary peritoneal cancer.

Patients will be randomly assigned to one of two groups. Patients in group one will receive thalidomide by mouth once a day. Patients in group two will receive tamoxifen by mouth twice a day. Treatment may continue for as long as benefit is shown. Patients will be evaluated every three months for two years, every six months for three years, and once a year thereafter.

PHASE III RANDOMIZED STUDY OF THE BENEFIT OF EARLY CHEMOTHERAPY BASED ON CA 125 LEVEL ONLY VERSUS DELAYED CHEMOTHERAPY BASED ON CONVENTIONAL CLINICAL INDICATORS IN PATIENTS WITH RELAPSED OVARIAN CANCER

This randomized Phase III trial is designed to compare early chemotherapy based on blood levels of CA 125 alone with chemotherapy based on conventional clinical indicators in patients who have recurrent ovarian epithelial cancer.

All patients will have their blood CA 125 levels measured. Patients with an elevated CA 125 level will be randomly assigned to one of two groups. Patients in group one will immediately have a second blood CA 125 level done to confirm the elevation. No more than four weeks after the first CA 125 elevation, patients with a confirmed elevation will receive chemotherapy. Patients in group two will be monitored and will receive chemotherapy when cancer recurrence is apparent. Quality of life will be assessed periodically in both groups. Patients will receive follow-up evaluations every three months.

PHASE III RANDOMIZED STUDY OF YTTRIUM Y 90 MONOCLONAL ANTIBODY HMFG1 VERSUS STANDARD THERAPY IN PATIENTS WITH OVARIAN EPITHELIAL CARCINOMA IN REMISSION AFTER DEBULKING SURGERY AND PLATINUM-BASED CHEMOTHERAPY

This randomized Phase III trial is designed to compare the effectiveness of monoclonal antibody therapy with that of observation in treating patients who have ovarian cancer or primary peritoneal cancer in remission following surgery and chemotherapy.

Patients will be randomly assigned to one of two groups. Patients in group one will be placed under observation. Patients in group two will receive an intraperitoneal infusion of the monoclonal antibody. Quality of life will be assessed before random assignment, at weeks 4 and 8, at three months, and every three months thereafter. Patients will be evaluated periodically.

PILOT DIAGNOSTIC STUDY OF PROTEOMIC EVALUATION IN PATIENTS WITH STAGE III OR IV PRIMARY PERITONEAL, FALLOPIAN TUBE, OR OVARIAN EPITHELIAL CANCER, OR STAGE IIC OVARIAN CLEAR CELL CYSTADENOCARCINOMA IN FIRST CLINICAL REMISSION TO DEVELOP A PROTEIN PROFILE ASSOCIATED WITH RELAPSE

This diagnostic trial is designed to study the effectiveness of protein evaluation in predicting disease relapse in patients who have stage III or stage IV primary peritoneal or fallopian tube cancer, or stage II, stage III, or stage IV ovarian epithelial cancer, or stage IIC ovarian clear cell cystadenocarcinoma, that is in remission.

Patients will be evaluated at one month and every three months until disease relapse. Protein samples will be collected and analyzed.

PILOT SCREENING STUDY FOR OVARIAN CANCER IN PARTICIPANTS WHO ARE AT HIGH GENETIC RISK FOR DEVELOPING OVARIAN CANCER

This screening trial is designed to determine the significance of CA 125 levels in detecting ovarian cancer in participants who have a high genetic risk of developing ovarian cancer.

Blood samples will be collected and patients will complete questionnaires every three months for up to two years. Some patients may also undergo transvaginal ultrasound. Patients will be evaluated periodically for one year after completing the study.

PILOT STUDY TO CORRELATE DNA SEQUENCE COPY NUMBER ABNORMALITIES WITH OUTCOME IN PATIENTS WITH ADVANCED EPITHELIAL OVARIAN CANCER

This genetic study is designed for patients who have stage III or stage IV ovarian cancer. A sample of the patient's tumor removed during previous surgery will be tested. Several genetic tests will be completed using the tumor sample.

PROSPECTIVE SCREENING STUDY OF RISK-REDUCING SALPINGO-OOPHERECTOMY AND LONGITUDINAL CA 125 SCREENING IN PARTICIPANTS AT INCREASED GENETIC RISK OF OVARIAN CANCER

This screening trial is designed to study the effectiveness of surgery to remove the fallopian tubes and ovaries combined with monitoring of CA 125 levels in participants who are at increased genetic risk for ovarian cancer. Surgery to remove the fallopian tubes and ovaries may decrease the risk of ovarian cancer and may improve quality of life in women who are at increased genetic risk. Monitoring CA 125 levels may help doctors detect cancer cells early and plan more effective treatment for ovarian cancer.

Participants will choose to be in one of two groups. All participants will complete questionnaires and undergo transvaginal ultrasound and measurement of CA 125 levels. Participants in group one will undergo measurement of CA 125 levels every three months and transvaginal ultrasound and mammography once a year. Some participants may undergo additional transvaginal ultrasound and laparotomy/laparoscopy. Participants in group two will undergo surgery to remove the fallopian tubes and ovaries. They will then have CA 125 levels measured every three months and undergo a mammogram once a year. Some participants may undergo additional transvaginal ultrasound and laparotomy/laparoscopy. Participants in group one may choose to undergo surgery to remove the fallopian tubes and ovaries at any time during the study. Quality of life will be assessed in both groups every six months for three years.

SCREENING STUDY FOR OVARIAN CANCER IN WOMEN WHO ARE AT HIGH GENETIC RISK FOR DEVELOPING OVARIAN CANCER

This screening trial is designed to determine the best procedure to detect ovarian cancer in women who have a high genetic risk for developing ovarian cancer.

Patients will undergo transvaginal ultrasound of the ovaries once a year, and blood samples will be collected every four months.

STUDY OF CLINICAL, GENETIC, BEHAVIORAL, LABORATORY, AND EPIDEMIOLOGIC CHARACTERISTICS OF INDIVIDUALS AND FAMILIES AT HIGH RISK OF BREAST OR OVARIAN CANCER

This study is designed to identify genetic, behavioral, and environmental factors related to cancer risk in individuals and families at high risk for breast or ovarian cancer.

Individuals will undergo a medical evaluation that may include a medical history, physical examination, imaging procedures, and collection of blood and/or tissue samples. One family member will complete a family history questionnaire. Some individuals may undergo a biopsy, other diagnostic procedures, and/or genetic testing and genetic counseling. Families will be evaluated once a year.

VAGINAL CANCER

PHASE II PILOT STUDY OF NONMYELOABLATIVE ALLOGENEIC PERIPHERAL BLOOD STEM CELL TRANSPLANTATION WITH FLUDARABINE AND LOW-DOSE TOTAL-BODY IRRADIATION FOLLOWED BY CYCLOSPORINE AND MYCOPHENOLATE MOFETIL FOLLOWED BY DONOR LYMPHOCYTE INFUSION IN PATIENTS WITH RECURRENT METASTATIC OR LOCALLY ADVANCED HUMAN PAPILLOMAVIRUS–ASSOCIATED CERVICAL OR VAGINAL CARCINOMA

This Phase II trial is designed to study the effectiveness of donor peripheral stem cell transplantation plus chemotherapy and total-body irradiation followed by donor white blood cell infusion in treating patients who have recurrent metastatic or locally advanced cancer of the cervix or vagina that is associated with human papillomavirus.

Patients will receive infusions of fludarabine on days 1 through 3, total-body irradiation on day 5, and an infusion of donor peripheral stem cells on day 5. Patients will also receive cyclosporine twice a day by infusion on days 4 and 5 and by mouth on days 6 through 61. They will receive mycophenolate mofetil by mouth twice a day on days 5 through 32. Some patients may receive donor white blood cell infusions on day 61 and then every 65 days for up to four doses. Patients will be evaluated once a week for three months, once a month for six months, every six months for two years, and once a year for five years.

VULVAR CANCER

PHASE II STUDY OF ANTINEOPLASTONS A10 AND AS2-1 IN PATIENTS WITH STAGE IV CARCINOMA OF THE UTERINE CERVIX AND/OR VULVA

This Phase II trial is designed to study the effectiveness of antineoplaston therapy in treating patients with stage IV cancer of the cervix and/or vulva.

Patients will receive infusions of antineoplastons six times a day. Treatment may be repeated for as long as benefit is shown. Patients will be evaluated every two months for a year and then every three months for a year.

PHASE II STUDY OF PACLITAXEL IN PATIENTS WITH LOCALLY ADVANCED, METASTATIC, OR RECURRENT SQUAMOUS CELL CARCINOMA OF THE VULVA

This Phase II trial is designed to study the effectiveness of paclitaxel in treating patients who have locally advanced, metastatic, or recurrent cancer of the vulva.

Patients will receive an infusion of paclitaxel. Treatment may be repeated every three weeks for up to 10 courses, and will then be evaluated every nine weeks.

PHASE III RANDOMIZED STUDY OF FIBRIN SEALANT TO REDUCE LYMPHEDEMA INCIDENCE AFTER LYMPH NODE DISSECTION IN PATIENTS WITH VULVAR MALIGNANCIES

This randomized Phase III trial is designed to determine the effectiveness of fibrin sealant in reducing lymphedema following surgical removal of lymph nodes in patients who have cancer of the vulva. Fibrin sealant may decrease lymphedema following surgery to remove lymph nodes in the groin by helping to seal the lymphatic vessels. It is not yet known if fibrin sealant is effective in decreasing lymphedema following surgery to remove lymph nodes.

Patients will be randomly assigned to one of two groups. Patients in both groups will undergo surgery to remove part or all of the vulva and lymph nodes in the groin area. Patients in group one will have the surgical site closed with stitches and fibrin sealant. Patients in group two will have the surgical site closed with stitches alone. Patients will be assessed for lymphedema at one week, six weeks, three months, and six months. Patients will be evaluated every three months for two years, every six months for three years, and once a year thereafter.

PHASE III STUDY OF INTRAOPERATIVE LYMPHATIC MAPPING IN PATIENTS WITH INVASIVE SQUAMOUS CELL CARCINOMA OF THE VULVA

This Phase III trial is designed to study the effectiveness of lymphatic mapping in treating patients with stage I or stage II cancer of the vulva.

Patients will receive injections of a blue dye near the tumor, and will then undergo surgery to remove affected lymph nodes and the primary tumor. Patients will receive follow-up evaluations every three months for two years, every six months for three years, and once a year thereafter.

APPENDIX IV
DRUGS USED TO TREAT REPRODUCTIVE CANCER

Actiq   See FENTANYL CITRATE.

Adriamycin   See DOXORUBICIN.

Adrucil   See 5-FU.

aldesleukin   See INTERLEUKIN-2.

alendronate sodium   A drug that affects bone metabolism. Alendronate sodium is being studied as a possible treatment for bone pain caused by secondary cancer that has spread to the bones. It belongs to the family of drugs called bisphosphonates.

Alkeran   See L-PHENYLALANINE MUSTARD.

allopurinol sodium (Zyloprim)   An oral drug given before chemotherapy to reduce some toxic side effects.

altretamine (Hexalen, hexamethylmelamine)   An oral chemotherapy drug sometimes used to treat persistent or recurrent ovarian cancer after other chemotherapy drugs have failed. This drug is an alkylating agent that disrupts the growth of cancer cells, which are then destroyed. It is given in three or four divided doses a day.

More common side effects include decreased platelet and white blood cell counts (causing increased risk of bleeding and infection), nausea and vomiting, and fetal abnormalities (when used by pregnant women). Less common side effects include fatigue, mood changes, appetite loss, diarrhea, and kidney function changes. Rarely, patients may experience skin rash or itching,

walking problems, nerve pain, or pins and needles sensations.

amethopterin   See METHOTREXATE.

amifostine (Ethyol)   An intravenous (IV) drug that can lower the cumulative kidney toxicity associated with repeated administration of cisplatin to patients who have advanced ovarian cancer. It is also being studied as a drug that can protect radiation therapy patients from side effects. This drug neutralizes the platinum in normal tissues so that DNA and RNA are not damaged and protects the kidneys from damage by platinum chemotherapy.

Side effects include nausea and vomiting, and low blood pressure. Less common side effects include facial flushing, chills, sneezing or hiccups, and sleepiness. Rarely, this drug may lower the blood calcium level.

9-aminocamptothecin (9-AC)   An investigational topoisomerase inhibitor that is being studied as a treatment for several cancers, including ovarian cancer. This drug disrupts the growth of cancer cells by preventing the development of certain elements necessary for cell division. The drug is given by intravenous infusion over 72 hours.

More common side effects include decreases in white blood cell and platelet counts (with an increased risk of infection or bleeding), fatigue, nausea and vomiting, diarrhea, hair loss, and anemia.

Anzemet   See DOLASETRON.

Aromasin   See EXEMESTANE.

atamestane A drug being studied for the treatment of cancer that blocks the production of estrogen in the body.

Biafine cream A topical preparation used to reduce the risk of, and treat skin reactions to, radiation therapy.

Blenoxane See BLEOMYCIN.

bleomycin A common chemotherapy drug that belongs to the family of drugs called antitumor antibiotics. Bleomycin is sometimes used to treat vulvar cancer and cervical cancer as well as cancers of the head and neck, penis, skin, testes, kidney, lung, and esophagus; and lymphomas, soft tissue sarcomas, Kaposi's sarcoma, and melanoma. This drug interferes with cell division, thereby killing the cell. It is given as an intravenous (IV) infusion over 20 to 30 minutes or as a continuous infusion. It also can be injected.

Side effects include fever and chills, appetite loss and nausea, hair loss, mouth sores, and skin changes. Less commonly, there may be pain at the injection or tumor site and irritation of lungs or in the vein where the drug was given. Rarely, it may cause an allergic reaction or lung fibrosis.

broxuridine A drug that makes cancer cells more sensitive to radiation and is also used as a diagnostic agent to determine the rate at which cancer cells grow.

carbogen An inhalant of oxygen and carbon dioxide that increases the sensitivity of tumor cells to the effects of radiation therapy.

carboplatin (Paraplatin) An intravenously administered platinum chemotherapy agent that belongs to the family of drugs called alkylating agents and is considered to be the drug of choice for ovarian cancer. It is also used for other cancers, including those of the lung and of the head and neck. Carboplatin disrupts cancer cell growth, destroying malignant cells.

Common side effects include decreased platelet and white blood cell counts (causing risk of bleeding and infection), brittle hair, altered kidney function at high dosages, and fetal abnormalities. Less common side effects include nausea and vomiting, appetite loss, diarrhea or constipation, taste changes, or "pins and needles" sensations. Rarely, it may cause confusion, visual changes, rash, tinnitus, severe allergic reaction, or dizziness.

carboxypeptidase G2 A bacterial enzyme used to neutralize the toxic effects of the chemotherapy drug methotrexate.

CBDCA See CARBOPLATIN.

CDC A combination of the chemotherapy drugs carboplatin, doxorubicin (Adriamycin), and Cytoxan (cyclophosphamide) sometimes used to treat ovarian cancer.

CDDP cis-Diamminedichloroplatinum See CISPLATIN.

celecoxib A nonsteroidal anti-inflammatory drug that reduces pain, currently being studied as a possible cancer prevention treatment.

cevimeline A substance that increases production of saliva and tears. Cevimeline is being studied as a treatment for dry mouth caused by radiation therapy to the head and neck. It belongs to the family of drugs called cholinergic enhancers.

CF A combination of the chemotherapy drugs cisplatin and 5-fluorouracil (5-FU) that may be used to treat gestational trophoblastic tumor.

CFL A combination of the chemotherapy drugs cisplatin, 5-fluorouracil (5-FU), and leucovorin calcium that may be used to treat gestational trophoblastic tumor.

CHAD A combination of the chemotherapy drugs cyclophosphamide, hexamethylmelamine, doxorubicin, and cisplatin that may be used to treat ovarian cancer.

Chex-Up   A combination of the chemotherapy drugs cyclophosphamide (Cytoxan), hexamethylmelamine, 5-fluorouracil (5-FU), and Platinol (cisplatin) that may be used to treat ovarian cancer.

chlorambucil (Leukeran)   A chemotherapy agent that belongs to the family of drugs called alkylating agents. Chlorambucil is sometimes used to treat ovarian cancer as well as cancers of the breast and testes and chronic lymphocytic leukemia, lymphomas, and choriocarcinoma. This drug disrupts the growth of cancer cells, destroying them.

Common side effects include decreased platelet and white blood cell counts (increasing the risk of bleeding or infection), fetal changes, and interruption of menstruation. Less common effects include appetite and weight loss; rarely, it may cause nausea and vomiting, liver damage, confusion or seizures, and visual problems.

cis-**diamminedichloroplatinum**   See CISPLATIN.

cisplatin (Platinol, *cis*-platinum)   A very commonly used platinum intravenous chemotherapy agent that belongs to the family of drugs called alkylating agents. Cisplatin is sometimes used to treat ovarian or cervical cancer. It is also used to treat lymphomas, myeloma, melanoma, and osteogenic sarcoma and cancers of the testes, head and neck, bladder, prostate, breast, lung, and esophagus. This drug disrupts the growth of cancer cells, destroying them.

More common side effects include nausea and vomiting, taste changes, "pins and needles" sensations, fetal changes, and kidney damage. Less common side effects include fatigue, appetite loss, hair thinning, diarrhea, and decreased platelet and white blood counts (causing risk of bleeding or infection). Rarely, this drug may cause chest pain and heart attack, severe allergic reaction, hearing loss, or gait problems.

CLB   See CHLORAMBUCIL.

clodronate   A drug used as treatment for abnormally high level of calcium in the blood (hypercalcemia) and for cancer that has spread to the bone (bone metastasis). It may decrease pain, risk of fractures, and development of new bone metastasis.

Compazine   See PROCHLORPERAZINE.

Cosmegen   See DACTINOMYCIN.

CP   A combination of the chemotherapy drugs Cytoxan (cyclophosphamide) and Platinol (cisplatin) sometimes used to treat ovarian cancer.

CYADIC   A combination of the chemotherapy drugs Cytoxan (cyclophosphamide), Adriamycin (doxorubicin), and dimethyl triazeno imidazole carboxamide (DTIC) sometimes used to treat soft tissue sarcoma.

cyclobutane dicarboxylate platinum   See CARBOPLATIN.

cyclophosphamide (Cytoxan)   One of the most commonly used chemotherapy drugs, in the treatment of endometrial and ovarian cancer, as well as lymphoma, leukemia, myeloma, neuroblastoma, Ewing's sarcoma, mycosis fungoides, rhabdomyosarcoma, and cancers of the breast, lung, and testes. It can be given either intravenously or orally; it belongs to the family of alkylating agents. It disrupts the growth of cancer cells, killing them.

Common side effects include hair loss, nausea and vomiting, appetite loss, mouth sores, diarrhea, interruption of menstruation, and decreased white blood cell count, causing an increased risk of infection. Less common side effects include a drop in platelet count (increasing risk of bleeding), presence of blood in urine, acne, fatigue, and fetal changes. Rarely, cyclophosphamide may cause heart problems at high dosages or lung fibrosis; it very rarely induces certain types of cancer.

cyclosporine   A drug used to help reduce the risk that organ and bone marrow transplants will be rejected by the body. Cyclosporine is also used in clinical trials to make cancer cells more sensitive to chemotherapy drugs.

Cytoxan   See CYCLOPHOSPHAMIDE.

DACT   See DACTINOMYCIN.

dactinomycin (Actinomycin D [Cosmegen])   An intravenous antibiotic chemotherapy drug sometimes used to treat choriocarcinoma and rhabdomyosarcoma as well as testicular cancer, melanoma, Wilms' tumor, neuroblastoma, Ewing's sarcoma, retinoblastoma, and Kaposi's sarcoma. It disrupts the growth of cancer cells, killing them.

More common side effects include decreased platelet and white blood cell counts (causing increased risk of bleeding or infection), hair loss, nausea and vomiting, appetite loss, mouth sores, diarrhea, rash, and radiation recall. Less common side effects include fatigue, fever, depression, muscle or bone aches, and fetal changes. Rarely, there may be liver or kidney damage, or rarely second malignancies.

danazol (Danocrine)   A synthetic androgen that is being evaluated in the treatment of endometrial cancer. It is also used to treat some cancer patients whose platelet count has dropped to below-normal levels.

Danocrine   See DANAZOL.

DBD   See DIBROMODULCITOL.

DDP   See CISPLATIN.

Decadron   See DEXAMETHASONE.

defibrotide   A drug under study for the prevention of veno-occlusive disease, a rare complication of high-dose chemotherapy and stem cell transplantation in which small veins in the liver become blocked.

Demerol   See MEPERIDINE.

2'-deoxycytidine   A drug that protects healthy tissues from the toxic effects of cancer drugs.

dexamethasone (Decadron)   An antinausea drug and synthetic adrenocorticoid that is very effective in preventing nausea and vomiting in chemotherapy patients. Because this pill can irritate the stomach, it must be taken with food.

More common side effects include weight gain, sodium or fluid retention, depression, increased blood sugar level and appetite, sleep problems, increased risk of infection, bruising, mood changes, or delayed wound healing. Less common side effects include thirst, increased urination, fungal infections, bone fractures, sweating, diarrhea, nausea, headache, increased heart rate, or calcium loss. Rarely, this drug may cause cataracts, personality changes, blurry vision, or stomach ulcer.

dexrazoxane (Zinecard)   A drug used to protect the heart from the toxic effects of anthracycline drugs, such as doxorubicin, although the exact mechanism is not known. One of the family of drugs called chemoprotective agents, it is given intravenously before the administration of doxorubicin or daunorubicin.

More common side effects include decreased white blood cell count or platelet counts, with increased risk of infection or bleeding. Less common side effects include fatigue.

dibromodulcitol (mitolactol [Elobromol])   An oral chemotherapy drug sometimes used to treat recurrent invasive cervical cancer.

Dilaudid   See HYDROMORPHONE.

dipyridamole   A drug that prevents blood cell clumping and enhances the effectiveness of fluorouracil and other chemotherapeutic agents.

DMC   A combination of the chemotherapy drugs dactinomycin (Cosmegen), methotrexate, and Cytoxan (cyclophosphamide) sometimes used to treat gestational trophoblastic tumor.

dolasetron (Anzemet)   A drug that prevents or reduces the nausea and vomiting that typically occur during chemotherapy. It can be given intravenously or orally and works by blocking the serotonin pathway by which chemotherapy stimulates the vomiting center in the brain.

Occasionally this drug may cause headache; rarely, it may cause fever, fatigue, bone pain, muscle aches, constipation, heartburn, appetite loss, pancreatic inflammation, electrical changes in the heart, flushing, abnormal dreams, sleep problems, confusion and anxiety, anaphylaxis, or itching.

donepezil A drug used to treat Alzheimer's disease being studied as a treatment for side effects of radiation therapy to the brain.

doxorubicin (Adriamycin) A major intravenous antibiotic chemotherapy drug used to treat many malignancies, including ovarian cancer as well as cancers of the breast, bladder, thyroid, and lung, and Wilms' tumor, neuroblastoma, rhabdomyosarcoma, Ewing's sarcoma, retinoblastoma, and Kaposi's sarcoma. This drug must be administered carefully, since it can cause severe skin damage if it leaks out into the surrounding area. Patients taking this drug should drink plenty of fluids to prevent kidney or bladder problems.

In addition to typical side effects common to many chemotherapy drugs (nausea and vomiting, hair loss, appetite loss, and decreased platelet and white blood cell counts), this drug can cause direct damage to the muscle cells of the heart (cardiomyopathy), which is related to total accumulative lifetime dosage. This drug also turns urine red, with potential to stain clothes. This reddening is not blood, but a normal appearance of the drug in urine, which lasts one or two days after the drug is given.

dronabinol (Marinol) A synthetic pill form of delta-9-tetrahydrocannabinol, an active ingredient in marijuana that is used to treat nausea and vomiting associated with cancer chemotherapy when the usual antinausea drugs are not effective.

More common side effects include mood changes, disorientation, drowsiness, muddled thinking, dizziness, perception changes, dry mouth, and increased appetite. Less common side effects include increased heart rate and decreased blood pressure when changing positions.

Efudex See 5-FU.

EHDP See ETIDRONATE.

Ellence See EPIRUBICIN.

Elobromol See DIBROMODULCITOL.

endostatin A drug that is being studied for its ability to prevent the growth of new blood vessels into a solid tumor. Endostatin belongs to the family of drugs called angiogenesis inhibitors.

eniluracil (ethynyluracil) A chemotherapy drug that increases the effectiveness of fluorouracil.

epirubicin (Ellence) An intravenous antibiotic chemotherapy drug sometimes used to treat ovarian cancer as well as soft tissue sarcoma, non-Hodgkin's lymphoma, and cancers of the breast, stomach, colon or rectum, pancreas, and head or neck.

Epogen See EPOIETIN ALFA.

epoietin (EPO [Epogen, Procrit], epoetin alfa [Eprex]) A colony-stimulating factor that increases the production of red blood cells. Erythropoietin is sometimes used to treat anemia of patients who have nonmyeloid cancer, or who are having chemotherapy. This drug is made by recombinant deoxyribonucleic acid (DNA) technology and is similar to hormones the body makes in the bone marrow to produce blood cells. Erythropoietin can be given by injection. Less common side effects include fever, fatigue, headache, and hives.

etanidazole (Nitrolmidazole) A drug that increases the effectiveness of radiation therapy. Cancer cells are injured more severely by radiation when they have adequate oxygen; this drug mimics oxygen, increasing the damaging effect of radiation. It also inhibits the capacity of cells to repair themselves.

More common side effects include decreased sensations in hands and feet or "pins and needles" feelings. Less common side effects include nausea and vomiting; rarely, this drug may cause a rash or muscle aches.

ethynyluracil (eniluracil)   An anticancer drug that increases the effectiveness of fluorouracil.

Ethyol   See AMIFOSTINE.

etidronate (Didronel)   An orally and intravenously administered drug that belongs to the family of drugs called bisphosphonates. Etidronate is used as treatment for cancer that has spread to the bone. It prevents bone from breaking down. This drug should not be given with milk, which interferes with its absorption.

Rarely, etidronate may cause diarrhea, nausea and vomiting, abdominal pain, or rash.

etoposide (Toposar, Etopophos, VePesid)   An important chemotherapy drug derived from podophyllotoxin that belongs to the family of drugs called mitotic inhibitors. Etoposide is sometimes used to treat uterine cancer as well as lymphomas, acute nonlymphocytic leukemia, hepatoma, rhabdomyosarcoma, Kaposi's sarcoma, and cancers of the testes, lung, and prostate. It can be given either orally or intravenously.

More common side effects include decreased platelet and white blood cell counts (causing increased risk of bleeding and infection), mild nausea and vomiting, appetite loss, taste changes, hair loss, and fetal changes. Less common side effects include constipation or diarrhea, stomach pain, and radiation recall. Rarely, this drug may cause a drop in blood pressure, breathing problems during infusion, rash or itching, heart problems, numbness, fever and chills, or allergic reactions.

exemestane (Aromasin)   An anticancer drug used to decrease estrogen production and suppress the growth of estrogen-dependent tumors.

fentanyl citrate (Actiq)   A narcotic pain medication in the form of a raspberry-flavored lollipop, prescribed for cancer patients whose extreme pain is not controlled by oral narcotics. Pain relief occurs while the patient sucks on (but does not chew) the lollipop and for several hours afterward. The patient should remove the lollipop if the pain is relieved or if a side effect occurs. When unused portions of this lollipop are discarded, it should be wrapped in toilet tissue with the stick removed and flushed down the toilet; it can seriously harm children who mistake it for candy.

This drug binds to opioid receptors in the brain and central nervous system, altering the perception of pain as well as the emotional response. Onset of relief occurs within about five minutes. Patients must be taking opioid drugs in order to take this drug, because it is very strong and can be dangerous if other opioid pain relievers have not been taken for at least a week. This short-acting drug is intended to give relief between doses of long-acting opioid pain relievers. The smallest effective dose should be used to prevent dependence or tolerance.

More common side effects include sleepiness, dizziness, headache, fever, fatigue, and constipation. Less common side effects include breathing problems, cough, sore throat, gait problems, anxiety and confusion, depression, sleeping problems, muscle aches, itching, rash, sweating, nausea and vomiting, appetite loss, or heartburn. Rarely, it may cause bowel rupture as a result of severe constipation, or vision changes.

filgrastim (Neupogen)   A substance that can increase numbers of white blood cells of women receiving chemotherapy. It belongs to the family of drugs called biological response modifiers and is given by injection at least 24 hours after chemotherapy, continuing for up to two weeks. The patient's blood count is monitored twice a week during treatment to determine the drug's effects on her white blood count. Common side effects include bone pain.

flecainide   A drug used to treat abnormal heart rhythms that may also relieve nerve pain—the burning, stabbing, or stinging pain that may arise from damage to nerves caused by some types of cancer or cancer treatment.

floxuridine (FUDR) A chemotherapy drug given as a continuous regional intraarterial infusion. FUDR is currently being studied as an intraperitoneal agent in treating ovarian cancer; however, use of FUDR may cause injuries to the bile duct system that result in death. This drug prevents cells from making deoxyribonucleic acid (DNA) and ribonucleic acid (RNA) by interfering with the synthesis of nucleic acids, disrupting the growth of cancer cells.

More common side effects include appetite loss, diarrhea, and numbness or tingling in hands or feet. Less common side effects include stomach cramps, mouth sores, and bleeding or infection at catheter site. Rarely, it may cause nausea and vomiting, sore throat, swallowing problems, rash and itching, seizures, depression, blurry vision, or decreased platelet and white blood cell counts (causing increased risk of bleeding and infection).

Fluoroplex See 5-FU.

fluorouracil See 5-FU.

5-fluorouracil See 5-FU.

5-Fluracil See 5-FU.

5-FU (5-fluorouracil, fluorouracil [Adrucil]) A standard intravenous (IV) chemotherapy agent that belongs to the family of drugs called antimetabolites, and is sometimes used to treat ovarian cancer. This drug may be administered by infusion over days or months. It prevents cells from making deoxyribonucleic acid (DNA) and ribonucleic acid (RNA) by interfering with the synthesis of nucleic acids, disrupting the growth of cancer cells. 5-FU is a very commonly used drug, often combined with other chemotherapy agents.

More common side effects include decreased platelet and white blood cell counts (causing increased risk of bleeding and infection), nausea and vomiting, mouth sores, thinning of hair, diarrhea, and increased sensitivity to the Sun. Less common side effects include appetite loss, headache, weakness, and muscle aches. Rarely, this drug may cause gait problems, eye irritation, and blurred vision.

Folex See METHOTREXATE.

FUDR See FLOXURIDINE.

gallium nitrate (Ganite, Cytovene) A drug that lowers the level of calcium in the blood. Gallium nitrate is used as treatment for cancer that has spread to the bone, blocking bone breakdown. It is given intravenously as a 24-hour infusion.

Less common side effects include diarrhea, nausea, or constipation. Rarely, this drug may cause kidney damage or vomiting.

Ganite See GALLIUM NITRATE.

G-CSF (granulocyte colony-stimulating factor, [Neupogen], filgrastim) Substance that stimulates the growth of a type of white blood cell (granulocyte) and serves as a growth factor for peripheral blood stem cells.

genistein An isoflavone found in soy products. Soy isoflavones are being studied for their potential to prevent cancer.

granisetron (Kytril) An antinausea drug given to chemotherapy patients to prevent or control nausea and vomiting, administered either intravenously or orally. It belongs to a general class of drugs called serotonin antagonists; it blocks two pathways of serotonin to prevent nausea and vomiting. It binds to the serotonin receptors in the lining of the stomach, preventing the stimulation of the vomiting center in the brain.

Less common side effects include headache, constipation, or diarrhea. Rarely, it may cause fatigue.

hematopoietin-1 See INTERLEUKIN-1.

Herceptin See TRASTUZUMAB.

Hexadrol See DEXAMETHASONE.

Hexalen See ALTRETAMINE.

hexamethylmelamine See ALTRETAMINE.

Hycamtin See TOPOTECAN.

hydromorphone (Dilaudid) A prescription narcotic painkiller that is stronger than heroin and lasts for up to six hours. It can be given to cancer patients in severe pain as either an oral medication, a rectal suppository, or an intramuscular injection. It binds to opioid receptors in the brain, altering the perception of pain as well as the emotional response to it.

More common side effects include constipation, drowsiness, sedation, dizziness, nausea, and dry mouth. Less common side effects include mood changes, euphoria, mental clouding, decreased breathing rate, vomiting, delayed digestion, and decreased heart rate and blood pressure. Rarely, this drug may cause seizures, urination problems, decreased sexual interest, and bowel rupture due to constipation.

hydroxyurea (Hydrea) An oral anticancer drug that belongs to the family of drugs called antimetabolites. Hydroxyurea is sometimes used to treat ovarian cancer as well as chronic myelogenous leukemia and acute leukemia, and cancers of the head, neck, and colon. This drug prevents cells from making DNA and RNA by interfering with the synthesis of nucleic acids, disrupting the growth of cancer cells.

More common side effects include decreased white blood cell count (causing increased risk of infection). Less common side effects include decreased platelet count (causing increased risk of bleeding), fatigue, and fetal changes. Rarely, hydroxyurea may cause nausea and vomiting, mouth sores, diarrhea, confusion, headache, appetite loss, and drowsiness.

ID A combination of the chemotherapy drugs ifosfamide and mesna and doxorubicin (Adriamycin). ID is sometimes used to treat soft tissue sarcoma.

ifosfamide (isophosphamide [Ifex]) An intravenous chemotherapy drug that belongs to the family of drugs called alkylating agents, used to treat ovarian cancer and non-Hodgkin's lymphoma, sarcoma, melanoma, acute lymphocytic leukemia, and cancers of the pancreas, testes, and lungs. Because the drug is very irritating to the bladder, it is combined with mesna to protect the bladder (sometimes called mesna rescue). It works by disrupting the growth of cancer cells, killing them.

More common side effects include nausea and vomiting, hair loss, bladder irritation, kidney function problems, and fetal changes. Less common side effects include decreased white blood cell count (causing increased risk of infection) and pain at the injection site. Rarely, ifosfamide may cause decreased platelet count (causing increased risk of bleeding), fatigue, confusion, dizziness, or fatigue.

indomethacin (Indocin, Indotech) A nonsteroidal anti-inflammatory drug that blocks the synthesis of prostaglandins, preventing pain receptors from passing the pain message to the brain, effectively decreasing pain.

More common side effects include headache, vomiting, tinnitus, tremor, and sleeplessness. Less common side effects include dizziness, depression, fatigue, nausea and appetite loss, heartburn, indigestion, and bleeding from the gastrointestinal tract. Rarely, indomethacin may cause kidney problems; increased heart rate; palpitations; high blood pressure; swelling; rash; itching; decreased platelet, white, and red blood cell counts (causing increased risk of bleeding and infection); allergic reactions; congestive heart failure; chest pain; nightmares; confusion; blurred vision; and hearing loss.

interleukin-1 (IL-1, hematopoietin-1) A type of biological response modifier (a substance that can improve the body's response to infection and disease) produced by a variety of cells, including the natural killer cells, T cells, and B cells. IL-1 stimulates inflammatory immune system cells to fight disease and triggers bone marrow growth. It is normally produced by the body, but it can also be made in the laboratory.

interleukin-2 (aldesleukin [Proleukin], teceleukin, recombinant IL-2 [rIL-2])   A protein produced by activated T cells that stimulates the immune system to kill tumor cells; it also may interfere with blood flow to the tumor. These substances are normally produced by the body. Aldesleukin is a form of interleukin-2 produced in the lab for use in treating cancer; it works by triggering the production of blood cells (especially platelets) during chemotherapy. It belongs to the family of drugs called hematopoietic (blood-forming) agents.

Most patients experience fever and chills within one to four hours after the drug is given. Other common side effects include decreased platelet and white blood cell counts (causing increased risk of bleeding and infection), confusion, depression, abnormal kidney or liver function test results, irritability, low blood pressure, increased heart rate, breathing problems, nausea and vomiting, diarrhea, decreased urine excretion, itching and rash, headache, fatigue, chest pain, or heart attack. Less common side effects include disorientation, mouth sores, memory problems, speech problems, and kidney damage. Rarely, this drug may cause severe breathing problems, irregular heartbeat, fluid in the lungs, and peeling skin.

interleukin-2/TIL (IL-2/TIL)   A new biological therapy combining IL-2 with tumor-infiltrating lymphocyte (TIL) cells to stimulate the immune system to fight cancer. This newer version of IL-2/LAK (lymphokine-activated killer cells) appears to be more effective and is being studied for use with a variety of cancers.

interleukin-3 (multi-CSF)   A type of biological response modifier (a substance that can improve the body's natural response to disease) that enhances the immune system's ability to fight tumor cells and stimulates the growth of many bone marrow cells. Biological response modifiers are normally produced by the body; they are also made in the laboratory for use in treating cancer and other diseases. They help the bone marrow stem cells grow and stimulate the production of white blood cells.

More common side effects include fever, headache, stiff neck, and facial flushing; less common side effects include mild bone pain and swollen feet. Rarely, this drug may cause a drop in blood pressure, rash, or bruising.

interleukin-4 (IL-4, B-cell stimulatory factor-1)   A type of biological response modifier that enhances B-cell growth and the production of antibodies. These substances are normally produced by the body; they are also made in the laboratory for use in treating cancer and other diseases.

interleukin-5 (IL-5, eosinophil CSF)   Biological response modifier that stimulates the production of blood cells called eosinophils, which kill bacteria.

interleukin-6 (IL-6, thrombopoietin)   A type of biological response modifier that can stimulate the body's B-cell growth and production of platelets, improving the natural response to infection and disease. IL-6 is normally produced by the body; it can also be made in the laboratory.

Flulike symptoms are common after this drug is given; patients may experience fever, chills, and a severe headache within one to four hours after administration. Other common side effects include a drop in red blood cell count, with higher risk of anemia. Less common side effects include appetite loss and joint aches; rarely, this drug may cause abnormal liver function test findings.

interleukin-11 (IL-11 oprelvekin [Neumega])   A type of biological response modifier that stimulates immune response and is used to prevent thrombocytopenia (low level of platelets). IL-11 also may reduce toxicity to the gastrointestinal system resulting from cancer therapy. These substances are normally produced by the body; they are also made in the laboratory for use in treating cancer and other diseases.

interleukin-12   A type of biological response modifier (a substance that can improve the body's natural response to disease) that enhances the ability of the immune system to kill tumor cells and may interfere with blood flow to the tumor. Biological response modifiers are normally produced by the body; they are also made in the laboratory for use in treating cancer and other diseases.

iseganan hydrochloride   A substance being studied as a treatment for painful mouth sores caused by chemotherapy. It belongs to the family of drugs called synthetic protegrin analogs.

keyhole limpet hemocyanin   One of a group of drugs called immune modulators given as a vaccine to help the body respond to cancer.

Kytril   See GRANISETRON.

Leukeran   See CHLORAMBUCIL.

Levo-Dromoran   See LEVORPHANOL.

levorphanol (Levo-Dromoran)   A narcotic injectible and oral drug, similar to morphine, used to control pain by binding to receptors in the brain so that the perception of pain is muted. More common side effects include constipation, drowsiness, sedation, nausea, and dry mouth. Less common side effects include mood changes, euphoria, depression, mental clouding, drop in breathing rate, vomiting, and decreased blood pressure and heart rate. Rarely, this drug may cause urination problems, facial flushing, itching, sweating, decreased sexual interest, and bowel rupture due to constipation.

L-phenylalanine mustard (Alkeran)   An oral alkylating chemotherapy drug sometimes used to treat ovarian cancer, breast cancer, or myeloma.

L-sarcolysin   See L-PHENYLALANINE MUSTARD.

Marinol   See DRONABINOL.

medroxyprogesterone (Provera, Depo-Provera)   A female sex hormone that has sometimes been used to treat endometrial cancer.

MEG   See MEGESTROL.

Megace   See MEGESTROL.

megestrol (Megace, MEG, Pallace)   A hormonal type of oral chemotherapy sometimes used to treat uterine cancer as well as cancers of the breast or kidney. It is often used in higher dosages to increase appetite. It is unclear how this drug stops cancer cells from growing; it appears to compete for certain receptor sites on the cell.

More common side effects include fluid retention; rarely, this drug may cause nausea or blood clots in legs or lungs.

meperidine (Demerol)   A strong narcotic used to treat severe pain for a short period (between two and three hours). For this reason, it is not given for chronic pain, but instead for occasional episodes of pain after surgery.

More common side effects include constipation, sedation, nausea and vomiting, dizziness, and dry mouth. Less common side effects include mood changes, including euphoria and mental clouding; and decreased breathing rate, blood pressure, and heart rate. Rarely, this drug may cause urination problems, seizures, and lack of sexual interest. Patients should drink fluids every hour to prevent constipation.

methotrexate (amethopterin [Mexate, Folex])   An important antimetabolite chemotherapy drug sometimes used to treat cervical cancer as well as cancers of the breast, head and neck, colon, lung, and testes, and acute leukemia, sarcoma, lymphoma, and mycosis fungoides. This drug can be administered intravenously or orally. Methotrexate prevents cells from making DNA and RNA by interfering with the synthesis of nucleic acids, disrupting the growth of cancer cells.

More common side effects include nausea and vomiting at high dosages, mouth sores, diarrhea, increased sunburn risk, radiation recall, and appetite loss. Less common side effects include decreased platelet and white blood cell counts (causing increased risk of bleeding and infection) and kidney damage at high dosages. Rarely, methotrexate may cause liver toxicity, lung collapse at high dosages, hair loss, rash or itching, dizziness, and blurred vision. Drinking alcohol while using the drug can increase the risk of liver damage.

metoclopramide (Reglan) An antinausea drug that may be given to chemotherapy patients before treatment to prevent nausea and vomiting, either intravenously or orally. When given in low dosages, it increases stomach emptying so that there is less chance of nausea and vomiting due to food in the stomach. At high dosages it blocks the messages to the part of the brain responsible for nausea and vomiting.

More common side effects include sedation, sleepiness, diarrhea, or dry mouth. Rarely, it may cause rash, hives, or a drop in blood pressure. Metoclopramide may have extrapyramidal side effects, which include restlessness, tongue protrusion, and involuntary movements, which stop when the patient is given diphenhydramine.

Mexate See METHOTREXATE.

mifepristone (RU486) A French abortion drug that is currently being studied as a possible chemotherapy drug to treat ovarian cancer as well as metastatic breast cancer, some brain tumors, and prostate cancer.

Mithracin See PLICAMYCIN.

mithramycin See PLICAMYCIN.

mitomycin (Mutamycin) An intravenous chemotherapy drug that is an antibiotic but acts as an alkylating agent. It is used to treat cervical cancer, as well as cancers of the breast, stomach, colon, pancreas, and bladder.

More common side effects include decreased platelet and white blood cell counts (causing increased risk of bleeding and infection), nausea and vomiting, appetite loss, fatigue and hair loss; mitomycin use may lead to the destruction of red blood cells (hemolysis), which can be fatal. Less common side effects include mouth sores; rarely, mitomycin may cause lung inflammation and kidney damage.

MTX See METHOTREXATE.

multi-CSF See INTERLEUKIN-3.

Mutamycin See MITOMYCIN.

MYX See METHOTREXATE.

neocarzinostatin (Zinostatin) An experimental intravenous drug used to prevent the onset of a heart muscle condition known as doxorubicin cardiomyopathy, which is linked to treatment with Adriamycin.

Neosar See CYCLOPHOSPHAMIDE.

Neumega See INTERLEUKIN-11.

Neupogen See G-CSF.

Oncovin See VINCRISTINE.

ondansetron (Zofran) A drug especially helpful for patients who are taking cisplatin, because it dramatically reduces nausea and vomiting. This drug blocks the serotonin pathway by which chemotherapy stimulates the vomiting center in the brain. It is given immediately before intravenous chemotherapy or within an hour of orally administered chemotherapy. Occasionally ondansetron may cause diarrhea, constipation, or headache.

oxaliplatin This experimental alkylating agent is being studied as a treatment for ovarian cancer as well as colon or breast cancer. It is given intravenously over one hour or as a continuous infusion.

More common side effects include nausea and vomiting, numbness of lips, or nerve toxicity. Less common side effects include walking problems or decreased platelet and white blood cell counts (causing increased risk of bleeding and infection).

oxycodone (Percodan, Percocet, Endodan, Oxy-Contin) A prescription narcotic drug used to ease moderate to severe pain that is given either orally or by injection. It binds to opioid receptors in the brain, altering the perception of pain and the emotional response to it. This drug may cause constipation, drowsiness or sedation, nausea, dizziness, or dry mouth. Less common side effects include vomiting, depression, euphoria, mental clouding, decreased breathing and heart rates, and a drop in blood pressure.

PAC   A combination of the chemotherapy drugs Platinol (cisplatin), Adriamycin (doxorubicin), and Cytoxan (cyclophosphamide) sometimes used to treat ovarian cancer.

Pallace   See MEGESTROL.

Paraplatin   See CARBOPLATIN.

Percodan   See OXYCODONE.

Phenoxodiol   A synthetic anticancer drug that has been found in laboratory studies to induce cell death in 100 percent of ovarian cancer cells, including those cells resistant to conventional agents such as paclitaxel and carboplatin. A Phase II trial using phenoxodiol is under way at Yale University for women who have chemoresistant ovarian cancer. Five Phase I human trials with phenoxodiol are complete and show few, if any, side effects. Preliminary results of a trial conducted at the Cleveland Clinic found that more than half of the 10 patients tested on the experimental drug showed some response. All of these patients had different types of advanced cancer that did not respond to chemotherapy.

Phenoxodiol is the first in a new class of chemotherapy drugs known as multiple signal transduction regulators (MSTRs). Under U.S. law, a new drug cannot be marketed until it has been investigated in clinical trials. After the results of these trials are submitted in an Investigational New Drug application to the U.S. Food and Drug Administration (FDA), the FDA must approve the drug as safe and effective before it can be sold.

Platinol   See CISPLATIN.

platinum   See CISPLATIN.

plicamycin (mithramycin, Mithracin)   An antibiotic chemotherapy drug administered occasionally as a means of lowering calcium level in patients with hypercalcemia, which occurs in a number of cancers. More common side effects include nausea and vomiting, hair loss, appetite loss, mouth sores, and decreased platelet and white blood cell counts (causing increased risk of bleeding and infection). Less common side effects include fetal changes.

prochlorperazine (Compazine)   A drug commonly prescribed for chemotherapy patients to control severe nausea and vomiting. Prochlorperazine works by blocking messages to the part of the brain responsible for these side effects. It can be given intravenously or orally.

More common side effects of this drug include dry mouth, constipation, sedation, and sleepiness. Less common side effects include blurred vision, restlessness, involuntary muscle movements, tremor, increased appetite, weight gain, increased heart rate, and decreased blood pressure. Rarely, prochlorperazine may cause jaundice, rash, or hives, and increased sensitivity to sunlight.

Proleukin   See INTERLEUKIN-2.

RU486   See MIFEPRISTONE.

sargramostim (Leukine)   A protein cytokine that belongs to the general class of synthetic substances called biological response modifiers, used to prevent fever or infection caused by low white blood cell counts after chemotherapy. It is given intravenously over two hours or as an injection and often causes flulike symptoms including fever, chills, fatigue, headache, and muscle aches. Less common symptoms include facial flushing or rash. Rarely, sargramostim causes breathing problems, swollen feet, and weight gain.

suramin   A drug currently used to treat certain infections that is being studied as a possible chemotherapy drug against ovarian cancer as well as cancers of the lung, bladder, and prostate. Many studies are currently assessing the usefulness of this drug in combination with other chemotherapy drugs.

teceleukin   See INTERLEUKIN-2.

teniposide (VM-26, Vumon)   An intravenous chemotherapy drug that is a plant alkaloid and topoisomerase inhibitor. It is being studied for use against ovarian cancer as well as cancers of the bladder, brain, breast, lung, and kidney. It works by disrupting and killing cancer cells.

More common side effects include decreased platelet and white blood cell counts (causing increased risk of bleeding and infection); less common side effects include nausea and vomiting, numbness and tingling, drop in blood pressure, and fetal changes. Rarely, teniposide may cause an allergic reaction, hair loss, mouth sores, or abnormal liver function test results.

thiotepa (TSPA, triethylenethiophosphoramide)   An injectable alkylating chemotherapy drug sometimes used to treat ovarian cancer as well as Hodgkin's disease or cancers of the breast and bladder. It works by disrupting and killing cancer cells.

More common side effects include decreased platelet and white blood cell counts (causing increased risk of bleeding and infection), nausea and vomiting, and stopping of menstruation. Less common side effects include fatigue, dizziness, headache, and fever. Rarely, thiotepa may cause appetite loss or allergic reaction; very rarely it can induce certain types of cancer, such as leukemia.

thrombopoietin   See INTERLEUKIN-6.

TOPO   See TOPOTECAN.

Toposar   See ETOPOSIDE.

topotecan hydrochloride (Hycamtin)   An intravenous chemotherapy drug derived from the bark of the Chinese *Camptotheca acuminata* tree used to treat metastatic ovarian cancer that has not responded to other drugs. This drug disrupts the growth of cancer cells by preventing the development of certain elements necessary for cell division.

More common side effects include decreased platelet and white blood cell counts (causing increased risk of bleeding and infection), severe anemia, fatigue, nausea and vomiting, diarrhea or constipation, and abdominal pain.

TPT   See TOPOTECAN.

trastuzumab (Herceptin)   An intravenous monoclonal antibody genetically engineered to attack the protein generated by the *HER-2/neu* gene, studied in combination with taxol to treat advanced ovarian cancer. Herceptin works best in the 20 percent of ovarian cancer patients whose tumors show high levels of this gene.

Trastuzumab often can cause an allergic reaction, with fever and chills. Rarely, it may cause a severe allergic reaction, generalized pain, breathing problems, abdominal pain, fatigue, nausea and vomiting, diarrhea, or liver failure.

VePesid   See ETOPOSIDE.

vincristine (Oncovin)   An intravenous chemotherapy drug sometimes used to treat cervical cancer as well as cancers of the brain, breast, and testes, and lymphoma, acute leukemia, Wilm's tumor, neuroblastoma, and rhabdomyosarcoma. Vincristine, derived from the periwinkle plant, disrupts and kills cancer cells.

This drug can cause constipation, hair loss and numbness or tingling. Less common side effects include weakness, muscle aches, cramping, and stomach pain. Rarely, vincristine can cause double vision, depression, taste changes, decreased platelet and white blood cell counts (causing increased risk of bleeding and infection), jaw pain, and headache.

Vumon   See TENIPOSIDE.

Zinecard   See DEXRAZOXANE.

zinostatin   See NEOCARZINOSTATIN.

Zofran   See ONDANSETRON.

Zyloprim   See ALLOPURINOL SODIUM.

GLOSSARY

ablative therapy   A treatment that removes or destroys the function of an organ, such as removal of the ovaries.

action studies   In cancer prevention clinical trials, studies that focus on finding out whether actions people take can prevent cancer.

adjuvant therapy   Treatment given after the primary treatment to increase the chance of a cure. Adjuvant therapy may include chemotherapy, radiation therapy, hormone therapy, or biological therapy.

agonists   Drugs that trigger an action from a cell or another drug.

agranulocyte   A type of white blood cell that includes monocytes and lymphocytes.

alkylating agent   A type of chemotherapy drug that works directly on DNA to prevent a cancer cell from reproducing at all phases of a cell's life. These drugs are used to treat ovarian cancer, among others.

allogeneic   Originating from another person.

anaplastic   A characteristic of cancer cells of dividing rapidly and bearing little or no resemblance to normal cells.

anemia   Low red blood cell count.

antibody   A protein in the blood that fights against an invading foreign agent (antigen). Each antibody bonds to a particular antigen.

antiemetic   Drug that prevents or eases nausea and vomiting.

antigen   A protein marker on the surface of a cell that identifies the cell.

antimetabolites   A class of drugs that interfere with DNA and RNA growth and are used to treat ovarian cancer, among others.

antitumor antibiotics   Drugs that kill bacteria and cells and interfere with DNA by inhibiting enzymes and altering cellular membranes. They are used to treat a wide variety of cancers.

apoptosis   Programmed cell death. Apoptosis is a normal part of cellular function, and is vital for proper cellular development, since programmed cell death can destroy cells that represent a threat to cellular integrity.

autologous   Originating from the same person.

axillary   Related to the armpit.

B cell   White blood cell that makes antibodies and is an important part of the immune system. The B cell is from bone marrow. Also called B lymphocyte.

biological response modifier   A natural substance, such as interferon, that can boost the body's immune system to fight cancer. These substances are often produced in the laboratory. Use of these drugs is also called biological therapy.

blood count   Total number of red and white blood cells in a given sample of blood.

B lymphocytes   See **B cell.**

cachexia   Severe malnutrition, emaciation, and debility, sometimes seen in cancer patients.

carcinoma   Cancer that begins in the tissues that line or cover an organ.

cell   The basic structural unit of all life. All living matter is composed of cells.

cervix   The lower, narrow end of the uterus that forms a canal between the uterus and vagina.

chromosome   Part of a cell that contains genetic information. Except the sperm and egg, every human cell contains 46 chromosomes.

coenzyme   A substance needed for the proper functioning of an enzyme.

colony-stimulating factors   Biological products (including erythropoietin, granulocyte colony-stimulating factor [G-CSF], and granulocyte-macrocyte CSF [GM-CSF]) that stimulate the growth of normal blood cells. CSFs are naturally produced in the body, but extra CSF may be given to ease or prevent side effects of chemotherapy.

cyst   An abnormal, saclike structure that contains liquid or semisolid material. A cyst may be benign or malignant.

cytokines   A class of substances produced by immune system cells that affect the immune response and that may cause regression of certain cancers. Cytokines can also be produced in the laboratory.

cytopenia   A reduction in the number of blood cells.

cytotoxic   Cell-killing.

differentiation   The extent of development of the cancer cells in a tumor. Differentiated tumor cells resemble normal cells and grow at a slower rate than undifferentiated tumor cells, which lack the structure and function of normal cells and grow uncontrollably.

diploid   The characteristic of having two sets of chromosomes in a cell.

DNA   One of two nucleic acids (the other is RNA) found in the nucleus of all cells. DNA contains genetic information on cell growth, division, and function.

drug resistance   The ability of cells to become resistant to the effects of chemotherapy drugs used to treat cancer.

dysplasia   Abnormal cells, usually atypical cells on the cervix.

endocrine glands   Glands that manufacture and secrete hormones into the blood. Endocrine glands include the pituitary, thyroid, parathyroid, adrenal, ovary and testes, placenta, and part of the pancreas.

endometrium   The lining of the uterus.

enzyme   A protein that promotes essential functions involved in cell growth and metabolism.

eosinophil   Type of white blood cell.

epithelium   A thin layer of tissue that covers organs, glands, and other structures in the body.

estrogen   Hormone that acts on the female reproductive tract.

estrogen receptor   A protein on some cells that attaches to the estrogen hormone. A tumor that is estrogen receptor positive has this protein on its cells and requires estrogen for its growth.

gene   A unit of heredity. Located in the nucleus of the cell, genes contain hereditary information that is transferred from cell to cell, and passed on from parent to child. Genes are series of ordered nucleotides located in a particular position on a chromosome.

granulocyte   A type of white blood cell that fights bacterial infection. Neutrophils, eosinophils, and basophils are granulocytes.

growth factors   Naturally occurring proteins that make cells grow and divide. Cancer cells that produce too much growth factor grow wildly; new treatments to block these growth factors are being tested. Other growth factors help normal cells recover from chemotherapy.

hemoglobin   A protein in red blood cells that carries oxygen from the lungs to the body's tissues.

hormone therapy   Treatment with hormones or with drugs that interfere with hormones to kill cancer cells or slow their growth.

hypercalcemia   An excessive level of calcium in the blood, which can lead to weakness, confusion, and heart rhythm dysfunction. This syndrome requires immediate medical attention.

hypoxia   A lack of oxygen to the tissues of the body.

hysteroscope   A lighted device that can be inserted through the cervix to visualize the inside of the uterus.

immunotherapy   Treatment that entails use of biological response modifiers to strengthen the body's immune system.

in situ   Presence of cancerous cells in the lining of an organ without any spreading to the interior of the tissue.

intraperitoneal chemotherapy   Administration of chemotherapy through a catheter into the space around the abdominal organs to bathe the tissues.

killer cells   White blood cells that attack tumor cells and body cells that have been invaded by foreign substances.

leukocytes   A white blood cell that does not contain hemoglobin. White blood cells include lymphocytes, neutrophils, eosinophils, macrophages, and mast cells, all of which are produced by bone marrow and help the body fight infection.

leukopenia Decrease in white blood cell count that often occurs during chemotherapy.

lymph The clear fluid of the lymphatic system through which cells travel as they fight infection and disease.

lymphocyte A type of white blood cell that helps produce antibodies and other substances that fight infection and diseases.

malignant ascites A condition in which fluid containing cancer cells collects in the abdomen.

mast cell A type of white blood cell.

metastasis Cancer that has spread from the site of origin to another part of the body, usually through the lymphatic system or the blood.

mitotic inhibitors Natural plant alkaloids that can inhibit cellular division or inhibit enzymes that prevent protein synthesis needed for cell reproduction.

monoclonal antibodies Substances produced in the lab that can locate and bind to cancer cells wherever they are in the body. Many monoclonal antibodies are used in cancer diagnosis or treatment. Each recognizes a different protein on certain cancer cells. Monoclonal antibodies can be used alone, or they can be used to deliver drugs, toxins, or radioactive material directly to a tumor.

monocyte A type of white blood cell.

myeloid Derived from or pertaining to bone marrow.

myometrium The muscular outer layer of the uterus.

natural killer cells (NK cells) White blood cells that can kill tumor cells and infected body cells. NK cells kill on contact by binding to the target cell and releasing a burst of toxic chemicals. Normal cells are not affected by NK cells, which play a major role in cancer prevention by destroying abnormal cells before they can become dangerous.

necrosis Tissue death.

neoplasm A new growth of tissue serving no physiological function.

neutrophil A type of white blood cell.

nodule A small, solid lump that can be detected by touch. This term usually refers to a lump that is malignant, although it may refer to one that is benign.

omentum The thin tissue covering the stomach and large intestine.

parathyroid glands Four pea-sized glands on the thyroid that produce parathyroid hormone, which increases calcium level in the blood.

peptide Any compound consisting of two or more amino acids, the building blocks of proteins.

peritoneal cavity The space within the abdomen that contains the intestines, the stomach, and the liver. It is bound by thin membranes.

peritoneum The tissue that lines the abdominal wall and covers most of the organs in the abdomen.

plasma The clear, yellowish fluid part of the blood that carries the blood cells.

platelets Blood cells that help prevent bleeding by causing formation of blood clots. Chemotherapy can cause a drop in platelets count and an increased risk of excess bleeding.

pleural cavity A space enclosed by the pleura (thin tissue covering the lungs and lining the interior wall of the chest cavity).

polyp A growth that protrudes from a mucous membrane.

precancerous Also called premalignant, an abnormal change in cells, indicating the potential for development of cancer.

protein A molecule made up of amino acid chains that the body needs for proper function. Proteins form the structure of skin, hair, enzymes, cytokines, and antibodies.

radiation sensitizer Chemical that makes a cell more susceptible to the effects of radiation therapy.

radioisotope An unstable element that releases radiation as it breaks down. Radioisotopes can be used in imaging tests and in cancer treatment.

receptor A molecule inside or on the surface of a cell that binds to a specific substance.

red blood cell A cell (also called an erythrocyte) that carries oxygen to all parts of the body.

regional involvement The spread of cancer from its original site to nearby areas.

serum The clear liquid part of the blood that remains after blood cells and clotting proteins have been removed.

stem cells Cells from which other types of cells can develop.

supraclavicular nodes The lymph nodes located above the collar bone in the area of the neck.

systemic Affecting the whole body.

T cell A type of white blood cell that attacks invaders such as cancer cells and that produces substances that regulate the immune response.

thyroid gland A gland located beneath the larynx that produces thyroid hormone and that helps regulate growth and metabolism.

white blood cell A blood cell, including lymphocytes, neutrophils, eosinophils, macrophages, and mast cells, that does not contain hemoglobin. These cells are made by bone marrow and help the body fight infection and disease.

BIBLIOGRAPHY

Abramova L., et al. "Sentinel Node Biopsy in Vulvar and Vagina Melanoma: Presentation of Six Cases and a Literature Review." *Annals of Surgical Oncology* 9, no. 9 (November 2002): 840–846.

Adami, H. O., et al. "Absence of Association between Reproductive Variables and the Risk of Breast Cancer in Young Women in Sweden and Norway." *British Journal of Cancer* 62 (1990): 122–126.

Adjetey, V., R. Ganesan, and G. P. Downey. "Primary Vaginal Endometrioid Carcinoma following Unopposed Estrogen Administration." *Journal of Obstetrics and Gynecology* 23, no. 3 (May 2003): 316–317.

Adlercreutz, H., et al. "Estrogen Excretion Patterns and Plasma Levels in Vegetarian and Omniverous Women." *New England Journal of Medicine* no. 307 (1982): 1,542–1,547.

Ah Lee, S., et al. "Multiple HPV Infection in Cervical Cancer Screened by HPVDNA Chip." *Cancer Letter* 198, no. 2 (August 2003): 187–192.

Albertazzi, P., et al. "Dietary Soy Supplementation and Phytoestrogen Levels." *Obstetrics and Gynecology* 94 (1999): 229–231.

Altman, R., and M. J. Sarg. *The Cancer Dictionary.* New York: Facts On File, 2000.

Ambrosone, C. B., et al. "Breast Cancer Risk, Meat Consumption, and N-acetyltransferase Genetic Polymorphisms." *International Journal of Cancer* 75 (1998): 30.

Anderson, J. J. B., and S. C. Garner. "Phytoestrogens and Human Function." *Nutrition Today* 32 (1997): 39.

Ardies, C. M., and C. Dee. "Xenoestrogens Significantly Enhance Risk for Breast Cancer during Growth and Adolescence." *Medical Hypotheses* 50 (1998): 457–464.

Armstrong, B. K., et al. "Diet and Reproductive Hormones: A Study of Vegetarian and Nonvegetarian Postmenopausal Women." *Journal of the National Cancer Institute* no. 67 (1981): 761–767.

Armstrong, C., C. Stern, and B. Corn. "Memory Performance Used to Detect Radiation Effects on Cognitive Functioning." *Applied Neuropsychology* 8 (2001): 129–139.

Atallah, D., G. Chahine, and I. A. Voutsadakis. "Brain Metastasis from Ovarian Cancer." *Journal of Clinical Oncology* 21, no. 15 (August 1, 2003): 2,996–2,998.

Austin H., C. Drews, and E. E. Partridge "A Case-control Study of Endometrial Cancer in Relation to Cigarette Smoking, Serum Estrogen Levels, and Alcohol Use." *American Journal of Obstetrics and Gynecology* 169 (1993): 1,086–1,091.

Barnes, M. N., et al. "Paradigms for Primary Prevention of Ovarian Carcinoma." *CA: Cancer Journal for Clinicians* 52 (2002): 216–225.

Beeson, W. L., et al. "Cancer Incidence among California Seventh-Day Adventists 1976–1982." *American Journal of Clinical Nutrition* 59 (1994): 1,136S–1,142S.

Berman, M. L., et al. "Reproductive, Menstrual and Medical Risk Factors for Endometrial Cancer: Results from a Case-control Study." *American Journal of Obstetrics and Gynecology* 167 (1993): 1,317–1,325.

Bingham, S. A., et al. "Phyto-oestrogens: Where Are We Now?" *British Journal of Nutrition* no. 79 (1998): 393–406.

Bocciolone, L., et al. "The Epidemiology of Endometrial Cancer." *Gynecologic Oncology* 41 (1991): 1–16.

Boran, N., F. Kayikcioglu, and M. Kir. "Sentinel Lymph Node Procedure in Early Vulvar Cancer." *Gynecologic Oncology* 90, no. 2 (August 2003): 492–493.

Bouker, K. B., and L. Hilakivi-Clarke. "Genistein: Does It Prevent or Promote Breast Cancer?" *Environmental Health Perspectives* no. 108 (2000): 701–708.

Bowlin, S. J., et al. "Breast Cancer Risk and Alcohol Consumption: Results from a Large Case-control Study." *International Journal of Epidemiology* 26 (1997): 915–923.

Braga, C., et al. "Intake of Selected Foods and Nutrients and Breast Cancer Risk: An Age- and Menopause-specific Analysis." *Nutrition and Cancer* 28 (1997): 258–263.

Brekelmans, C. T., et al. "Rotterdam Committee for Medical and Genetic Counseling: Effectiveness of Breast Cancer Surveillance in *BRCA1/2* Gene Mutation Carriers and Women with High Familial Risk." *Journal of Clinical Oncology* 19, no. 4 (2001): 924–930.

Brown, S., and L. Degner. "Delirium in the Terminally Ill Cancer Patient: Aetiology, Symptoms and Management." *International Journal of Palliative Nursing* 7 (2001): 266–272.

Calle, E. E., et al. "Estrogen Replacement Therapy and Ovarian Cancer Mortality in a Large Prospective Study of U.S. Women." *Journal of the American Medical Association* 185, no. 11 (March 2001): 1,460–1,465.

Cedars-Sinai Medical Center. "Possible Effects of Plant Compounds on Uterus." Media Advisory (July 31, 1999).

Chang, S., and H. A. Risch. "Perineal Talc Exposure and Risk of Ovarian Carcinoma." *Cancer* 79, no. 12 (June 15, 1997): 2,396–2,401.

Chang, Hsueh-Wei. "Assessment of Plasma DNA Levels, Allelic Imbalance, and CA125 as Diagnostic Tests for Cancer." *Journal of the National Cancer Institute* 94/22 (November 20, 2002): 1,697–1,703.

Cox, J. T. "The Clinician's View: Role of Human Papillomavirus Testing in the American Society for Colposcopy and Cervical Pathology Guidelines for the Management of Abnormal Cervical Cytology and Cervical Cancer Precursors." *Archives of Pathology and Laboratory Medicine* 127, no. 8 (August 2003): 950–958.

Cramer, D. W., et al. "Genital Talc Exposure and Risk of Ovarian Cancer." *International Journal of Cancer* 81, no. 3 (May 5, 1999): 351–356.

Cryns P., N. J. Roofthooft, and W. A. Tjalma. "Ovarian Sex Cord-stromal Tumors in Children and Adolescents." *Journal of Clinical Oncology* 15, no. 21 (June 12, 2003): 2,357ff.

Daling, J. R., et al. "The Relationship of Human Papillomavirus-related Cervical Tumors to Cigarette Smoking, Oral Contraceptive Use, and Prior Herpes Simplex Virus Type 2 Infection." *Cancer Epidemiology, Biomarkers, and Prevention* 5, no. 7 (1996): 541–548.

D'Avanzo, B., et al. "Alcohol and Endometrial Cancer Risk: Findings from an Italian Case-control Study." *Nutritional Cancer* 23 (1995): 55–62.

Davidson, E. J., et al. "Human Papillomavirus Type 16 E2- and L1-specific Serological and T-cell Responses in Women with Vulval Intraepithelial Neoplasia." *Journal of General Virology* 84, pt. 8 (August 2003): 2,089–2,097.

Decarli, A., et al. "Nutrition and Diet in the Etiology of Endometrial Cancer." *Cancer* 57 (1986): 1,248–1,253.

Duenas-Gonzalez, A., et al. "Modern Management of Locally Advanced Cervical Carcinoma." *Cancer Treat Review* 29, no. 5 (October 2003): 389–399.

Elit, L. "Familial Ovarian Cancer." *Canadian Family Physician* 47 (April 2001): 778–784.

Fiorica, J. V. "The Role of Topotecan in the Treatment of Advanced Cervical Cancer." *Gynecologic Oncology* 90, no. 3, pt. 2 (September 2003): S16–S21.

Folsom, A. R., et al. "Association of Incident Carcinoma of the Endometrium with Body Weight and Fat Distribution in Older Women: Early Findings of the Iowa Women's Health Study." *Cancer Research* 49 (1989): 6,828–6,831.

Foth, D., and M. J. Cline. "Effects of Mammalian and Plant Estrogens on Mammary Glands and Uteri of Macaques." *American Journal of Clinical Nutrition* no. 68 (1998): 1,413S–1,417S.

Frank, T. S. "Testing for Hereditary Risk of Ovarian Cancer." *Cancer Control* 6, no. 4 (July 1999): 327–334.

Frank, S. J., et al. "Definitive Treatment of Vaginal Cancer with Radiation Therapy." *International Journal of Radiation Oncology and Biological Physics* 57 (suppl. 2) (October 2003): S194.

Gapstur, S. M., et al. "Alcohol Consumption and Postmenopausal Endometrial Cancer: Results from the Iowa Women's Health Study." *Cancer Control* 4 (1993): 323–329.

Gavaler, J. S. "Protective Effect of Alcohol against Endometrial Cancer." *Lancet* 2, no. 983 (1983): 627.

Goldin, B., et al. "The Effect of a Low Fat Diet on Estrogen Metabolism." *Journal of Clinical Endocrinology and Metabolism* 64 (1987): 1,246–1,250.

Goodman, M. T., et al. "Association of Soy and Fiber Consumption with the Risk of Endometrial Cancer." *American Journal of Epidemiology* no. 146 (1997): 294–306.

Grady, D., et al. "Cardiovascular Disease Outcomes During 6.8 Years of Hormone Therapy: Heart and Estrogen/Progestin Replacement Study Follow-up (HERS II)." *Journal of the American Medical Association* no. 288 (2002): 49–57.

Gray, S., and O. I. Olopade. "Direct-to-consumer Marketing of Genetic Tests for Cancer: Buyer Beware." *Journal of Clinical Oncology* no. 21 (2003): 3,191–3,193.

Hammes, B., and C. J. Laitman. "Diethylstilbestrol (DES) Update: Recommendations for the Identification and Management of DES-exposed Individuals." *Journal of Midwifery and Women's Health* 48, no. 1 (January–February 2003): 19–29.

Hartge, P., et al. "Rates and Risks of Ovarian Cancer in Subgroups of White Women in the United States." The Collaborative Ovarian Cancer Group. *Obstetrics and Gynecology* 84, no. 5 (November 1994): 760–764.

Hertel, H., et al. "Laparoscopic-assisted Radical Vaginal Hysterectomy (LARVH): Prospective Evaluation of 200 Patients with Cervical Cancer." *Gynecologic Oncology* 90, no. 3 (September 2003): 505–511.

Herzog, T. J. "New Approaches for the Management of Cervical Cancer." *Gynecologic Oncology* 90, no. 3 (pt. 2) (September 2003): S22–S27.

Holschneider C. H., and J. S. Berek. "Ovarian Cancer: Epidemiology, Biology, and Prognostic Factors." *Seminar in Surgical Oncology* 19, no. 1 (July–August 2000): 3–10.

Hulley, S., et al. "Noncardiovascular Disease Outcomes During 6.8 Years of Hormone Therapy: Heart and Estrogen/Progestin Replacement Study Follow-up (HERS II)." *Journal of the American Medical Association* 288 (2002): 58–66.

Kalandidi, A., et al. "Case-control Study of Endometrial Cancer in Relation to Reproductive, Omatometric, and Life-style Variables." *Oncology* 53 (1996): 354–359.

Kaminski, J. M., et al. "Primary Small Cell Carcinoma of the Vagina." *Gynecologic Oncology* 88, no. 3 (March 2003): 451–455.

Kattlove, H., and R. J. Winn. "Ongoing Care of Patients after Primary Treatment for Their Cancer." *CA: A Cancer Journal for Clinicians* 53 (2003): 172–196.

Kauff, N. D., et al. "Risk-reducing Salpingo-oophorectomy in Women with a *BRCA1* or *BRCA2* Mutation." *New England Journal of Medicine* 346, no. 21 (May 23, 2002): 1,609–1,615.

Lacey, J. V., et al. "Menopausal Hormone Replacement Therapy and Risk of Ovarian Cancer." *Journal of the American Medical Association* 288 (2002): 334–341.

Lantz, P., et al. "Implementing Women's Cancer Screening Programs in American Indian and Alaska Native Populations." *Health Care Women International* 24, no. 8 (September 2003): 674–696.

Lawlor, P. "The Panorama of Opioid-related Cognitive Dysfunction in Patients with Cancer: A Critical Literature Appraisal." *Cancer* no. 94 (2002): 1,836–1,863.

Leiserowitz, G. S., et al. "Endometriosis-related Malignancies." *International Journal of Gynecologic Cancer* 13, no. 4 (July–August 2003): 466–471.

Levi, F., et al. "Dietary Factors and the Risk of Endometrial Cancer." *Cancer* no. 71 (1983): 3,575–3,581.

Long, H. J., et al. "Long-term Survival of Patients with Advanced/Recurrent Carcinoma of Cervix and Vagina after Neoadjuvant Treatment with Methotrexate, Vinblastine, Doxorubicin, and Cisplatin with or without the Addition of Molgramostim, and Review of the Literature." *American Journal of Clinical Oncology* 25, no. 6 (December 2002): 547–551.

Lynch, H. T., J. A. Ens, and J. F. Lynch. "The Lynch Syndrome II and Urological Malignancies." *Journal of Urology* 143, no. 1 (January 1990): 24–28.

Martin, A. M., et al. "Germline Mutation in *BRCA1* and *BRCA2* in Breast-Ovarian Families from a Breast Cancer Risk Evaluation Clinic." *Journal of Clinical Oncology* 19, no. 8 (April 15, 2001): 2,247–2,253.

McGinn, K. A., and P. J. Haylock. *Women's Cancers: How to Prevent Them, How To Treat Them, How To Beat Them.* Alameda, Calif.: Hunter House, 1998.

Meijers-Heijboer, H., C. T. M. Brekelmans, and M. Menke-Pluymers. "Use of Genetic Testing and Prophylactic Mastectomy and Oophorectomy in Women with Breast or Ovarian Cancer from Families with a *BRCA1* or *BRCA2* Mutation." *Journal of Clinical Oncology* no. 21 (2003): 1,675–1,681.

Menczer, J., et al. "Frequency of BRCA Mutations in Primary Peritoneal Carcinoma in Israeli Jewish women." *Gynecologic Oncology* 88, no. 1 (January 2003): 58–61.

Mirhashemi, R., et al. "Papillary Squamous Cell Carcinoma of the Uterine Cervix: An Immunophenotypic Appraisal of 12 Cases." *Gynecologic Oncology* 90, no. 3 (September 2003): 657–661.

Modan, B., et al. "Oral Contraceptives, and the Risk of Ovarian Cancer among Carriers and Noncarriers of a *BRCA1* or *BRCA2* Mutation." *New England Journal of Medicine* 345, no. 4 (July 26, 2001): 235–240.

Mohamed, A. A., and S. D. Sharma. "Fallopian Tube Hydatidiform Mole." *Journal of Obstetrics and Gynaecology* 23, no. 3 (May 2003): 330–331.

Moslehi, R., et al. "Oral Contraceptives and Hereditary Ovarian Cancer." *New England Journal of Medicine* 340, no. 1 (January 7, 1999): 59.

Mullineaux, L., et al. "Impact of *BRCA-1* Testing on Women with Cancer: A Pilot Study." *Genetic Testing* 4, no. 3 (2000): 265–272.

Narod, S. A. "Oral Contraceptives and the Risk of Ovarian Cancer." *New England Journal of Medicine* 339 (1998): 424–428.

Narod S. A., et al. "Oral Contraceptives and Hereditary Ovarian Cancer." *New England Journal of Medicine* 340, no. 1 (January 7, 1999): 59.

Neto, A. G., et al. "Metastatic Tumors of the Vulva: A Clinicopathologic Study of 66 Cases." *American Journal of Surgical Pathology* 27, no. 6 (June 2003): 799–804.

Newcomb, P. A., B. E. Storer, and A. Trentham-Dietz. "Alcohol Consumption in Relation to Endometrial Cancer Risk." *Cancer Epidemiology, Biomarkers, and Prevention* no. 6 (1997): 773–778.

Peterson, E. P. "Endometrial Carcinoma in Young Women." *Obstetrics and Gynecology* 31 (1968): 702–707.

Pichert, G., et al. "Evidence-based Management Options for Women at Increased Breast/Ovarian Cancer Risk." *Annals of Oncology* no. 14 (2003): 9–19.

Piek, J. M., et al. "*BRCA1/2*-related Ovarian Cancers Are of Tubal Origin: A Hypothesis." *Gynecologic Oncology* 90, no. 2 (August 2003): 491.

Piver, M. S., et al. "Primary Peritoneal Carcinoma after Prophylactic Oophorectomy in Women with a Family History of Ovarian Cancer: A Report of the Gilda Radner Familial Ovarian Cancer Registry." *Cancer* 71, no. 9 (May 1, 1993): 2,751–2,755.

Powell, J. L. "Extramammary Paget's Disease." *Journal of the American College of Surgeons* 196, no. 5 (May 2003): 824.

Rebbeck, T. R. "Prophylactic Oophorectomy in *BRCA1* and *BRCA2* Mutation Carriers." *Journal of Clinical Oncology* 18, no. 21 (suppl.) (November 1, 2000): 100S–103S.

Riggs, B. L., and L. C. Hartmann. "Selective Estrogen-receptor Modulators—Mechanisms of Action and Application to Clinical Practice." *New England Journal of Medicine* no. 348 (2003): 618–629.

Rodriguez, C., et al. "Estrogen Replacement Therapy and Ovarian Cancer Mortality in a Large Prospective Study of U.S. Women." *Journal of the American Medical Association* 285, no. 11 (March 2001): 1,460–1,465.

Rosenberg, L., et al. "Breast Cancer and Alcoholic Beverage Consumption." *Lancet* (1982): 267–271.

Roukos, D. H., A. M. Kappas, and E. Tsianos. (2002). "Role of Surgery in the Prophylaxis of Hereditary Cancer Syndromes." *Annals of Surgical Oncology* no. 9, 607–609.

Rozario, D., et al. "Is Incidental Prophylactic Oophorectomy an Acceptable Means to Reduce the Incidence of Ovarian Cancer?" *American Journal of Surgery* 173, no. 6 (June 1997): 495–498.

Ruffin, M. T., 4th. "Family Physicians' Knowledge of Risk Factors for Cervical Cancer." *Journal of Women's Health* 2, no. 6 (July–August 2003): 561–567.

Rutter, J. L., et al. "Gynecologic Surgeries and Risk of Ovarian Cancer in Women with *BRCA1* and *BRCA2* Ashkenazi Founder Mutations: An Israeli Population-based Case-control Study." *Journal of the National Cancer Institute* no. 95 (2003): 1,072–1,078.

Satagopan, J. M., et al. "Ovarian Cancer Risk in Ashkenazi Jewish Carriers of *BRCA1* and *BRCA2* Mutations." *Clinical Cancer Research* 8 (2002): 3,776–3,781.

Schagen, S., et al. "Neurophysiological Evaluation of Late Effects of Adjuvant High-dose Chemotherapy on Cognitive Function." *Journal of Neurooncology* no. 51 (2001): 159–162.

Schneider, D. T., et al. "A Population-based Case-control Study of Endometrial Cancer in Shanghai, China." *International Journal of Cancer* no. 49 (1991): 38–43.

Snijders, P. J., A. J. Van Den Brule, and C. J. Meijer. "The Clinical Relevance of Human Papillomavirus Testing: Relationship between Analytical and Clinical Sensitivity." *Journal of Pathology* 201, no. 1 (September 23, 2003): 1–6.

Swanson, C. A., et al. "Moderate Alcohol Consumption and the Risk of Endometrial Cancer." *Epidemiology* 4 (1993): 530–536.

Teeley, P., and P. Bashe. *The Complete Cancer Survival Guide.* New York: Doubleday, 2000.

Webster L. A., N. S. Weiss, and The Cancer and Steroid Hormone Study Group. "Alcoholic Beverage Consumption and the Risk of Endometrial Cancer." *International Journal of Epidemiology* 18 (1989): 786–791.

Weiderpass, E., et al. "Low-potency Estrogen and Risk of Endometrial Cancer: A Case-control Study." *Lancet* no. 353 (May 29, 1999): 1,824–1,828.

Wideroff, L., A. N. Freedman, and L. Olson. "Physician Use of Genetic Testing for Cancer Susceptibility: Results of a National Survey." *Cancer Epidemiology, Biomarkers & Prevention* 12 (2003): 295–303.

Wilkes, G. M., T. B. Ades, and I. Krakoff. *American Cancer Society' Consumer's Guide to Cancer Drugs.* Sudbury, Mass.: Jones & Bartlett, 2000.

Writing Group for the Women's Health Initiative Investigators. "Risks and Benefits of Estrogen plus Progestin in Healthy Postmenopausal Women: Principal Results from the Women's Health Initiative Randomized Controlled Trial." *Journal of the American Medical Association* 28 (2002): 321–333.

Zhuang, S. H., G. D. Leonard, and S. M. Swain. "Oophorectomy in Carriers of *BRCA* Mutations." *New England Journal of Medicine* 47 (2002): 1,037–1,040.

INDEX

Boldface page numbers
denote extensive treatment
of a topic.

A

abdominal swelling **1,** 197
ablative therapy 131–132, 275
absolute neutrophil count
(ANC) 122
ACS. *See* American Cancer
Society
Actinomycin C 264. *See also*
Cosmegen
action studies 275
Actiq **1,** 266
acupressure **1**
acupuncture **1–2,** 114, 144
acustimulation **2**
adenocarcinoma **2,** 30
cervical 30–31
clear cell **47**
endometrial 2, 30, 86,
236, 238
fallopian tube 69
ovarian 2, 248
vaginal 30, 188
vulvar 193
adenoma, ovarian 66
adenomatous hyperplasia **2**
atypical 65
without atypical cells 65
adenosquamous carcinoma 31
adjuvant treatment **2,** 40, 144,
275
adnexal mass **2–4**
diagnosis of 3

symptoms of 3
treatment of 3–4
adrenal steroid inhibitors 9
Adriamycin **4,** 265
for cervical cancer 230,
233–234
in combination regimens
12, 29, 39, 262–263,
268, 272
for endometrial cancer
40, 63, 183, 236–240
for fallopian tube cancer
241–243
with hyaluronic acid
15–16
with hyperthermia ther-
apy 233–234, 238–239,
243–244, 253
for ovarian cancer 4, 247,
252–255
side effects of 4, 42, 46,
49, 103, 265
for uterine cancer 183
Adrucil 12, **75,** 267
for cervical cancer 37, 39,
230, 233–234
in combination regimens
39, 47, 262
with hyperthermia ther-
apy 233–234, 238–239,
253
side effects of 44, 267
topical 40, 75, 192, 195
advance directives **4,** 57, 59,
83
advocacy groups 203

African-American women
4–5, 32, 60, 217–218
age **5**
and cervical cancer 5, 32
and endometrial cancer 5,
59–60
and ovarian cancer 133
and ovarian cysts 140
and uterine cancer 179
and uterine sarcoma 185
and vaginal cancer 189
and vulvar cancer 5, 194
agonists 275
agranulocyte 275
AICT2 genes 127
Air Care Alliance **5–6,** 203
AirLifeLine **6,** 203
air transportation 5–6, 73,
121, 203–204, 210–211
Alaska Natives 96, **121,**
217–218
Albert Einstein Comprehensive
Cancer Center 226
alcohol and endometrial cancer
6
aldesleukin. *See* Proleukin
alendronate sodium **6,** 261
alkaline phosphatase **6,** 21
placental **151**
alkaline phosphatase test **6**
Alkeran 270
alkylating agents **6,** 29, 47,
263, 275
allicin **6,** 77
allium 77, 148–149
allogeneic 275

DATE DUE
